T0229315

Pancreatic Cancer

Editor

BRIAN M. WOLPIN

HEMATOLOGY/ONCOLOGY CLINICS OF NORTH AMERICA

www.hemonc.theclinics.com

Consulting Editors
GEORGE P. CANELLOS
H. FRANKLIN BUNN

August 2015 • Volume 29 • Number 4

ELSEVIER

1600 John F. Kennedy Boulevard • Suite 1800 • Philadelphia, Pennsylvania, 19103-2899

http://www.theclinics.com

HEMATOLOGY/ONCOLOGY CLINICS OF NORTH AMERICA Volume 29, Number 4
August 2015 ISSN 0889-8588, ISBN 13: 978-0-323-39336-2

Editor: Jennifer Flynn-Briggs
Developmental Editor: Donald Mumford

Hematology/Oncology Clinics (ISSN 0889-8588) is published bimonthly by Elsevier Inc., 360 Park Avenue South, New York, NY 10010-1710. Months of issue are February, April, June, August, October, and December. Business and Editorial Offices: 1600 John F. Kennedy Blvd., Ste. 1800, Philadelphia, PA 19103–2899. Customer Service Office: 3251 Riverport Lane, Maryland Heights, MO 63043. Periodicals postage paid at New York, NY and at additional mailing offices. Subscription prices are $385.00 per year (domestic individuals), $633.00 per year (domestic institutions), $190.00 per year (domestic students/residents), $440.00 per year (Canadian individuals), $783.00 per year (Canadian institutions), $520.00 per year (international individuals), $783.00 per year (international institutions), and $255.00 per year (international and Canadian students/residents). International air speed delivery is included in all *Clinics* subscription prices. All prices are subject to change without notice. **POSTMASTER:** Send address changes to *Hematology/Oncology Clinics of North America*, Elsevier Health Sciences Division, Subscription Customer Service, 3251 Riverport Lane, Maryland Heights, MO 63043. Customer Service (orders, claims, online, change of address): Elsevier Health Sciences Division, Subscription **Customer Service, 3251 Riverport Lane, Maryland Heights, MO 63043. Tel: 1-800-654-2452 (U.S. and Canada); 314-447-8871 (outside U.S. and Canada). Fax: 314-447-8029. E-mail: journalscustomerservice-usa@elsevier.com (for print support); journalsonlinesupport-usa@elsevier.com (for online support).**

Reprints. For copies of 100 or more, of articles in this publication, please contact the Commercial Reprints Department, Elsevier Inc., 360 Park Avenue South, New York, New York 10010-1710; Tel.: 212-633-3874, Fax: 212-633-3820, E-mail: reprints@elsevier.com.

Hematology/Oncology Clinics of North America is covered in *MEDLINE/PubMed (Index Medicus), EMBASE/ Excerpta Medica, and BIOSIS.*

Contributors

CONSULTING EDITORS

GEORGE P. CANELLOS, MD
William Rosenberg Professor of Medicine, Department of Medical Oncology, Dana-Farber Cancer Institute, Boston, Massachusetts

H. FRANKLIN BUNN, MD
Professor of Medicine, Division of Hematology, Brigham and Women's Hospital, Harvard Medical School, Boston, Massachusetts

EDITOR

BRIAN M. WOLPIN, MD, MPH
Co-Director, Pancreas and Biliary Tumor Center, Department of Medical Oncology, Dana-Farber Cancer Institute; Assistant Professor of Medicine, Harvard Medical School, Boston, Massachusetts

AUTHORS

LAUFEY T. AMUNDADOTTIR, PhD
Laboratory of Translational Genomics, Division of Cancer Epidemiology and Genetics, National Cancer Institute, National Institutes of Health, Bethesda, Maryland

THOMAS E. CLANCY, MD
Division of Surgical Oncology, Brigham and Women's Hospital; Co-Director, Pancreas and Biliary Tumor Center, Dana-Farber/Brigham and Women's Cancer Center; Assistant Professor of Surgery, Harvard Medical School, Boston, Massachusetts

MELISSA DEFOE, MD
Department of Internal Medicine, Washington University School of Medicine, St Louis, Missouri

LINGLING DU, MD
Division of Oncology, Department of Internal Medicine; Division of Medical Oncology, Alvin J. Siteman Cancer Center, Washington University School of Medicine, St Louis, Missouri

RICHARD F. DUNNE, MD
Division of Hematology/Oncology, Wilmot Cancer Institute, University of Rochester Medical Center, Rochester, New York

CARLOS FERNANDEZ-DEL CASTILLO, MD
Professor, Director of Pancreas and Biliary Surgery Program, Department of Surgery, Massachusetts General Hospital, Boston, Massachusetts

ARAM F. HEZEL, MD
Division of Hematology/Oncology, Wilmot Cancer Institute, University of Rochester Medical Center, Rochester, New York

KUNAL JAJOO, MD
Associate Physician, Division of Gastroenterology, Department of Medicine, Brigham and Women's Hospital; Assistant Professor of Medicine, Harvard Medical School, Boston, Massachusetts

MATTHEW HAROLD G. KATZ, MD, FACS
Assistant Professor of Clinical Oncology, Department of Surgical Oncology, The University of Texas MD Anderson Cancer Center, Houston, Texas

TERESA S. KIM, MD
General Surgery Resident, Department of Surgery, Massachusetts General Hospital, Boston, Massachusetts

ANDREW H. KO, MD
Division of Hematology/Oncology, University of California San Francisco, San Francisco, California

ALBERT C. KOONG, MD, PhD
Department of Radiation Oncology, Stanford Cancer Center, Stanford University, Stanford, California

ALEXANDER LEE, MD
Advanced Endoscopy Fellow, Division of Gastroenterology, Department of Medicine, Brigham and Women's Hospital; Harvard Medical School, Boston, Massachusetts

MAEVE A. LOWERY, MD
Assistant Attending Physician, Gastrointestinal Oncology Service, Department of Medicine, Memorial Sloan Kettering Cancer Center; Assistant Professor of Medicine, Weill Medical College of Cornell University, New York, New York

EILEEN M. O'REILLY, MD
Associate Director, Clinical Research, Gastrointestinal Oncology Service, Department of Medicine, Rubenstein Center for Pancreatic Cancer Research, Memorial Sloan Kettering Cancer Center; Associate Professor of Medicine, Weill Medical College of Cornell University, New York, New York

JEFFREY R. OLSEN, MD
Department of Radiation Oncology, Washington University School of Medicine, St Louis, Missouri

GLORIA M. PETERSEN, PhD
Consultant and Professor of Epidemiology, Department of Health Sciences Research, Mayo Clinic Cancer Center, Mayo Clinic, Rochester, Minnesota

ERQI L. POLLOM, MD
Department of Radiation Oncology, Stanford Cancer Center, Stanford University, Stanford, California

MARIANO PONZ-SARVISE, MD, PhD
Clinical Fellow, Cancer Biology, Cold Spring Harbor Laboratory, Cold Spring Harbor, New York

MICHAEL H. ROSENTHAL, MD, PhD
Staff Physician, Department of Imaging, Dana-Farber Cancer Institute; Associate
Radiologist, Department of Radiology, Brigham and Women's Hospital; Instructor in
Radiology, Harvard Medical School, Boston, Massachusetts

DOUGLAS A. RUBINSON, MD, PhD
Department of Medical Oncology, Dana-Farber Cancer Institute; Instructor of Medicine,
Harvard Medical School, Boston, Massachusetts

MARIANNA B. RUZINOVA, MD, PhD
Department of Pathology and Immunology, Washington University School of Medicine,
St Louis, Missouri

LILIAN SCHWARZ, MD
Research Resident, Department of Surgical Oncology, The University of Texas MD
Anderson Cancer Center, Houston, Texas

RACHAEL Z. STOLZENBERG-SOLOMON, PhD, MPH, RD
Nutritional Epidemiology Branch, Division of Cancer Epidemiology and Genetics, National
Cancer Institute, National Institutes of Health, Rockville, Maryland

DAVID A. TUVESON, MD, PhD
Professor, Cold Spring Harbor Laboratory, Cold Spring Harbor, New York; Memorial
Sloan Kettering Cancer Center, New York, New York

ANDREA WANG-GILLAM, MD, PhD
Division of Medical Oncology, Department of Internal Medicine; Alvin J. Siteman Cancer
Center, Washington University School of Medicine, St Louis, Missouri

BRIAN M. WOLPIN, MD, MPH
Co-Director, Pancreas and Biliary Tumor Center, Department of Medical Oncology,
Dana-Farber Cancer Institute; Assistant Professor of Medicine, Harvard Medical School,
Boston, Massachusetts

KENNETH H. YU, MD, MSc
Clinical Fellow, Cold Spring Harbor Laboratory, Cold Spring Harbor, New York; Assistant
Professor, Memorial Sloan Kettering Cancer Center; Weill Medical College, Cornell
University, New York, New York

Contents

genetically high risk. Research reveals that a half dozen known hereditary syndromes or genes are associated with increased risk of developing pancreatic cancer, the most prominent of which are *BRCA2* and *CDKN2A*. Genetic risk assessment and testing is already available. Owing to limited experience worldwide, guidance is often based on expert opinion, although all agree that research is needed to improve the shaping of options.

Incidentally discovered pancreatic cystic lesions are increasingly common, affecting up to 10% to 15% of patients undergoing cross-sectional imaging. Although some pancreatic cystic neoplasms harbor invasive malignancy or the potential to progress over time, a majority are benign and can be observed safely. Accurate diagnosis is key to appropriate management. Diagnosis requires a multidisciplinary and multimodal approach. This review discusses each type of pancreatic cystic neoplasm and the current data on diagnosis and treatment.

Imaging and endoscopy both play important and complementary roles in the initial diagnosis, staging, monitoring, and symptomatic management of pancreatic cancer. This article provides an overview of the uses of each of the diagnostic modalities, common imaging findings, alternative considerations, and areas of ongoing work in diagnostic imaging. This article also provides details of the uses of endoscopy for diagnosis, staging, and intervention throughout the course of a patient's care. These modalities each play important roles in the complex multidisciplinary care of patients with pancreatic cancer.

Surgical resection remains the only potentially curative therapy for pancreatic cancer, despite a high rate of systemic recurrence. Because of local invasion or distant spread, a minority of patients presenting with pancreatic cancer are candidates for surgery. Although perioperative mortality is low in high-volume settings, pancreatic surgery remains associated with considerable morbidity. Minimally invasive and robotic surgical techniques are increasingly used for pancreatic resection, although not always applicable to all patients. Strategies to extend the benefits of margin-negative surgical resection to more patients include surgery with vascular resection and reconstruction for locally invasive tumors, and resection after neoadjuvant therapy.

It is estimated that 10% to 20% of patients with pancreatic cancer present with resectable disease. Although surgery offers curative intent, the median survival after curative resection is less than 2 years. To improve clinical outcomes in this patient population, clinical studies have investigated the role of perioperative therapy, including neoadjuvant and adjuvant treatment in resectable pancreatic cancer. The role of adjuvant therapy has been well established by large randomized phase III studies, whereas benefit of the neoadjuvant approach remains inconclusive. Here, we review various treatment modalities and their clinical benefits in resectable pancreatic cancer.

Lilian Schwarz and Matthew Harold G. Katz

Borderline resectable pancreatic cancer represents a subcategory of advanced cancer that is typically defined by limited involvement of the major mesenteric vasculature. Such involvement is associated with a high likelihood of microscopically incomplete resection if surgery is used as the primary therapeutic modality. Increasing data support the role of neoadjuvant therapy as part of multimodality management but there is no uniformly accepted standard of care. This review discusses, based on recent literature and the experience of the Pancreatic Tumor Study Group at The University of Texas MD Anderson Cancer Center, the classification, definition, diagnosis, and management of borderline resectable pancreatic cancer.

Erqi L. Pollom, Albert C. Koong, and Andrew H. Ko

This article focuses on the management of locally advanced pancreatic cancer, which should be treated as a distinct entity separate from metastatic disease and borderline resectable disease. Although the role, timing, and sequencing of radiation relative to systemic therapy in this disease are controversial, an emerging treatment paradigm involves induction chemotherapy, followed by consolidative chemoradiation in patients who do not progress. In addition, new chemotherapy regimens as well as novel radiosensitizers have shown promise and need to be tested further in the locally advanced setting. Advances in radiotherapy have enabled stereotactic body radiotherapy and should continue to be prospectively evaluated.

Douglas A. Rubinson and Brian M. Wolpin

Since the US Food and Drug Administration's approval of gemcitabine in 1996, numerous randomized trials have investigated treatment programs to further improve the quality of life and survival of patients with advanced pancreatic cancer. After little progress over the ensuing 15 years, 2 combination treatment programs recently conferred improved survival compared with gemcitabine monotherapy in patients with metastatic pancreatic cancer: FOLFIRINOX (folinic acid, 5-fluorouracil, irinotecan, oxaliplatin) and gemcitabine plus nab-paclitaxel. Importantly, our understanding of the biology of pancreatic cancer continues to grow. This improved biologic understanding holds great promise for integrating new targeted and immune-modifying therapies into current treatment programs.

The last decade has seen significant developments in the use of combination systemic therapy for advanced pancreatic ductal adenocarcinoma (PDAC), with median survival approaching 1 year for select patients treated with FOLFIRINOX in the metastatic setting. However, it is sobering that these developments have been achieved with the use of traditional cytotoxics rather than from successes in the more modern fields of molecularly targeted therapies or immunotherapy. This article highlights several promising therapeutic approaches to PDAC currently under clinical evaluation, including immune therapies, molecularly targeted therapies, strategies for stromal depletion, and targeted therapy for genetically selected patients.

HEMATOLOGY/ONCOLOGY CLINICS OF NORTH AMERICA

THE CLINICS ARE AVAILABLE ONLINE!
Access your subscription at:
www.theclinics.com

Preface

Pancreatic Cancer

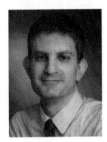

Brian M. Wolpin, MD, MPH
Editor

Although pancreatic cancer remains a leading cause of cancer death, steady progress is being made in understanding the biology of the disease and optimal treatment approaches for patients. This issue of *Hematology/Oncology Clinics of North America* brings together experts in the field to discuss a wide range of topics in pancreatic cancer, including work at the bench, emerging concepts related to cancer risk, current treatment approaches at the bedside, and future directions in research and patient care. This issue is dedicated primarily to pancreatic ductal adenocarcinoma (PDAC) and its precursors, with discussion of neuroendocrine tumors and other less common histologies left for future issues.

The issue begins with a comprehensive overview of the biology of PDAC by Drs Dunne and Hezel, describing the critical role of mutant KRAS, additional intracellular pathways contributing to malignant progression, the importance of the tumor microenvironment, and the unique metabolic dependencies of PDAC. In the second article, Drs Ponz-Sarvise, Tuveson, and Yu discuss how mouse models of PDAC can be leveraged to expand our understanding of disease biology and facilitate preclinical testing of new therapeutic strategies. The next three articles turn attention to predisposition to PDAC. Drs Stolzenberg-Solomon and Amundadottir discuss genetic predisposition to sporadic PDAC and risk factors for the disease, including cigarette smoking, obesity, diabetes, and chronic pancreatitis. Dr Petersen discusses familial pancreatic cancer, hereditary syndromes with defined germline mutations, and the complexities of translating these discoveries into clinical management of patients. Drs Kim and Fernandez-del Castillo then provide a valuable overview of diagnosis and treatment of cystic neoplasms of the pancreas, lesions increasingly detected incidentally on high-resolution abdominal imaging and with varying risk for malignant transformation.

The subsequent articles in the issue thoroughly discuss current strategies for diagnosis and management of patients with PDAC, finishing with an article on emerging treatment approaches. In article 6, Drs Rosenthal, Lee, and Jajoo provide a beautifully annotated guide to the radiologic and endoscopic assessment of

Hematol Oncol Clin N Am 29 (2015) xiii–xiv
http://dx.doi.org/10.1016/j.hoc.2015.06.002
0889-8588/15/$ – see front matter © 2015 Published by Elsevier Inc.

hemonc.theclinics.com

pancreatic tumors, with additional discussion of endoscopic interventions. In the following two articles, Dr Clancy describes technical considerations and new approaches to pancreatic resections, and Dr Wang-Gillam and colleagues discuss perioperative chemotherapy and radiation to improve cure rates in patients with resectable PDAC. Drs Schwarz and Katz then provide an outstanding overview of a still emerging and complex entity, borderline-resectable pancreatic cancer, highlighting the need for multidisciplinary collaboration for optimal management. The care of patients with locally advanced PDAC is then discussed by Drs Pollom, Koong, and Ko, with a thorough consideration of the roles and sequencing of chemotherapy and radiation and an interesting discussion of newer radiation approaches. Drs Rubinson and Wolpin then discuss the diagnosis and management of patients with metastatic PDAC, highlighting recent studies that have defined new standards of care for these patients. The final article of the issue is contributed by Drs Lowery and O'Reilly and provides an exciting overview of therapeutic approaches currently under study, including disruption of key intracellular signaling pathways, modulation of the tumor microenvironment, enhanced immune cell engagement, and exploitation of defective tumor DNA repair mechanisms. Thus, the issue ends as it began, with a focus on the biology of pancreatic cancer and how we can leverage a better mechanistic understanding of the disease to improve the care of our patients.

Although pancreatic cancer continues to challenge scientists, clinicians, and patients alike, a diverse community of talented individuals is dedicated to overcoming this highly lethal disease—at the bench, at the bedside, and with advocacy efforts. With their creativity, commitment, courage, and collaboration, we are certain to see additional progress for patients in the near term. The individuals at risk for and with this disease deserve nothing less.

Brian M. Wolpin, MD, MPH
Center for Gastrointestinal Oncology
Dana-Farber Cancer Institute
Harvard Medical School
450 Brookline Avenue
Boston, MA 02215, USA

E-mail address:
bwolpin@partners.org

Genetics and Biology of Pancreatic Ductal Adenocarcinoma

Richard F. Dunne, MD, Aram F. Hezel, MD*

KEYWORDS

- Pancreatic Cancer • KRAS • Microenvironment • Stroma • Immunomodulation
- Autophagy

KEY POINTS

- Pancreatic ductal adenocarcinoma remains a clinical challenge.
- Thus far, enlightenment on the downstream activities of Kras, the tumor's unique metabolic needs, and how the stroma and immune system affect it have remained untranslated to the clinical practice.
- Given the numbers of diverse therapies in development and a growing knowledge about how to evaluate these systems preclinically and clinically, this is expected to change significantly and for the better over the next 5 years.

Pancreatic ductal adenocarcinoma (PDA) is an aggressive malignancy that carries a poor prognosis with a 5-year survival on the order of 6%[1]; new and innovative treatments are needed. Several factors underlie its aggressive nature and resistance to treatment: the genetic framework, early metastasis, a dense stroma, propensity for growth in a nutrient-deplete environment, and immunomodulation have all made therapeutic progress a challenge.[2] This article focuses on recent advances in understanding the tumor genetics and cell biology of pancreatic cancer. It reviews the established genetic hallmarks, examines more recently described mutations and altered pathways, and highlights key biological principles identified in PDA with a focus on those most likely to lead to future therapeutic targets.

GENETICS

Pancreatic adenocarcinoma shows genetic homogeneity on one level with mutations in *KRAS*, found in anywhere from 90% to 95% of advanced pancreatic cancers, and

Funding sources: Dr A.F. Hezel, NCI (172302) and Pancreatic Cancer Association of Western NY. Dr R.F. Dunne, nil.
Conflicts of interest: Nil.
Division of Hematology/Oncology, Wilmot Cancer Institute, University of Rochester Medical Center, 601 Elmwood Avenue, Box 704, Rochester, NY 14642, USA
* Corresponding author.
E-mail address: aram_hezel@urmc.rochester.edu

Hematol Oncol Clin N Am 29 (2015) 595–608
http://dx.doi.org/10.1016/j.hoc.2015.04.003
0889-8588/15/$ – see front matter © 2015 Elsevier Inc. All rights reserved.

hemonc.theclinics.com

additional frequent and well-characterized mutations in the key tumor suppressor pathways *TP53/p19ARF*, *RB/CDKN2A/INK4A*, and *TGFBeta/SMAD4*.[3] The biological significance of many of these mutations has been investigated in numerous contexts and model systems and the main impact of each on the disease is briefly highlighted later. Beyond this element of genetic homogeneity, PDA is broadly characterized by general genetic instability with widespread mutations and chromosomal translocations, including the recent discovery of many additional mutated loci and classes of genes whose full cancer-specific functions have yet to be fully explored. These genes include members of the SWI/SNF family, MLLs, and the DNA damage repair system, including *ATM*. The genetic hallmarks of PDA are described below and the broad implications of recent tumor genetic analyses are discussed later with regard to understanding of the natural history of the disease (**Box 1**).

Box 1
Genetics of PDA

- *KRAS* is the most common mutational hallmark of PDA and can activate the RAF/MEK/ERK and PI3K pathways.
- Mouse models with K-RAS mutations typically require subsequent genetic events, such as loss of tumor suppressor genes INK4A, P53, or SMAD4, to develop tumors similar to human PDA.
- Finding that loss of SMAD4 has a greater propensity for metastatic spread is an example of how genetic sequencing may help tailor future therapy to the individual.

KRAS

KRAS is a member of the RAS family of GTP-binding proteins that controls cellular proliferation and survival. Inactivation of RAS occurs via GTP hydrolysis with the aid of GTPase-activating proteins (GAPs). Activating *KRAS* point mutations at codon 12, the most common in PDA, occur near the nucleotide binding site, desensitizing RAS to GAPs and inhibiting GTP hydrolysis,[4–6] resulting in a constitutively active RAS. This process leads to a unique genetic/biochemical/signaling paradigm compared with other oncogenes, because *KRAS* is not so much biochemically turned on via mutation, but rather cannot be turned off. Consequently, mutant RAS is a difficult therapeutic target because the loss of its GTPase enzymatic activity is not easily pharmacologically restored. This challenge has shifted efforts from targeting *KRAS* directly to focusing on downstream signaling pathways of *KRAS*.

KRAS mutation leads to constitutive activations of key mitogenic and survival signaling pathways, including RAF/MEK/ERK and phosphatidylinositol 3 kinase (PI3K). The relative importance of each of these has been evaluated in several *in vitro* and *in vivo* systems. In vitro studies revealed that RAS activates RAF and mitogen-activated protein (MAP) kinases, crucial for DNA synthesis, in the absence of other growth factors,[7,8] and that its activities could also be abrogated with PI3K dominant negatives.[9] Mouse models have provided further insight into the relative importance of PI3K and RAF/MAP/MEK pathways. PI3K-activated models without *Kras* mutation showed no pancreatic abnormalities, whereas *Braf*-mutated models developed PanIn (pancreatic intraepithelial neoplasms; these are discussed later), leading investigators to conclude that this may be the dominant branch of *KRAS*-mediated signaling in PDA.[10] Furthermore, a *Braf* and *Tp53* mutated model showed clear evidence of PDA with extensive metastasis. Treatment with MEK inhibitors suppressed phosphorylation of ERK but led to increased levels of phosphorylated AKT, a marker of PI3K activation, and cell lines treated with both MEK and AKT inhibition led to a synergistic antitumor effect. This antitumor effect, albeit modest, is also seen in dual MEK/PI3K treatment studies in mouse models.[11,12] Thus, although RAF/MEK/ERK activation may be a dominant effector of KRAS activity, its pharmacologic inhibition led to activation of other compensatory downstream pathways driving survival and proliferation, explaining PDA's resistance to single-agent MEK inhibition clinically.[13]

Oncogene addiction has been described as a process in which effector proteins are involved in an intricate network of synergistic positive-feedback and negative-feedback loops to maintain tumor growth, homeostasis, and structural integrity; a process that is not simply a summation of the effects of acquired mutations.[14] The addiction of subsets of PDAs to KRAS has been well described, shown by tumor regression with mutant *Kras* extinction.[15] Dependence on mutant KRAS can be overcome, however, similar to the mechanisms of resistance described in many targeted therapies, and was recently described via amplification and overexpression of YAP-1.[16] Yap-1 is a transcriptional coactivator involved in cell proliferation, epithelial-to-mesenchymal transition (EMT), and metastasis, previously linked to liver and esophageal tumors.[17,18] Other routes to KRAS independence are also described,[19] suggesting that there may be additional molecular routes by which KRAS-independent growth of PDA may be sustained.

INK4a/CDKN2A/P16

Loss of *INK4a* function brought about by mutation, deletion, or promoter hypermethylation occurs in about 80% to 95% of sporadic PDA.[20,21] The INK4a gene encodes the tumor suppressor protein p16, which inhibits CDK4/6-mediated phosphorylation of RB, thereby blocking entry into the S phase (DNA synthesis) of the cell cycle (for a more in-depth review of *INK4a/ARF*, see Sharpless[22]). The 9q21 locus that contains *INK4a* also encodes the tumor suppressor gene *ARF*, whose protein product p19 stabilizes p53 by inhibiting MDM2-dependent proteolysis. Pancreatic cancers with mutations at this locus may sustain loss of both *INK4a* and *ARF* tumor suppression pathways, although some mutations have been found to affect loss of p16 alone. The importance of Ink4a in restraining PDA has been shown in murine models with engineered mutations in this locus designed to affect both *p16Ink4a* and *p19Arf* genes or *p16Ink4a* alone.[23,24]

TP53 Tumor Suppressor Pathway

Mutations, predominantly missense, in the *TP53* tumor suppressor gene occur in approximately 75% to 80% of human PDA cases.[21,25,26] In normal unstressed cells, p53 is bound to MDM2, which targets p53 for proteasomal degradation. In response to cell stress and/or oncogene activation, p53 protein is stabilized and targets activation of genes involved in cell cycle arrest, apoptosis, DNA damage repair, and cellular metabolism.[27] The role of *TP53* loss in cancer is well established in that its mutation has been described in most human cancers and germline mutation of *TP53* leads to the early development of sarcomas and carcinomas, also known as the Li-Fraumeni syndrome[28] (for in-depth review of p53, see "The p53 Family," subject collection in *CSH Perspectives in Biology*, 2010). Evidence from PDA precursor lesions (PanINs) suggests that loss or mutation of *TP53* is a late event possibly caused by selective pressure after the collective accumulation of genetic aberrations, reactive oxygen species (ROS), and telomere erosion.[4,29] The loss of *p19ARF* coexists with *TP53* mutations in only about 40% of tumors, whereas the loss of *TP53* or inactivation of this pathway is a more common feature of PDA, leading many to believe that these tumor suppressors have some overlapping function as well as independent capabilities.[30,31]

DPC4/SMAD4/Transforming Growth Factor Beta

The *SMAD4* (*DPC4*) gene is located within chromosome 18q21 and is a key transcriptional regulator of the transforming growth factor beta (TGF-β) signaling cascade, a pathway that mediates proliferation, cell migration, apoptosis, and EMT.[32–34] Loss of *SMAD4* function has been reported in ~50% to 60% of tumors and is associated with poor outcome in surgical patients.[26,32] In a rapid-autopsy program examining 76 cases of PDA, *SMAD4* loss was reported in only 22% of locally advanced cases with no metastatic disease at autopsy, but in 78% of those with widespread metastatic disease.[26] These clinical findings, along with associated poor outcome in patients with *SMAD4* loss, imply that intact *SMAD4* function may help constrain metastatic spread, and investigators suggest that such patients with functional *SMAD4* may benefit from intensive locoregional therapies.[26]

Somatic mutation of *Smad4*, as well as the type 2 TGF-β receptor[35] in the murine pancreatic epithelium, neither disrupted pancreatic development nor induced malignancy, but hastened PDA development when coupled with *Kras* mutation.[36] Although *SMAD4* is mutated in about 50%, almost all tumors express high levels of both receptor and TGF-β ligands. In both human and murine model systems, activation of this pathway has been found to underlie cellular migration, metastasis, and EMT,[37] raising the question of TGF-β inhibition as a therapy. Studies have been mixed depending on models used and underlying tumor genetics.[38]

Advanced Genetic Sequencing Reveals Novel Mutations

The application of whole-genome sequencing to PDA has revealed additional new mutations in genes and pathways not previously recognized as being important in its pathogenesis as well as insights into its genetic evolution. Exon sequencing of 24 PDAs uncovered 1562 somatic mutations in 1327 genes[39] and investigators organized these into a collection of 12 core signaling pathways (**Table 1**). Although most of the 1327 genes identified were mutated in a small minority of cases, each core

Table 1
Core signaling pathways in PDA as described by Jones and colleagues[39] and highlighted mutations of each pathway

Core Pathway	Key Mutated Genes
KRAS signaling	KRAS, MAP2K4, RASGRP3
Regulation of G1/S phase	CDKN2A, FBXW7, CHD1, APC2
TGF-β signaling	SMAD4, SMAD3, TGFBR2, BMPR2
DNA damage control	TP53, ERCC4, ERCC6, RANBP2
Hedgehog signaling	TBX5, SOX3, LPR2, GL1, BOC, CREBBP
WNT/Notch signaling	MYC, GATA6, WNT9A, TCF4, MAP2, TSC2
Apoptosis	CASP10, VCP, CAD, HIP1
C-Jun N-terminal kinase signaling	MAP4K3, TNF, ATF2, NFATC3
Regulation of invasion	ADAM11, DPP6, MEP1A, PCSK6, APG4A, PRSS23
Homophilic cell adhesion	CDH1, CDH10, PCDH15, PCDH17, FAT
Small GTPase-dependent signaling (non-KRAS)	AGHGEF7, CDC42BPA, DEPDC2, PLCB3
Integrin signaling	ITGA4, ITGA9, LAM1, FN1, ILK

Data from Jones S, Zhang X, Parsons DW, et al. Core signaling pathways in human pancreatic cancers revealed by global genomic analyses. Science 2008;321:1801–6.

pathway was mutated in 67% to 100% of the 24 tumor specimens, suggesting that, although the mutational spectrum may be broad and heterogeneous, the physiologic result is distilled down to effects on conserved pathways.[39] Separately, whole-exon sequencing of 99 patients[40] confirmed these described mutations and identified novel mutations in PDA, including the axon guidance pathway genes SLIT and ROBO, previously known to be important in embryogenesis and central nervous system development **(Table 2)**.[41] SLIT2/ROBO2 inactivating mutations were present in 5% of the cohort with copy number losses in ROBO1 and SLIT2 in another 15% of the population. The biological impact of SLIT/ROBO mutations in PDA is unexplored but, in other contexts, affects both MET and WNT signaling.[41] In addition, novel mutations were discovered in EPC1 (3%) and ARID2 (3%), which affect chromatin modification, and in ATM (5%), with likely more of the cohort affected because of copy number variation losses in a small percentage of each gene.[40] ATM, which encodes for a serine/threonine kinase DNA damage repair protein, has already been linked to familial cases of PDA along with BRCA2 and PALB2[42]; this finding supports a role in sporadic PDA as well.

Beyond the identification of genes harboring mutations that may be causal to the disease, these studies have offered more global insights into the genetic landscape and trajectory of the disease. In order to understand the relationship of a primary tumor to its attendant metastatic sites, somatic genetic rearrangements in 13 primary PDA tumors were compared with metastases.[43] Although most of the 206 rearrangements were found in the primary tumor and all metastatic sites, supporting a conserved origin, clonal evolution was also identified. Furthermore, some genetic aberrations found in metastatic sites were organ specific, including mutations in MYC and CCNE1 that were found exclusively in lung metastases, suggesting that certain subclones may evolve in an organ-specific manner.[43]

Genetic Pathogenesis

PDA may arise from at least 3 types of precursor lesions: PanIN, intraductal papillary mucinous neoplasm (IPMN), and mucinous cystic neoplasm (MCN). The most prevalent precursor is PanIN, a microscopic lesion graded I to III, encompassing a spectrum of increasing dysplasia and architectural disruption.[44] High-grade PanIN lesions are commonly found in association with invasive PDA. Furthermore, advanced PanINs harbor many of the same genetic mutations as PDA, linking these entities molecularly as

Table 2
Significant novel mutations identified by genetic sequencing of human PDA samples in studies in by Jones and colleagues[39] and Biankin and colleagues[40]

Jones et al,[39] 2008	Biankin et al,[40] 2012
MLL3 (transcriptional activator)	ARID2 (chromatin modification)
CDH10, PCDH15, PCDH18 (cadherin homologs)	ATM (DNA damage repair)
CTNNA2 (alpha-catenin)	ZIM2 (transcriptional regulator)
DPP6 (dipeptidyl-peptidase)	NALCN (Na-channel activity)
BAI3 (angiogenesis inhibitor)	MAGEA6 (protein binding)
GPR133 (G protein–coupled receptor)	MAP2K4 (toll-like receptor signaling pathway)
GUCY1A2 (guanylate cyclase)	SLC16A4 (monocarboxylate transporter)
PRKCG (protein kinase)	SLIT2, ROBO1, ROBO2 (axon guidance pathway genes)
Q9H5F0 (unknown function)	SEMA3A, SEMA3E (semaphorins, axon guidance)

well as pathologically.[45] IpMNs are less common precursors and PDA derived from IpMNs are thought by some clinicians to represent a different disease process, especially given its better prognosis and 5-year survival rate of 42% in those surgically resectable patients.[46] Sixty-six percent of IpMNs harbor mutations in *GNAS*.[47] Furthermore, investigation of 95 surgical PDA specimens without IpMN yielded no mutations in *GNAS*. These findings were corroborated through sequencing of 48 IpMNs that identified *GNAS* mutations in 79% of patients; only 50% harbored *KRAS* mutations and fewer showed loss of p16 (36%) and *SMAD4* (24%).[48] The genetics of MCNs are not clearly delineated, but a presentation in young women, mainly in the body and tail of the pancreas, suggests potential differing biology.[49] Although there are key shared genetic traits between PanINs, PDA, and the lesser common precursors IpMNs and MCNs,[4] these recent studies show how different genetic events may explain the divergent phenotypes of the malignancies arising from each type of precursor (**Box 2**).

MICROENVIRONMENT

The pancreatic cancer microenvironment, referred to as stroma, or desmoplasia, is composed of fibroblasts, myofibroblasts, immune cells, vascular components, and a dense extracellular matrix (ECM).[50] The role of the tumor stroma has been alternatively viewed as either shielding tumor cells from treatment through the creation of a hypoxic and high-tensile environment impenetrable by current available therapies or, more recently, functioning to constrain tumor cells through the facilitation of immune response or impaired vascular access.[51–53] Several signaling pathways active in PDA can modulate this environment, including TGF-β (discussed earlier), notch, and Sonic Hedgehog (Shh). The Shh pathway, identified as frequently activated in PDA,[39] promotes stromal desmoplasia,[54–57] and is being evaluated as a potential therapeutic target. Administration of IPI-926, an inhibitor of the Shh pathway,[58] in murine models has been shown to reduce tumor-associated stromal tissue burden, promote angiogenesis, and enhance drug delivery, and combining IPI-926 with gemcitabine resulted in doubling of overall survival compared with those mice treated with gemcitabine alone.[59]

The ECM of the stroma found in PDA contains a large proportion of hyaluronic acid (HA), a large glycosaminoglycan,[51] crucial to normal tissue homeostasis via its influence on cell shape and malleability.[60] In PDA and other tumors in which there is an abundance of HA, which is thought to affect interstitial fluid pressures (IFPs) leading to relative hypovascularity, itself a major hindrance to treatment delivery, levels have been associated with tumor metastasis, drug resistance, angiogenesis, and poor prognosis.[61–64] By administering pegylated hyaluronidase (PEGPH20), tumors

---

Box 2
Advanced genetic sequencing efforts in PDA

- More than 1500 mutations have been identified to occur in PDA; focusing on the core signaling cascades these affect may show greater promise than focusing on individual mutations.

- Next-generation sequencing efforts have identified many novel genetic aberrations in PDA, such as those in axon guidance pathways and chromatin modification, which require further investigation.

- PanINs are precursor lesions that have tight genetic linkage with PDA; IpMNs are less common PDA precursor lesions found to have frequent mutation of *GNAS* and slightly better outcomes, suggesting a potential divergent phenotype.

showed decreased IFP, increased chemotherapy delivery, and greater patency of the vasculature that previously collapsed amid increased interstitial pressures. Furthermore, improved response rates and overall survival were seen with mouse models when combining PEGPH20 with gemcitabine compared with gemcitabine alone. These findings, combined with improved outcomes found using Shh inhibitors described earlier, strengthened the argument that desmoplasia was a significant culprit in PDA's poor prognosis and drug resistance.[51,59,65]

Although previous work showed prolonged survival in mice with PDA with pharmacologic inhibition of Shh,[66] the somatic deletion of Shh in a murine PDA model conversely led to more aggressive pancreatic tumors with an increased metastatic burden.[52] On histology, Shh knockout PDA is predictably fibroblast deplete, but undifferentiated, with a more prominent vasculature and high expression of Zeb1 and SLUG, both transcription factors that are important for EMT.[67,68] Further supporting a protective role for the stroma, elimination of myofibroblasts in PDA models led to a decreasing number of T effector cells and an increase in T regulatory cells (T_{reg}), representing weakened immune surveillance (immunomodulation, as discussed later).[53]

The studies described earlier have created a therapeutic dilemma as to whether the stroma should be targeted and eliminated, to enable drug delivery, or promoted to bolster its antitumoral immune response. Pegylated hyaluronidase is currently being studied as an adjunct to gemcitabine and nab-paclitaxel in a phase II clinical trial (clinicaltrials.gov NCT01839487). It is possible that although some stromal elements function to constrain tumor growth (via enhanced immunity and so forth), others may enhance malignant behavior (ie, conferring chemoresistance; discussed later regarding tumor macrophages) and that a greater understanding of the interplay between the tumor cells and the host will ultimately be necessary to design therapies that target the tumor stroma.

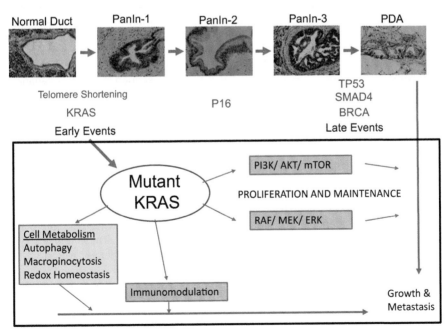

Fig. 1. Evolution of PanIN (pancreatic intraepithelial neoplasms) to PDA and the many mechanisms by which RAS influences tumor growth.

IMMUNE RESPONSE

Immunosuppression in cancer, specifically in PDA, that is promoted by cancer-associated inflammation is now recognized to foster tumor development and growth.[69] The microenvironment of PDA is crucial to this process because it harbors a range of immunosuppressive cells, including tumor-associated macrophages (TAMs), myeloid-derived suppressor cells (MDSCs), and T_{reg} (see review by Vonderheide and Bayne[69]). Current understanding is that these leukocytes help to deplete T effector cells, which are an integral part of antitumoral immunity,[70] via several underlying mechanisms, including oncogenic activation of KRAS and granulocyte-macrophage colony-stimulating factor (GM-CSF)[71,72] and the CCL2/CCR chemokine axis.[73] Recent developments in understanding these systems are described later, as well as how targeting the immune response, or lack thereof, in PDA may provide clinical benefit.

In a Kras-mutant mouse model, an intense desmoplastic reaction with a prominent leukocytic infiltration was observed that was predominantly made up of T_{reg} cells, which can abrogate the immune response,[74] MDSCs, and TAMs and lacked effector T cells.[70] After an inverse relationship was discovered between MDSCs and T effector cells, it was found in vitro that MDSCs are capable of driving down T-cell proliferation.[70] In addition, investigators found that these immunosuppressive cells are present in PanINs and throughout progression to PDA, indicating that immunomodulation and suppression are possibly early events of PDA development.

GR-1+ CD11b+ immature myeloid cells are MDSCs that are precursors to macrophages, dendritic cells, and granulocytes and have been found to infiltrate PanIN and PDA lesions in mouse models.[69] Upregulation of GM-CSF, which has been found to be Kras dependent in mice, drives the accumulation of these immunosuppressive cells in PDA.[71,72] When GM-CSF is knocked down in Kras-mutated grafts, GR-1+ CD11b+ cells are scarce, there is an increase in CD8+ T cells, and orthotopic engrafted pancreatic tumor cells are subsequently eliminated.[72] CD8+ T-cell immunity was proved to be a dominant force in this response as tumor growth was restored when CD8+ T cells were ultimately eradicated by anti-CD8 antibody injection into the host.

Depleted numbers of CD8+ T cells in PDA was also described in a study examining the CCL2/CCR chemokine axis and its ability to regulate antitumor immunity.[73] The CCL2/CCR chemokine axis is an important modulator of inflammatory monocyte (IM) recruitment from the bone marrow to the peripheral blood and tumor sites where they are destined to become immunosuppressive TAMs.[75,76] CCR+ TAMs, which made up 28% of tumor-infiltrating leukocytes,[73] were suppressed in tumor-bearing mice with a CCR2 antagonist leading to an increase in the number of T effector cells, and diminished T_{reg} cell numbers and associated decreased tumor growth.[73] Furthermore, combining the CCR2 antagonist with gemcitabine had a synergistic effect in reducing tumor growth. In addition, they observed that treating these mice with gemcitabine led to persistent levels of IMs and an increase in TAMs, which could provide some insight into why PDA becomes resistant to chemotherapy. These findings provide the basis for an open-phase Ib/II trial combining chemotherapy with a CCR2 antagonist (NCT01413022; clinicaltrials.gov).

METABOLIC REQUIREMENTS

The recognition that PDA has unique metabolic requirements, compared with untransformed epithelial cells, has emerged from the basic study of mutations associated with the disease (eg, KRAS, TP53) as well as direct attention paid to metabolites that promote the tumor's growth.[77–79] Beyond metabolic pathways identified downstream of KRAS, PDA uses evolutionary-conserved cellular survival mechanisms (specifically, autophagy and macropinocytosis) to meet its heightened metabolic demands.[79,80] Furthermore, the hypoxic and metabolically active environment of PDA requires an increased capacity to contend with sequelae such as increased ROS stress.

Autophagy is a catabolic pathway that recycles damaged organelles and proteins for use as an alternative energy source in response to starvation.[81] Although autophagy has been described previously as a tumor suppressor involved in cell death in other contexts,[82,83] levels of autophagic markers are increased in PDA.[84] Autophagic flux was found to be upregulated in PDA cell lines at baseline, nutrient-rich conditions, and not only when under stress,[80] suggesting that autophagy is an essential metabolic process for PDA cell sustainability. Autophagy in pancreatic cancers seems in part to be driven by a constitutively active RAS.[81] When autophagy genes *Atg5* or *Atg7* were knocked down, RAS-expressing cells died in nutrient-deplete conditions; cells were found lacking substrates for tricarboxylic acid (TCA) cycle metabolism normally produced in the mitochondria. Furthermore, *Ras*-mutated mice had suppressed tumor growth with these same genes knocked down. Inhibition of autophagy in PDA cell lines using chloroquine, which increases lysosomal pH and blocks fusion with the phagosome,[85,86] led to diminished oxidative phosphorylation and decreased cellular proliferation.[80] Further supporting a role for autophagy in PDA tumor progression, Plac8, a protein upregulated by oncogenic mutations, is important to lysosomal/autophagosomal fusion and its absence hampers tumor growth. The role of p53 in mediating autophagy dependence is a matter of some debate with a dichotomous effect depending on the context studied.[86–88] Taken together, these studies support the critical role of autophagy in PDA cell nutrition, growth, and survival (possibly related to attenuation of ROS stress) and have prompted further investigation of autophagy as a therapeutic target.

RAS mutation has also been found to be pivotal in other metabolic pathways responsible for sustaining growth, including broadly reprogramming glucose use and glutamine metabolism to maintain optimal reduction and oxidation (REDOX) balance as well as via direct transcriptional upregulation of NRF2 pathways.[77,89,90] Glutamine consumption is increased in cancer as well as other highly proliferative, nonmalignant cells.[78,91] In healthy cells, glutamine can be converted to α-ketoglutarate to refuel the TCA cycle[92] through 2 distinct enzymatic processes: glutamate dehydrogenase 1 or transaminases including glutamic-oxaloacetic transaminase 1 (GOT1), an enzyme critical to glutamine metabolism in PDA and upregulated transcriptionally with *Kras* mutation. Loss of GOT1 function in PDA led to an increase in ROS and decreased ratio of NADPH/NADP+. PDA cells deprived of glutamine fail to thrive, likely because it plays a part in preventing accumulation of ROS and ensuring REDOX homeostasis. Macropinocytosis, a conserved signal-dependent endocytic process by which extracellular solutes and nutrients are transmitted into the cell,[93] is active in PDA and downstream of RAS, contributing to intracellular glutamine replenishment.[79]

KRAS mutations lead to a coordinated acquisition of macromolecules, via both internal scavenging, through autophagy, and from the external environment, via macropinocytosis, and then use of pathways that optimize cellular REDOX balance can be appreciated. Because KRAS has proved to be an elusive therapeutic target, attacking these adaptive metabolic pathways may be efficacious with minimal toxicity because they are likely to be less crucial in benign functional tissues (**Box 3**).

Box 3
Adaptive mechanisms for invasion and growth

- The PDA microenvironment is shifted to favor immunosuppressive leukocytes like TAMs, MDSCs, and T_{reg} rather than cells like T effector cells, which stimulate an immune response.
- Autophagy is a KRAS-driven process upregulated in PDA that provides alternate means for nutrition and growth that may be a therapeutic target and is under investigation.
- Glutamine metabolism is essential in PDA cells for protection against ROS; glutamine stores are replenished by macropinocytosis.

SUMMARY

PDA remains a clinical challenge and although treatments options have changed over the past 5 years, most of these advances have been through the novel combinations of previously established and known chemotherapeutics.[94,95] Thus far, enlightenment on the downstream activities of Kras, the tumor's unique metabolic needs, and how the stroma and immune system affect it has remained untranslated to clinical practice (**Fig. 1**). Given the numbers of diverse therapies in development and a growing knowledge about how to evaluate these systems preclinically and clinically, this is expected to change significantly and for the better over the next 5 years.

REFERENCES

1. Siegel R, Ma J, Zou Z, et al. Cancer statistics, 2014. CA Cancer J Clin 2014;64:9–29.
2. Ryan DP, Hong TS, Bardeesy N. Pancreatic adenocarcinoma. N Engl J Med 2014;371:1039–49.
3. Caldas C, Kern SE. K-ras mutation and pancreatic adenocarcinoma. Int J Pancreatol 1995;18:1–6.
4. Hezel AF, Kimmelman AC, Stanger BZ, et al. Genetics and biology of pancreatic ductal adenocarcinoma. Genes Dev 2006;20:1218–49.
5. McCormick F. Going for the GAP. Curr Biol 1998;8:R673–4.
6. Wittinghofer A, Scheffzek K, Ahmadian MR. The interaction of Ras with GTPase-activating proteins. FEBS Lett 1997;410:63–7.
7. Leevers SJ, Marshall CJ. MAP kinase regulation–the oncogene connection. Trends Cell Biol 1992;2:283–6.
8. Wood KW, Sarnecki C, Roberts TM, et al. Ras mediates nerve growth factor receptor modulation of three signal-transducing protein kinases: MAP kinase, Raf-1, and RSK. Cell 1992;68:1041–50.
9. Rodriguez-Viciana P, Warne PH, Khwaja A, et al. Role of phosphoinositide 3-OH kinase in cell transformation and control of the actin cytoskeleton by Ras. Cell 1997;89:457–67.
10. Collisson EA, Trejo CL, Silva JM, et al. A central role for RAF→MEK→ERK signaling in the genesis of pancreatic ductal adenocarcinoma. Cancer Discov 2012;2:685–93.
11. Alagesan B, Contino G, Guimaraes AR, et al. Combined MEK and PI3K inhibition in a mouse model of pancreatic cancer. Clin Cancer Res 2015;21(2):396–404.
12. Junttila MR, Devasthali V, Cheng JH, et al. Modeling targeted inhibition of MEK and PI3 kinase in human pancreatic cancer. Mol Cancer Ther 2015;14(1):40–7.
13. Rinehart J, Adjei AA, Lorusso PM, et al. Multicenter phase II study of the oral MEK inhibitor, CI-1040, in patients with advanced non-small-cell lung, breast, colon, and pancreatic cancer. J Clin Oncol 2004;22:4456–62.

14. Weinstein IB. Cancer. Addiction to oncogenes–the Achilles heal of cancer. Science 2002;297:63–4.
15. Collins MA, Bednar F, Zhang Y, et al. Oncogenic Kras is required for both the initiation and maintenance of pancreatic cancer in mice. J Clin Invest 2012;122: 639–53.
16. Kapoor A, Yao W, Ying H, et al. Yap1 activation enables bypass of oncogenic Kras addiction in pancreatic cancer. Cell 2014;158:185–97.
17. Zender L, Spector MS, Xue W, et al. Identification and validation of oncogenes in liver cancer using an integrative oncogenomic approach. Cell 2006;125:1253–67.
18. Muramatsu T, Imoto I, Matsui T, et al. YAP is a candidate oncogene for esophageal squamous cell carcinoma. Carcinogenesis 2011;32:389–98.
19. Lee HJ, Zhuang G, Cao Y, et al. Drug resistance via feedback activation of Stat3 in oncogene-addicted cancer cells. Cancer Cell 2014;26:207–21.
20. Hustinx SR, Leoni LM, Yeo CJ, et al. Concordant loss of MTAP and p16/CDKN2A expression in pancreatic intraepithelial neoplasia: evidence of homozygous deletion in a noninvasive precursor lesion. Mod Pathol 2005;18:959–63.
21. Rozenblum E, Schutte M, Goggins M, et al. Tumor-suppressive pathways in pancreatic carcinoma. Cancer Res 1997;57:1731–4.
22. Sharpless NE. INK4a/ARF: a multifunctional tumor suppressor locus. Mutat Res 2005;576:22–38.
23. Bardeesy N, Aguirre AJ, Chu GC, et al. Both p16(Ink4a) and the p19(Arf)-p53 pathway constrain progression of pancreatic adenocarcinoma in the mouse. Proc Natl Acad Sci U S A 2006;103:5947–52.
24. Aguirre AJ, Bardeesy N, Sinha M, et al. Activated Kras and Ink4a/Arf deficiency cooperate to produce metastatic pancreatic ductal adenocarcinoma. Genes Dev 2003;17:3112–26.
25. Scarpa A, Capelli P, Mukai K, et al. Pancreatic adenocarcinomas frequently show p53 gene mutations. Am J Pathol 1993;142:1534–43.
26. Iacobuzio-Donahue CA, Fu B, Yachida S, et al. DPC4 gene status of the primary carcinoma correlates with patterns of failure in patients with pancreatic cancer. J Clin Oncol 2009;27:1806–13.
27. Beckerman R, Prives C. Transcriptional regulation by p53. Cold Spring Harb Perspect Biol 2010;2:a000935.
28. Olivier M, Hollstein M, Hainaut P. TP53 mutations in human cancers: origins, consequences, and clinical use. Cold Spring Harb Perspect Biol 2010;2:a001008.
29. Maitra A, Adsay NV, Argani P, et al. Multicomponent analysis of the pancreatic adenocarcinoma progression model using a pancreatic intraepithelial neoplasia tissue microarray. Mod Pathol 2003;16:902–12.
30. Weber JD, Jeffers JR, Rehg JE, et al. p53-independent functions of the p19(ARF) tumor suppressor. Genes Dev 2000;14:2358–65.
31. Pomerantz J, Schreiber-Agus N, Liegeois NJ, et al. The Ink4a tumor suppressor gene product, p19Arf, interacts with MDM2 and neutralizes MDM2's inhibition of p53. Cell 1998;92:713–23.
32. Hahn SA, Schutte M, Hoque AT, et al. DPC4, a candidate tumor suppressor gene at human chromosome 18q21.1. Science 1996;271:350–3.
33. Massague J, Blain SW, Lo RS. TGFbeta signaling in growth control, cancer, and heritable disorders. Cell 2000;103:295–309.
34. Siegel PM, Massague J. Cytostatic and apoptotic actions of TGF-beta in homeostasis and cancer. Nat Rev Cancer 2003;3:807–21.
35. Ijichi H, Chytil A, Gorska AE, et al. Aggressive pancreatic ductal adenocarcinoma in mice caused by pancreas-specific blockade of transforming growth

factor-beta signaling in cooperation with active Kras expression. Genes Dev 2006;20:3147–60.

36. Bardeesy N, Cheng KH, Berger JH, et al. Smad4 is dispensable for normal pancreas development yet critical in progression and tumor biology of pancreas cancer. Genes Dev 2006;20:3130–46.

37. Horiguchi K, Shirakihara T, Nakano A, et al. Role of Ras signaling in the induction of snail by transforming growth factor-beta. J Biol Chem 2009;284:245–53.

38. Hezel AF, Deshpande V, Zimmerman SM, et al. TGF-beta and alphavbeta6 integrin act in a common pathway to suppress pancreatic cancer progression. Cancer Res 2012;72:4840–5.

39. Jones S, Zhang X, Parsons DW, et al. Core signaling pathways in human pancreatic cancers revealed by global genomic analyses. Science 2008;321:1801–6.

40. Biankin AV, Waddell N, Kassahn KS, et al. Pancreatic cancer genomes reveal aberrations in axon guidance pathway genes. Nature 2012;491:399–405.

41. Mehlen P, Delloye-Bourgeois C, Chedotal A. Novel roles for Slits and netrins: axon guidance cues as anticancer targets? Nat Rev Cancer 2011;11:188–97.

42. Roberts NJ, Jiao Y, Yu J, et al. ATM mutations in patients with hereditary pancreatic cancer. Cancer Discov 2012;2:41–6.

43. Campbell PJ, Yachida S, Mudie LJ, et al. The patterns and dynamics of genomic instability in metastatic pancreatic cancer. Nature 2010;467:1109–13.

44. Hruban RH, Adsay NV, Albores-Saavedra J, et al. Pancreatic intraepithelial neoplasia: a new nomenclature and classification system for pancreatic duct lesions. Am J Surg Pathol 2001;25:579–86.

45. Maitra A, Kern SE, Hruban RH. Molecular pathogenesis of pancreatic cancer. Best Pract Res Clin Gastroenterol 2006;20:211–26.

46. Poultsides GA, Reddy S, Cameron JL, et al. Histopathologic basis for the favorable survival after resection of intraductal papillary mucinous neoplasm-associated invasive adenocarcinoma of the pancreas. Ann Surg 2010;251:470–6.

47. Wu J, Matthaei H, Maitra A, et al. Recurrent GNAS mutations define an unexpected pathway for pancreatic cyst development. Sci Transl Med 2011;3:92ra66.

48. Amato E, Molin MD, Mafficini A, et al. Targeted next-generation sequencing of cancer genes dissects the molecular profiles of intraductal papillary neoplasms of the pancreas. J Pathol 2014;233:217–27.

49. Crippa S, Fernandez-Del Castillo C, Salvia R, et al. Mucin-producing neoplasms of the pancreas: an analysis of distinguishing clinical and epidemiologic characteristics. Clin Gastroenterol Hepatol 2010;8:213–9.

50. Feig C, Gopinathan A, Neesse A, et al. The pancreas cancer microenvironment. Clin Cancer Res 2012;18:4266–76.

51. Provenzano PP, Cuevas C, Chang AE, et al. Enzymatic targeting of the stroma ablates physical barriers to treatment of pancreatic ductal adenocarcinoma. Cancer Cell 2012;21:418–29.

52. Rhim AD, Oberstein PE, Thomas DH, et al. Stromal elements act to restrain, rather than support, pancreatic ductal adenocarcinoma. Cancer Cell 2014;25:735–47.

53. Ozdemir BC, Pentcheva-Hoang T, Carstens JL, et al. Depletion of carcinoma-associated fibroblasts and fibrosis induces immunosuppression and accelerates pancreas cancer with reduced survival. Cancer Cell 2014;25:719–34.

54. Berman DM, Karhadkar SS, Maitra A, et al. Widespread requirement for Hedgehog ligand stimulation in growth of digestive tract tumours. Nature 2003;425:846–51.

55. Thayer SP, di Magliano MP, Heiser PW, et al. Hedgehog is an early and late mediator of pancreatic cancer tumorigenesis. Nature 2003;425:851–6.

56. Yauch RL, Gould SE, Scales SJ, et al. A paracrine requirement for hedgehog signalling in cancer. Nature 2008;455:406–10.
57. Bailey JM, Swanson BJ, Hamada T, et al. Sonic hedgehog promotes desmoplasia in pancreatic cancer. Clin Cancer Res 2008;14:5995–6004.
58. Feldmann G, Fendrich V, McGovern K, et al. An orally bioavailable small-molecule inhibitor of Hedgehog signaling inhibits tumor initiation and metastasis in pancreatic cancer. Mol Cancer Ther 2008;7:2725–35.
59. Olive KP, Jacobetz MA, Davidson CJ, et al. Inhibition of Hedgehog signaling enhances delivery of chemotherapy in a mouse model of pancreatic cancer. Science 2009;324:1457–61.
60. Toole BP. Hyaluronan: from extracellular glue to pericellular cue. Nat Rev Cancer 2004;4:528–39.
61. Anttila MA, Tammi RH, Tammi MI, et al. High levels of stromal hyaluronan predict poor disease outcome in epithelial ovarian cancer. Cancer Res 2000;60:150–5.
62. Itano N, Sawai T, Miyaishi O, et al. Relationship between hyaluronan production and metastatic potential of mouse mammary carcinoma cells. Cancer Res 1999;59:2499–504.
63. Misra S, Ghatak S, Zoltan-Jones A, et al. Regulation of multidrug resistance in cancer cells by hyaluronan. J Biol Chem 2003;278:25285–8.
64. West DC, Hampson IN, Arnold F, et al. Angiogenesis induced by degradation products of hyaluronic acid. Science 1985;228:1324–6.
65. Hanahan D, Weinberg RA. Hallmarks of cancer: the next generation. Cell 2011; 144:646–74.
66. Feldmann G, Habbe N, Dhara S, et al. Hedgehog inhibition prolongs survival in a genetically engineered mouse model of pancreatic cancer. Gut 2008;57: 1420–30.
67. Eger A, Aigner K, Sonдеregger S, et al. DeltaEF1 is a transcriptional repressor of E-cadherin and regulates epithelial plasticity in breast cancer cells. Oncogene 2005;24:2375–85.
68. Cano A, Perez-Moreno MA, Rodrigo I, et al. The transcription factor snail controls epithelial-mesenchymal transitions by repressing E-cadherin expression. Nat Cell Biol 2000;2:76–83.
69. Vonderheide RH, Bayne LJ. Inflammatory networks and immune surveillance of pancreatic carcinoma. Curr Opin Immunol 2013;25:200–5.
70. Clark CE, Hingorani SR, Mick R, et al. Dynamics of the immune reaction to pancreatic cancer from inception to invasion. Cancer Res 2007;67:9518–27.
71. Bayne LJ, Beatty GL, Jhala N, et al. Tumor-derived granulocyte-macrophage colony-stimulating factor regulates myeloid inflammation and T cell immunity in pancreatic cancer. Cancer Cell 2012;21:822–35.
72. Pylayeva-Gupta Y, Lee KE, Hajdu CH, et al. Oncogenic Kras-induced GM-CSF production promotes the development of pancreatic neoplasia. Cancer Cell 2012;21:836–47.
73. Sanford DE, Belt BA, Panni RZ, et al. Inflammatory monocyte mobilization decreases patient survival in pancreatic cancer: a role for targeting the CCL2/CCR2 axis. Clin Cancer Res 2013;19:3404–15.
74. Sakaguchi S, Sakaguchi N, Shimizu J, et al. Immunologic tolerance maintained by CD25+ CD4+ regulatory T cells: their common role in controlling autoimmunity, tumor immunity, and transplantation tolerance. Immunol Rev 2001;182: 18–32.
75. Shi C, Pamer EG. Monocyte recruitment during infection and inflammation. Nat Rev Immunol 2011;11:762–74.

76. Qian BZ, Pollard JW. Macrophage diversity enhances tumor progression and metastasis. Cell 2010;141:39–51.
77. Son J, Lyssiotis CA, Ying H, et al. Glutamine supports pancreatic cancer growth through a KRAS-regulated metabolic pathway. Nature 2013;496:101–5.
78. Wise DR, Thompson CB. Glutamine addiction: a new therapeutic target in cancer. Trends Biochem Sci 2010;35:427–33.
79. Commisso C, Davidson SM, Soydaner-Azeloglu RG, et al. Macropinocytosis of protein is an amino acid supply route in Ras-transformed cells. Nature 2013; 497:633–7.
80. Yang S, Wang X, Contino G, et al. Pancreatic cancers require autophagy for tumor growth. Genes Dev 2011;25:717–29.
81. Guo JY, Chen HY, Mathew R, et al. Activated Ras requires autophagy to maintain oxidative metabolism and tumorigenesis. Genes Dev 2011;25:460–70.
82. Qu X, Yu J, Bhagat G, et al. Promotion of tumorigenesis by heterozygous disruption of the beclin 1 autophagy gene. J Clin Invest 2003;112:1809–20.
83. Liang XH, Jackson S, Seaman M, et al. Induction of autophagy and inhibition of tumorigenesis by beclin 1. Nature 1999;402:672–6.
84. Fujii S, Mitsunaga S, Yamazaki M, et al. Autophagy is activated in pancreatic cancer cells and correlates with poor patient outcome. Cancer Sci 2008;99:1813–9.
85. Rubinsztein DC, Gestwicki JE, Murphy LO, et al. Potential therapeutic applications of autophagy. Nat Rev Drug Discov 2007;6:304–12.
86. Yang A, Rajeshkumar NV, Wang X, et al. Autophagy is critical for pancreatic tumor growth and progression in tumors with p53 alterations. Cancer Discov 2014;4: 905–13.
87. Kinsey C, Balakrishnan V, O'Dell MR, et al. Plac8 links oncogenic mutations to regulation of autophagy and is critical to pancreatic cancer progression. Cell Rep 2014;7:1143–55.
88. Rosenfeldt MT, O'Prey J, Morton JP, et al. p53 status determines the role of autophagy in pancreatic tumour development. Nature 2013;504:296–300.
89. DeNicola GM, Karreth FA, Humpton TJ, et al. Oncogene-induced Nrf2 transcription promotes ROS detoxification and tumorigenesis. Nature 2011;475:106–9.
90. Ying H, Kimmelman AC, Lyssiotis CA, et al. Oncogenic Kras maintains pancreatic tumors through regulation of anabolic glucose metabolism. Cell 2012;149: 656–70.
91. Eagle H. Nutrition needs of mammalian cells in tissue culture. Science 1955;122: 501–14.
92. Vander Heiden MG, Cantley LC, Thompson CB. Understanding the Warburg effect: the metabolic requirements of cell proliferation. Science 2009;324:1029–33.
93. Lim JP, Gleeson PA. Macropinocytosis: an endocytic pathway for internalising large gulps. Immunol Cell Biol 2011;89:836–43.
94. Conroy T, Desseigne F, Ychou M, et al. FOLFIRINOX versus gemcitabine for metastatic pancreatic cancer. N Engl J Med 2011;364:1817–25.
95. Von Hoff DD, Ervin T, Arena FP, et al. Increased survival in pancreatic cancer with nab-paclitaxel plus gemcitabine. N Engl J Med 2013;369:1691–703.

Mouse Models of Pancreatic Ductal Adenocarcinoma

 CrossMark

Mariano Ponz-Sarvise, MD, PhD[a], David A. Tuveson, MD, PhD[a,b,*],
Kenneth H. Yu, MD, MSc[a,b,c,*]

KEYWORDS

- Genetic engineered mouse models • Pancreatic cancer • Kras • Therapeutics
- Models of cancer

KEY POINTS

- The use of genetic engineered mouse models in pancreatic cancer has helped to advance the knowledge of this disease.
- It is important to use mouse models that faithfully recapitulate the disease. This should be achieved by doing a thorough analysis, both at the molecular level and at the pathologic level.
- A model is just another tool to use. It does not represent the full spectrum of the disease.
- New genetically engineered mouse models are needed to address the genetic heterogeneity seen in human patients.

INTRODUCTION

Mortality due to pancreatic cancer is projected to surpass that of breast and colorectal cancers by 2030 in the United States.[1] This dire scenario reflects an aging population, improving outcomes for breast and colorectal cancer patients, the advanced stage of pancreatic cancer at presentation, and a lack of durable treatment responses in pancreatic cancer patients. Indeed, only 10% to 15% of patients with pancreatic ductal adenocarcinoma (PDAC), the most common type of pancreatic cancer, are candidates for potentially curative surgery due to the location or spread of disease at the time of diagnosis.[1,2]

Conflict of Interests: The authors declare no conflict of interests.
[a] Cancer Biology, Cold Spring Harbor Laboratory, One Bungtown Road, Cold Spring Harbor, NY 11724, USA; [b] Memorial Sloan Kettering Cancer Center, New York, NY 10065, USA; [c] Weill Medical College, Cornell University, New York, NY 10065, USA
* Corresponding authors. Cold Spring Harbor Laboratory, Cold Spring Harbor, NY 11724.
E-mail addresses: dtuveson@cshl.edu; yuk1@mskcc.org

Hematol Oncol Clin N Am 29 (2015) 609–617
http://dx.doi.org/10.1016/j.hoc.2015.04.010
0889-8588/15/$ – see front matter © 2015 Elsevier Inc. All rights reserved.

hemonc.theclinics.com

Despite rapid progress in the understanding of the molecular mechanisms underlying pancreatic ductal adenocarcinoma, translation to effective therapies has been modest at best. One of the key tools available for studying biology and developing more effective therapeutics is the laboratory mouse, *mus musculus*. In this sense there are some characteristics that mouse models should have in order to be useful for the advancement in a disease. Those characteristics are discussed in **Box 1**.

Modeling PDAC in the mouse offers certain clear benefits. The mouse is small, reproduces rapidly, and has a lifespan of 3 years. The mouse genome has been completely sequenced and bears strong homology to that of people. This review discusses current approaches for leveraging the mouse to model PDAC, weighs the relative benefits and shortcomings of each approach, and provides examples for how each approach has been utilized. The article also explores new and innovative approaches to mouse modeling and how these approaches can be utilized to move the field forward.

MOUSE XENOGRAFT MODELS

Historically cancer cell lines derived from human patients have been used in vitro and in vivo to study PDAC. To this day, cell lines remain widely used for initial screenings of drugs or to try to more clearly understand mechanisms in PDAC cell biology. **Table 1** summarizes some of the main characteristics of cell lines compared with the different models that will be discussed in this article. One key shortcoming of studying cell lines is a potential selection process that the tumor epithelial cells undergo to survive and replicate on a monolayer. This selection may impact the neoplastic cell properties and therefore confound one's ability to model the disease of a given patient.

The Immunocompromised Mouse

Transplantation of human cancer cell lines or primary human tumors into a host mouse to create a xenograft was one of the first models developed to study PDAC. This approach became possible with the discovery of mice incapable of rejecting the transplanted human cells, first with the T-cell deficient nude athymic mouse,[3] followed by the B- and T-cell deficient severe combined immunodeficient, or SCID, mouse,[4] and the nonobese diabetic, or NOD/SCID mouse.[5] With regards to modeling cancer, the major difference among these mice involves their immune competence and their ability to model the human immune response to cancer. Compared with the SCID mouse, the athymic mouse maintains intact granulocytes, macrophages, B-, NK- and dendritic cell components. Though not often utilized because of expense and technical complexity, NOD/SCID mice can be engrafted with human bone marrow cells to emulate the native immune response.[6,7]

Box 1
Characteristics for a mouse model to truthfully recapitulate a disease

1. Genetics should try to mimic what happens in humans.

2. Histology assessment by a pathologist should indicate the similarity with the human disease.

3. Molecular pathways (tumor phenotype at the molecular level) in the mice should reflect the molecular pathways in human patients.

Table 1
Characteristics of different preclinical models used in pancreatic ductal adenocarcinoma

	Cell Lines	Xenografts	GEMMs
Cost of maintenance	+++	++	+
Success rate of initiation	+	++	+++
Biological stability	+	++	+++
Expansion	+++	+	+
Genetic manipulation	+++	+	++
3-dimensional growth	−	++	+++
Tumor–stroma interaction	−	+	+++
High throughput drug screens	+++	−	−
Immune system	−	+	+++
Dose-limiting organ toxicity	−	++	+++

Cell Line Derived Xenografts

Xenografts can be derived either from established cell lines or directly from human tumors. Cells or tumor tissue can be implanted subcutaneously (heterotopically) or into the mouse pancreas (orthotopically). Each approach has certain advantages and disadvantages. Use of cell lines implanted heterotopically remains a primary tool for pharmaceutical development. This approach is convenient, less expensive, and allows for relatively rapid screening of a large number of candidate molecules to assess efficacy and safety. Unfortunately, this represents the least biologically faithful model. Immortalized cell lines may not emulate the genetic and cellular heterogeneity present in the human disease. Whole exome sequencing studies have shown that there is great genetic diversity, not only among tumors from different individuals, but also within a single tumor and across metastatic sites from the same individual.[8] Although implantation subcutaneously allows for convenient tumor size assessment, growth of the tumor outside of the pancreas and in the absence of tumor stroma does not reflect the human disease; for example, these tumors rarely metastasize.[9] The immunodeficient mouse also is not capable of generating the same immune response seen in human patients. Together, these factors contribute to the outcome that drugs predicted to be effective based on PDAC cell line xenografts often do not translate in the clinical setting.[10]

Patient Derived Xenografts

Patient derived xenografts (PDXs) are generated by transplantation of PDAC tumor tissue directly into mice, either subcutaneously or in the subrenal capsule. PDX tumors may reflect more of the genetic heterogeneity and stromal abundance present in the original tumor.[11] Despite serial passaging in mice, PDX tumors have been shown to maintain some of these features, as well as responses to cytotoxic chemotherapeutic agents.[12,13] Like standard xenografts, the PDX approach can be used to generate large numbers of mice, serving as a platform upon which therapeutic candidates can be screened. With the advent of gene expression profiling and genomic sequencing, specific gene mutations present in a specific tumor can be studied and response assessed to targeted drugs, administered either as a single agent or in combination. The genetic heterogeneity among PDXs derived from different tumors can be used to model differential responses to chemotherapeutic agents, as seen in patients. For example, a pharmacogenomics model incorporating gene expression profiles and treatment responses was developed with 32 different PDX models of PDAC. These data were used to support a clinical trial further validating the model's ability to predict treatment response, resistance, and survival in patients with metastatic PDAC.[14]

Many of the disadvantages present in standard xenografts are also problematic in PDXs (eg, an immunodeficient host mouse and subcutaneous tumors implanted distantly from the tissue of origin). Nevertheless, generation and drug screening of xenografts from individual patients has recently been put forward as an approach toward personalized medicine.[12] Overall, this approach is challenging, due to the time and effort required to generate PDXs and to perform drug screening, and the limited availability of effective cytotoxic and targeted agents. The prototypical example of how such an approach could work involves a patient who underwent resection with curative intent for PDAC.[15] The patient's tumor was used to generate PDXs. Drug screening against these PDXs revealed profound sensitivity to cisplatin and mitomycin C, but relative resistance to gemcitabine. The patient subsequently experienced disease recurrence, which did not respond to gemcitabine. By contrast, when the patient was treated with mitomycin C, a nonstandard approach, the tumor responded dramatically and for a long duration. Ultimately, the patient was found to have a rare germline mutation in the *PALB2* gene. Although a terrific example of the potential power of PDX models, it is currently unclear whether such an approach can be applied in patients without uncommon genetic susceptibilities.

GENETICALLY ENGINEERED MOUSE MODELS

The genetically engineered mouse model (GEMM) was developed to address many of the key weaknesses of the xenograft approach. The GEMM attempts to recapitulate the PDAC phenotype by introducing into the mouse pancreas the specific genetic mutations present in human PDAC. The most common of these are activating mutations in *KRAS*, followed by inactivating mutations in *CDKN2A* (*P16/INK4A*), *TP53*, and *SMAD4*.[8] Successful engineering of the *LSL-Kras^{G12D}* and the *LSL-Kras$^{G12V-bGeo}$* mouse was a key development that launched the field.[16–18]

LSL-Kras^{G12D} Model

The original GEMM, the *LSL-Kras^{G12D}* mouse, was generated by targeting expression of the endogenous oncogenic *LSL-Kras^{G12D}* allele to the developing pancreas through the use of pancreas-specific Cre recombinase alleles.[17] Such *PDX1-Cre, LSL-Kras^{G12D}*, or *P48$^{+/-Cre}$, LSL-Kras^{G12D}* (KC) GEMMs develop a spectrum of pre-invasive ductal lesions that mirror human pancreatic intraepithelial neoplasia (PanIN), and upon aging, KC mice stochastically develop primary and metastatic PDAC. The KC GEMM develops PanIN with 100% penetrance. The median survival of this model is around 1 year, and not all KC mice develop PDAC. The KC GEMM represents a suitable platform for the study of PanIN biology and the development of diagnostic and therapeutic approaches.

LSL-Trp53$^{R172H/-}$ Model

To promote the rapid onset of PDAC, additional mutations in tumor suppressor genes were incorporated.[19–22] As an example, the *PDX-1-Cre, LSL-Kras^{G12D}, LSL-Trp53$^{R172H/-}$* (KPC) GEMM incorporates inactivation of the *TP53* suppressor gene, and consequently, rapidly develops PDA. The median survival is approximately 5 months, and most mice (96%) develop PDAC at the time of death. Further studies demonstrated that the KPC GEMM possessed properties necessary to serve as a useful tool to study and develop new therapies to treat PDAC, including the histopathologic resemblance to the human PDAC. The KPC GEMM was shown to be deficient in vasculature, similar to the human disease, and resulting in impaired drug delivery.[10,23] KPC tumors proved resistant to standard chemotherapeutic agents, such as gemcitabine, similar to the human disease.[10] Therefore, unlike the xenograft model, GEMMs can be used to study and develop therapeutic approaches against the tumor microenvironment and tumor stroma.

Translational uses of the LSL-Trp53[R172H/-] model

Initial testing of the hedgehog signaling pathway inhibitor, IPI-926, demonstrated promising transient effects on the tumor microenvironment, leading to improved drug delivery, and associated improved survival in mice treated with both IPI-926 and gemcitabine. Unfortunately, IPI-926 combined with gemcitabine was ineffective when tested in PDAC patients in a randomized clinical trial.[24] Importantly, the GEMM paradigm could be used to study why targeting of the hedgehog pathway was unsuccessful. By developing a GEMM deficient in sonic hedgehog, $Shh^{fl/fl}$;$Pdx1$-Cre;$Kras^{LSL-G12D/+}$;$p53^{fl/+}$;$Rosa26^{LSL-YFP}$, Rhim and colleagues[24] performed studies demonstrating that hedgehog inhibition led to an absence of tumor stroma and an abundance of intratumoral blood vessels, similar to the previous findings of Olive and colleagues. However, prolonged hedgehog inhibition as a monotherapy, paradoxically, led to more aggressive tumor behavior. These studies illustrate the utility of GEMMs to study the complex interaction between cancer cells and the tumor microenvironment, particularly in response to pharmacologic perturbations.

The tumor microenvironment remains an intriguing area of study for developing novel therapeutics in PDAC. The glycosaminoglycan hyaluronan (HA) has been shown to be overrepresented in PDAC stroma.[25] HA may signal through hyaladherins such as CD44 to regulate receptor tyrosine kinase and small GTPase activity, and it is implicated in the processes of angiogenesis, epithelial–mesenchymal transition, and chemoresistance.[26] Moreover, HA's anionic repeats also sequester mobile cations and solvate water, resulting in osmotic swelling that provides structural support in HA-rich normal and malignant tissues.[27] HA can be degraded by the enzyme hyaluronidase. PEGPH20, a PEGylated human recombinant PH20 hyaluronidase, induces a rapid perfusion increase in xenograft tumors.[28] Like in the human disease, there is high HA expression in KPC GEMM PDAC tumors. In the KPC GEMM,[23] PEGPH20 was shown to rapidly and sustainably deplete HA, induce re-expansion of PDAC blood vessels, and increase intratumoral delivery of 2 chemotherapeutic agents, doxorubicin and gemcitabine. PEGPH20 caused fenestrations and interendothelial junction gaps in PDAC tumor blood vessels, and promoted a tumor-specific increase in macromolecular permeability. Finally, combination therapy with PEGPH20 and gemcitabine led to inhibition of PDAC tumor growth and prolonged survival over gemcitabine monotherapy, suggesting immediate clinical utility. These promising preclinical studies have led to phase 1 studies in people demonstrating safety (ClinicalTrials. gov Identifiers NCT00834704, NCT01170897) and a randomized phase 2 clinical trial in metastatic PDAC (ClinicalTrials.gov Identifier NCT01839487) studying the addition of PEGPH20 to the standard chemotherapy regimen of gemcitabine and nab-paclitaxel, currently ongoing.

One of the hallmarks of PDAC is the propensity of tumors to metastasize, even when the primary tumor is resected, or in the setting of a small primary tumor. Rhim and colleagues investigated this phenomenon by lineage tagging pancreatic epithelial cells using the $Rosa^{YFP}$ allele, crossed with the KPC GEMM. Importantly, circulating pancreatic cells were found to be present in the bloodstream early in PDAC development, prior to formation of invasive lesions. These tagged cells exhibited mesenchymal and stem cell properties and possessed the ability to seed the liver. Although these studies provide a plausible explanation for observations made in the human disease, and have important implications for strategies of early detection and treatment of early stage disease, it should be noted that the presence of disseminated cells does not mean that those cells are competent to form metastases.

Unlike xenograft models, the GEMMs have an intact immune system; therefore, they provide a tool to study the immune response in PDAC. CD40, a tumor necrosis factor receptor superfamily member, has been shown to play an important role in the development of a T cell antitumor response.[29] Beatty and colleagues studied the effects of the agonist CD40 mAb FGK45 in KPC GEMMs. These studies demonstrated some tumor responses; however, rather than a T cell response, macrophage infiltration appeared to be important, a finding confirmed in patients who responded to FGK45 treatment. More recently, the KPC GEMM has been utilized to further elucidate the complex mechanisms by which PDAC evades immune surveillance.[30] Although antagonism of immune checkpoints anticytotoxic T-lymphocyte-associated protein 4 (α-CTLA-4) and α-programmed cell death 1 ligand 1 (α-PD-L1) have been effective therapeutic strategies in other malignancies such as malignant melanoma and non-small cell lung adenocarcinoma, such approaches have thus far proven ineffective for PDAC. Feig and colleagues found that PDAC in KPC GEMMs also did not respond to checkpoint antagonists. Interestingly, when carcinoma-associated fibroblasts were depleted, checkpoint antagonists were able to control tumor growth. The chemokine CXCL12 was identified as a candidate molecule preventing T cell accumulation in PDAC tumors, a phenomenon that could be overcome with the CXCL12 receptor inhibitor, AMD3100. These studies demonstrate the potential for GEMMs, for studying disease biology and developmental therapeutics, particularly focused on tumor microenvironment and immune surveillance.

FUTURE DIRECTIONS

Looking to the future, ever more sophisticated murine models of PDAC are being developed. One example is the doxycycline-inducible $Kras^{G12D}$ GEMM, allowing investigators to readily turn oncogenic $KRAS$ expression on or off, and study the downstream effects.[31] A recent study published by this group using the inducible $KRAS$ model showed that Yap1 could be a potential mechanism of escape once $KRAS$ is turned off.[32] This finding implies that YAP might be a mechanism of resistance to therapies targeting $KRAS$ in PDAC. Clearly, there remains room for improved and innovative models to increase knowledge of this disease.

Several technologies are now available to improve the efficiency of engineering mouse models. One prominent example involves using transgenic RNAi as opposed to homologous recombination to rapidly and efficiently create GEMMs to study any mammalian gene.[33] This embryonic stem cell (ESC) targeted approach has several advantages, including the ability to engineer complex genotypes without the need for extensive cross-breeding and maintenance of large mouse colonies. This approach was used to create a PDAC GEMM containing the conditional LSL-$Kras^{G12D}$ mutation, and a homing cassette allowing for easy insertion of fluorescence-coupled shRNA under tetracycline control for rapidly and cost-effectively asking numerous biological and therapeutic targeting questions.[34]

Another important line of research focuses on trying to model the heterogeneous behavior of human PDAC. While studying a large number of PDXs can effectively address this issue, individual GEMMs generally do not. Collisson and colleagues[35] recently proposed 3 subtypes of PDAC—classical, quasimesenchymal and exocrine-like—with associated transcriptional profiles. Developing models of each subtype of PDAC may lead to better understand of PDAC subtypes not adequately modeled by existing GEMMs.

Recently developed technologies have allowed for rapid, reliable culture and expansion of human normal pancreas and PDAC tissue in vitro in a 3-dimensional culture. Originally described in intestinal epithelium, Sato and colleagues[36] used special culture conditions including the Wnt agonist, R-spondin1, to generate self-organizing structures, termed organoids, suspended in Matrigel. These organoids proliferated and could be passaged indefinitely. More recently, this approach has proven successful for generating in vitro models of pancreatic tissue[37] and PDAC.[38] The authors' laboratory, in collaboration with Clevers' laboratory, has been able to grow both mouse and human PDAC with this technique. These mice and human organoids can also be transplanted in mice, giving rise to the full spectrum of PDAC in those animals.[38] These results open the door to the design of exciting experiments that will shed light on the biology of both early and late PanIN, as well as frank PDAC.

Use of organoids and other techniques described to generate a next generation of mouse models will hopefully lead to a better understanding and effective therapeutics for a still intractable disease.

REFERENCES

1. Rahib L, Smith BD, Aizenberg R, et al. Projecting cancer incidence and deaths to 2030: the unexpected burden of thyroid, liver, and pancreas cancers in the United States. Cancer Res 2014;74(11):2913–21.

2. Ryan DP, Hong TS, Bardeesy N. Pancreatic adenocarcinoma. N Engl J Med 2014;371(22):2140–1.

3. Flanagan SP. 'Nude', a new hairless gene with pleiotropic effects in the mouse. Genet Res 1966;8(3):295–309.

4. Bosma GC, Custer RP, Bosma MJ. A severe combined immunodeficiency mutation in the mouse. Nature 1983;301(5900):527–30.

5. Shultz LD, Schweitzer PA, Christianson SW, et al. Multiple defects in innate and adaptive immunologic function in NOD/LtSz-scid mice. J Immunol 1995;154(1): 180–91.

6. McCune JM, Namikawa R, Kaneshima H, et al. The SCID-hu mouse: murine model for the analysis of human hematolymphoid differentiation and function. Science 1988;241(4873):1632–9.

7. Greiner DL, Shultz LD, Yates J, et al. Improved engraftment of human spleen cells in NOD/LtSz-scid/scid mice as compared with C.B-17-scid/scid mice. Am J Pathol 1995;146(4):888–902.

8. Jones S, Zhang X, Parsons DW, et al. Core signaling pathways in human pancreatic cancers revealed by global genomic analyses. Science 2008;321(5897): 1801–6.

9. Fidler IJ. Critical factors in the biology of human cancer metastasis: twenty-eighth G.H.A. Clowes Memorial Award Lecture. Cancer Res 1990;50(19):6130–8.

10. Olive KP, Jacobetz MA, Davidson CJ, et al. Inhibition of Hedgehog signaling enhances delivery of chemotherapy in a mouse model of pancreatic cancer. Science 2009;324(5933):1457–61.

11. Yachida S, Jones S, Bozic I, et al. Distant metastasis occurs late during the genetic evolution of pancreatic cancer. Nature 2010;467(7319):1114–7.

12. Rubio-Viqueira B, Jimeno A, Cusatis G, et al. An in vivo platform for translational drug development in pancreatic cancer. Clin Cancer Res 2006;12(15):4652–61.
13. Rubio-Viqueira B, Hidalgo M. Direct in vivo xenograft tumor model for predicting chemotherapeutic drug response in cancer patients. Clin Pharmacol Ther 2009; 85(2):217–21.
14. Yu KH, Ricigliano M, Hidalgo M, et al. Pharmacogenomic modeling of circulating tumor and invasive cells for prediction of chemotherapy response and resistance in pancreatic cancer. Clin Cancer Res 2014;20(20):5281–9.
15. Villarroel MC, Rajeshkumar NV, Garrido-Laguna I, et al. Personalizing cancer treatment in the age of global genomic analyses: PALB2 gene mutations and the response to DNA damaging agents in pancreatic cancer. Mol Cancer Ther 2011;10(1):3–8.
16. Jackson EL, Willis N, Mercer K, et al. Analysis of lung tumor initiation and progression using conditional expression of oncogenic K-ras. Genes Dev 2001;15(24): 3243–8.
17. Hingorani SR, Petricoin EF, Maitra A, et al. Preinvasive and invasive ductal pancreatic cancer and its early detection in the mouse. Cancer Cell 2003;4(6): 437–50.
18. Guerra C, Schuhmacher AJ, Canamero M, et al. Chronic pancreatitis is essential for induction of pancreatic ductal adenocarcinoma by K-Ras oncogenes in adult mice. Cancer Cell 2007;11(3):291–302.
19. Aguirre AJ, Bardeesy N, Sinha M, et al. Activated Kras and Ink4a/Arf deficiency cooperate to produce metastatic pancreatic ductal adenocarcinoma. Genes Dev 2003;17(24):3112–26.
20. Bardeesy N, Cheng KH, Berger JH, et al. Smad4 is dispensable for normal pancreas development yet critical in progression and tumor biology of pancreas cancer. Genes Dev 2006;20(22):3130–46.
21. Hingorani SR, Wang L, Multani AS, et al. Trp53R172H and KrasG12D cooperate to promote chromosomal instability and widely metastatic pancreatic ductal adenocarcinoma in mice. Cancer Cell 2005;7(5):469–83.
22. Ijichi H, Chytil A, Gorska AE, et al. Aggressive pancreatic ductal adenocarcinoma in mice caused by pancreas-specific blockade of transforming growth factor-beta signaling in cooperation with active Kras expression. Genes Dev 2006; 20(22):3147–60.
23. Jacobetz MA, Chan DS, Neesse A, et al. Hyaluronan impairs vascular function and drug delivery in a mouse model of pancreatic cancer. Gut 2013;62(1): 112–20.
24. Rhim AD, Oberstein PE, Thomas DH, et al. Stromal elements act to restrain, rather than support, pancreatic ductal adenocarcinoma. Cancer Cell 2014;25(6): 735–47.
25. Theocharis AD, Tsara ME, Papageorgacopoulou N, et al. Pancreatic carcinoma is characterized by elevated content of hyaluronan and chondroitin sulfate with altered disaccharide composition. Biochim Biophys Acta 2000;1502(2):201–6.
26. Toole BP, Slomiany MG. Hyaluronan: a constitutive regulator of chemoresistance and malignancy in cancer cells. Semin Cancer Biol 2008;18(4):244–50.
27. Chahine NO, Chen FH, Hung CT, et al. Direct measurement of osmotic pressure of glycosaminoglycan solutions by membrane osmometry at room temperature. Biophys J 2005;89(3):1543–50.
28. Thompson CB, Shepard HM, O'Connor PM, et al. Enzymatic depletion of tumor hyaluronan induces antitumor responses in preclinical animal models. Mol Cancer Ther 2010;9(11):3052–64.

29. Beatty GL, Chiorean EG, Fishman MP, et al. CD40 agonists alter tumor stroma and show efficacy against pancreatic carcinoma in mice and humans. Science 2011;331(6024):1612–6.
30. Feig C, Jones JO, Kraman M, et al. Targeting CXCL12 from FAP-expressing carcinoma-associated fibroblasts synergizes with anti-PD-L1 immunotherapy in pancreatic cancer. Proc Natl Acad Sci U S A 2013;110(50):20212–7.
31. Ying H, Kimmelman AC, Lyssiotis CA, et al. Oncogenic Kras maintains pancreatic tumors through regulation of anabolic glucose metabolism. Cell 2012;149(3): 656–70.
32. Kapoor A, Yao W, Ying H, et al. Yap1 activation enables bypass of oncogenic Kras addiction in pancreatic cancer. Cell 2014;158(1):185–97.
33. Premsrirut PK, Dow LE, Kim SY, et al. A rapid and scalable system for studying gene function in mice using conditional RNA interference. Cell 2011;145(1): 145–58.
34. Saborowski M, Saborowski A, Morris JP, et al. A modular and flexible ESC-based mouse model of pancreatic cancer. Genes Dev 2014;28(1):85–97.
35. Collisson EA, Sadanandam A, Olson P, et al. Subtypes of pancreatic ductal adenocarcinoma and their differing responses to therapy. Nat Med 2011;17(4): 500–3.
36. Sato T, Vries RG, Snippert HJ, et al. Single Lgr5 stem cells build crypt-villus structures in vitro without a mesenchymal niche. Nature 2009;459(7244):262–5.
37. Huch M, Bonfanti P, Boj SF, et al. Unlimited in vitro expansion of adult bi-potent pancreas progenitors through the Lgr5/R-spondin axis. EMBO J 2013;32(20): 2708–21.
38. Boj SF, Hwang C-I, Baker LA, et al. Organoid models of human and mouse ductal pancreatic cancer. Cell 2015;160:1–15.

Epidemiology and Inherited Predisposition for Sporadic Pancreatic Adenocarcinoma

Rachael Z. Stolzenberg-Solomon, PhD, MPH, RD[a,*],
Laufey T. Amundadottir, PhD[b,*]

KEYWORDS

- Pancreatic cancer • Diabetes • Etiology • Genome-wide association studies

KEY POINTS

- Given the changing demographics of Western populations, the numbers of pancreatic cancer cases are projected to increase during the next decade.
- Diabetes, recent cigarette smoking, and excess body weight are the most consistent risk factors of pancreatic cancer.
- The search for common and rare germline variants that influence risk of pancreatic cancer through genome-wide association studies (GWAS) and high-throughput-sequencing–based studies is underway and holds the promise of increasing the knowledge of variants and genes that play a role in inherited susceptibility of this devastating disease.
- Although research gaps remain, research reported in this review has advanced the understanding of pancreatic cancer.

EPIDEMIOLOGY FOR PANCREATIC ADENOCARCINOMA

Descriptive Epidemiology

Although pancreatic cancer accounts for less than 3% of cancer incidence, it ranks seventh for cancer mortality globally[1] and fourth in the United States.[2] Annually an

Both authors contributed equally to this review.

This work was supported by the Intramural Research Program of the National Institutes of Health, Division of Cancer Epidemiology and Genetics, National Cancer Institute, Department of Health and Human Services.

[a] Nutritional Epidemiology Branch, Division of Cancer Epidemiology and Genetics, National Cancer Institute, National Institutes of Health, 9609 Medical Center Drive, Room 6E420, Rockville, MD 20850, USA; [b] Laboratory of Translational Genomics, Division of Cancer Epidemiology and Genetics, National Cancer Institute, National Institutes of Health, 8717 Grovemont Circle, Bethesda, MD 20892, USA

* Corresponding authors. Nutritional Epidemiology Branch and Laboratory of Translational Genomics, National Cancer Institute, National Institutes of Health, Bethesda, MD.

E-mail addresses: rs221z@nih.gov; amundadottirl@mail.nih.gov

Hematol Oncol Clin N Am 29 (2015) 619–640

http://dx.doi.org/10.1016/j.hoc.2015.04.009

0889-8588/15/$ – see front matter Published by Elsevier Inc.

hemonc.theclinics.com

estimated 338,000 and 46,420 people will be diagnosed with pancreatic cancer and 331,000 and 39,590 will die from the disease, worldwide and in the United States, respectively.[1,2] There is no effective screening test for the malignancy; therefore, it is most often diagnosed at advanced stages with metastatic disease, which contributes to its high fatality with a mortality to incidence ratio of 0.98.[1] The 5-year survival rate is 6.7%, which is poorer than that of other cancers.[2] Only 9% of pancreatic cancer cases are diagnosed with localized disease when surgical resection may be an option for a cure.[3] Those with localized disease have a 5-year survival of 25.8%.[3] More than 90% of pancreatic cancers are ductal adenocarcinomas, with neuroendocrine tumors constituting about 5%.[4]

Internationally, rates of pancreatic cancer vary by 7-fold, with higher rates in developed than in developing countries.[1] In part the variation in incidence and mortality patterns worldwide may be explained by underascertainment of the disease and imperfect mortality data.[1] Pancreatic cancer occurs slightly more often in men than in women and in African Americans than in Caucasians and other ethnicities in the United States.[2] Its incidence and mortality rates increase with age. More than 88% of pancreatic cancer is diagnosed among people aged 55 years or older, with the median age at diagnosis of 71 years.[3] In the United States, incidence and mortality rates for pancreatic cancer either decreased or remained stable during the latter part of the twentieth century but increased slightly since 2000 (**Figs. 1** and **2**).[2,5] Given the changing demographics in the United States, namely, the aging population and minority distribution, one recent study has projected that the number of pancreatic cancer deaths will surpass that of breast and colorectal cancer by the year 2030.[6]

Risk Factors

Diabetes
Diabetes is associated with approximately a 2-fold risk for pancreatic cancer overall.[7–9] Excess risks tend to be particularly high (2.5- to 10-fold) for diabetes diagnosed within 5 years of pancreatic cancer diagnosis and become attenuated with long duration of diabetes.[7–9] A large pooled case-control study showed that the association with pancreatic cancer remained significant among those having diabetes for 20 years or more; however, the excess risk was diminished to 30%.[9]

Biomarkers for diabetes and insulin resistance Although diabetes as defined by fasting glucose, glucose intolerance,[7] or hemoglobin A(1c),[10,11] a marker for glucose control, has consistently been associated with pancreatic cancer in prospective epidemiologic studies, studies of other biomarkers hypothesized to mediate the diabetes-pancreatic cancer relationship have shown no association or inconsistent results (**Table 1**).[10–17] Insulin is a mitogen and has growth-promoting activity on pancreatic cancer cells, and patients with type 2 diabetes exhibit hyperinsulinemia during the early stages of the disease.[18] Two studies that examined insulin and subsequent risk of pancreatic cancer showed significant elevated risks that were graded with significant trends across increasing categories of insulin. In both studies, the associations were stronger among cases occurring 10 years or more after their blood collection.[11,12] These findings support that the positive associations observed among the later occurring cases are not the consequence of subclinical pancreatic cancer and that insulin resistance may play a role in pancreatic cancer etiology.

A nested case-control study of 4 cohorts examined the association between 83 metabolites and pancreatic cancer.[19] The investigators observed significant positive associations between plasma branched-chain amino acids (ie, isoleucine, leucine, and valine) and subsequent risk of pancreatic cancer in both humans and in a mutant

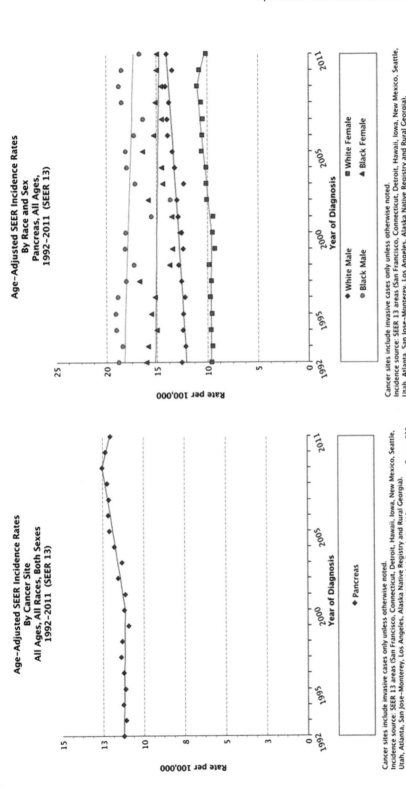

Fig. 1. Incidence rates for pancreatic cancer in the United States overall and by sex and race, 1992 to 2011. (*Data from* Fast Stats: An interactive tool for access to SEER cancer statistics. Surveillance Research Program, National Cancer Institute. http://seer.cancer.gov/faststats. Accessed February, 2015).

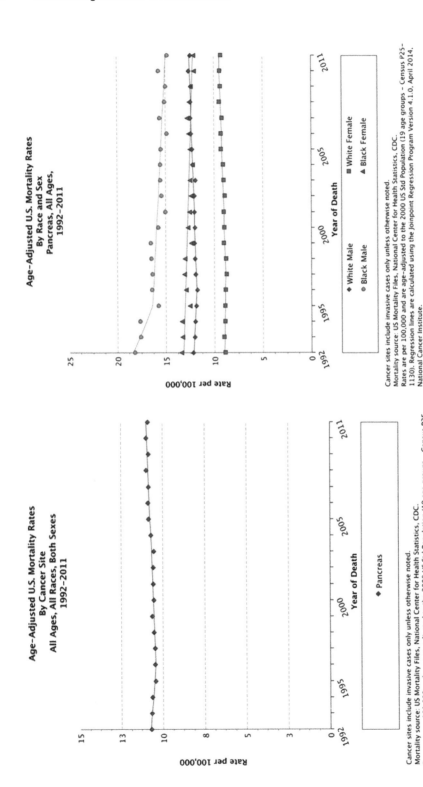

Fig. 2. Mortality rates for pancreatic cancer in the United States overall and by sex and race, 1992 to 2011. (*Data from* Fast Stats: An interactive tool for access to SEER cancer statistics. Surveillance Research Program, National Cancer Institute. http://seer.cancer.gov/faststats. Accessed February, 2015.)

Table 1
Prediagnostic diabetes or inflammation-related biomarkers measured in peripheral blood and pancreatic cancer risk

Biomarker	Number of Studies	Association for Higher Concentration Compared with Lower Concentration[a]
HbA(1c)[10,11]	2	↑↑
Insulin[11,12] or proinsulin[11]	2	↑↑ Overall, stronger among cases occurring >10 y after blood collection
C-peptide[10,147]	2	↑↑ But not significant
Adiponectin (high)[17,148,149]	3	↓↓ Null
IGF-1, IGFBP-3[13,150–152]	4	Null
IGFBP-1 (low)[153]	1	↑
IGF-2[13]	1	Null
sRAGE[15,16]	2	↓ Null
CML-AGE[15,16]	2	Null
C-reactive protein[14,154,155]	4	Null or ↓ in male smokers
IL6, sTNF-R1, sTNF-R2[154,155]	2	Null (↑sTNF-R1 but not significant in women only)
TGF-B[156]	1	↑ Among cases occurring >10 y after blood collection

[a] Each arrow or null represents one study.

KRAS mouse model.[19] The associations were independent of body mass index (BMI) and biomarkers related to insulin resistance and diabetes. Circulating branched-chain amino acid levels are elevated with obesity, glucose intolerance, and insulin resistance.[20] The strongest association for these metabolites in this nested case-control study, however, was among subjects with samples collected between 2 and 5 years before pancreatic cancer diagnosis.[19] The investigators hypothesized that this association was explained by breakdown of tissue protein that occurs in early-stage pancreatic cancer.

These studies support diabetes being an early manifestation of the malignancy as well as a risk factor involved in the cause of pancreatic cancer.

Pancreatitis and type 3c diabetes Chronic pancreatitis is a known risk factor for pancreatic cancer, with risks ranging from 2- to 3-fold.[21,22] The risk is particularly strong for familial pancreatitis. A large pooled analysis of 10 case-control studies estimated pancreatitis to account for approximately 1.34% of pancreatic cancer.[21]

Type 3c diabetes (T3cDM) due to exocrine pancreatic disease has been recognized to play a role in pancreatic carcinogenesis.[23,24] T3cDM is estimated to account for 5% to 10% of diabetes in Western populations.[23] Patients with T3cDM have pancreatic inflammation, with 78% of patients having pancreatitis and 8% pancreatic cancer.[23] Although pancreatic cancer contributes to T3cDM,[23] it is also plausible that the pancreatitis associated with T3cDM participates in the development of the malignancy.

Maturity-onset diabetes of the young Maturity-onset diabetes of the young (MODY) is estimated to account for 1% to 5% of all diabetes.[25] Although MODY is typically diagnosed in young adults, it can be diagnosed at older ages also.[25] MODY is caused by autosomal dominant gene mutations that alter islet beta-cell function.[25]

Loci in genes linked to MODY have been associated with pancreatic cancer in studies using genome-wide genotyping data (see later section).[26–28] In particular, common variants in 3 genes HNF1A, HNF1B, and PDX1 were associated with pancreatic cancer in individuals of European descent.[26–28] These genes are also important components for transcriptional networks governing embryonic pancreatic development and differentiation, in addition to maintaining pancreatic homeostasis in adults.[27,29,30]

Antidiabetic drugs Several studies have examined the association between antidiabetic drugs and pancreatic cancer.[9,31,32] Metformin works by suppressing glucose production in the liver, so there has been a particular interest in whether metformin has antitumor effects by decreasing circulating insulin concentrations.[31] In contrast to metformin, sulfonylureas lower blood glucose levels by increasing the release of insulin from the pancreas. A large well-conducted case-control study that used drug prescription and other data derived from the UK General Practice Research Database showed that compared with those with no prior respective drug treatment, no associations were observed for metformin use, whereas significant positive associations were observed overall for long duration of sulfonylureas and insulin use as quantified by the number of recorded prescriptions.[31] The same pattern of association was observed when this analysis was restricted to participants with a history of diabetes.[31] A meta-analysis of clinical trials and observational studies similarly showed no association between metformin use and pancreatic cancer.[32] In contrast, a large pooled case-control study showed a significant inverse association with long duration (15 years or more) of oral antidiabetic drug use and positive association for less than 10 years duration of insulin treatment compared with their respective nontreatment groups.[9] A limitation of these studies is that the referent group for the observation studies includes participants receiving treatment of the other antidiabetic drugs, which could potentially influence the individual drug risk estimates.[32]

Modifiable risk factors

Tobacco use Current cigarette smoking is the most consistent potentially modifiable factor associated with pancreatic cancer with a close to a 2-fold elevated risk observed in most studies[33–35] and has been estimated to account for up to 24% of pancreatic cancer. Compared with never smokers, the risk starts to decrease 10 years after smoking cessation, with the risk approaching that of never smokers 15 or more years after smoking cessation.[33,34] Cigar and pipe smoking and smokeless tobacco are also associated with increased risk for pancreatic cancer[34] in some but not all studies.[35]

Overweight and obesity Obesity is known to contribute to insulin resistance and type 2 diabetes. Most prospective studies show positive associations between middle-aged and older adult BMI and pancreatic cancer, with risk stronger among non-smokers.[36,37] Cigarette smoke contains a multitude of carcinogens, so it is possible that obesity does not play a substantial role in the cause of pancreatic cancer in smokers. A meta-analysis of 23 prospective cohort studies, totaling 9500 cases, showed that per 5 unit increase in BMI was associated with a significant 10% increased risk for pancreatic cancer.[37] There was some evidence for a nonlinear relationship between BMI and pancreatic cancer, with the most pronounced increased risk being among participants with a BMI greater than 35 kg/m^2.[37] Waist circumference and waist to hip ratio are measures of abdominal adiposity that have consistently been associated with type 2 diabetes and are also associated with pancreatic cancer.[37]

Adiposity at younger ages and across a lifetime in the same individuals and risk of pancreatic cancer has not been examined extensively. Ten studies, 5 case-control[38–42] and 5 prospective,[36,43–46] examined BMI during adolescence or early adulthood and risk of pancreatic cancer, with 6 showing statistically significant positive associations with excess risks ranging from 20% to 2-fold.[36,38,40,42,45,46] Three studies showed significant positive associations between adiposity in early, middle, or older age in the same individuals and subsequent pancreatic cancer.[36,40,42,45,46] One large prospective study of AARP members indicated longer duration of overweight was significantly associated with pancreatic cancer such that for every 10 years of having a BMI 25 kg/m^2 or more, pancreatic cancer risk increased 6% overall and 18% among those diagnosed with diabetes.[46] The association was not as strong among participants without diabetes.[46] This pattern of association with long duration of adiposity and diabetes supports the notion that diabetes may be on the causal pathway between obesity and pancreatic cancer. The proportion of pancreatic cancer explained by ever being overweight or obese at any age was substantial in the AARP population, 14% overall and 21% in never smokers.[46]

Although weight change has inconsistently been associated with pancreatic cancer, one pooled study of 14 cohorts showed that compared with subjects who maintained their BMI from early adulthood to older age, those who gained more than 10 kg/m^2 had a significantly elevated risk of pancreatic cancer.[36] The National Institutes of Health AARP study showed that a BMI gain of more than 10 kg/m^2 after age 50 years was associated with pancreatic cancer but not gain earlier in life.[46] A BMI gain of 10 kg/m^2 corresponds to an increase from normal weight to obese.

Maintaining a normal BMI and avoiding adiposity at any age may prevent pancreatic cancer.

Dietary exposures The low incidence and rapid fatality of pancreatic cancer have made it difficult for epidemiologists to examine dietary risk factors. Pancreatic cancer cases often have gastrointestinal problems, weight loss, or diabetes before being diagnosed because of subclinical cancer, which can influence dietary intake and related biomarkers. Retrospective ascertainment of diet for this cancer site in particular may have biases including control selection, recall, and proxy reporting that can result in inaccurate risk estimates. Prospective studies are less likely subject to these methodological problems. Dietary exposures are also subject to measurement error. Large prospective studies, including pooled efforts that harmonize data, have provided adequately powered analyses to detect small magnitudes of risk that are typical of nutritional exposures.

Among dietary exposures, coffee consumption is consistently not associated with pancreatic cancer.[47] There is suggestive evidence for heavy alcohol use (>3 drinks per day) and high red meat, total and saturated fat, and fructose intake playing a role in pancreatic cancer.[47] Some but not all studies have shown protective associations between healthier lifestyle and dietary patterns and pancreatic cancer.[48–51]

Heavy alcohol use is the most common cause of both acute and chronic pancreatitis, and high levels of alcohol use could plausibly contribute to pancreatic cancer development via pancreatitis. Large studies have observed 35% to 80% increased risk between heavy alcohol use and pancreatic cancer.[52–55] Individuals who are heavy drinkers often tend to also smoke cigarettes, and there is a concern about residual confounding by smoking. One large prospective study with more than 6500 cases that was conducted for 24 years showed a significant increased pancreatic cancer risk for participants who consumed more than 3 drinks per day compared with non-drinkers, with the association remaining significant in never smokers.[53]

Several nested case-control studies that examined the association between vitamin D status and subsequent pancreatic cancer have shown varying results.[56–59] 25-Hydroxyvitamin D [25(OH)D] is the best measure of vitamin D exposure, as it represents that from both the diet and that synthesized endogenously from solar ultraviolet

B light exposure. A large pooled analysis of 8 cohorts showed a statistically significant 2-fold increased risk among participants with circulating 25(OH)D concentrations greater than 100 nmol/L compared with those with concentrations of 50 to 75 nmol/L and no association for concentrations less than 50 nmol/L.[58] A subsequent pooled study using comparable clinically relevant 25(OH)D cut points and referent category observed a statistically significant 40% increased risk for participants with concentrations 37.5 to less than 50 nmol/L but did not observe associations for participants with concentrations less than 37.5 nmol/L or greater than or equal to 75 nmol/L.[59]

Other nutrition-related exposures, such as glycemic load and index; total carbohydrate, sucrose, fiber, folate, vitamin C, vitamin E, sweetened beverage, soft drink, and cholesterol intake; and folate and multivitamin supplement use, and physical activity are not consistently associated with pancreatic cancer.[48]

INHERITED PREDISPOSITION FOR SPORADIC PANCREATIC ADENOCARCINOMA
Common Low-Risk Pancreatic Cancer Susceptibility Loci

The first pancreatic cancer GWAS were performed by the Pancreatic Cancer Cohort Consortium and the Pancreatic Cancer Case-Control Consortium with the aim of identifying common susceptibility markers for this deadly disease. Three phases of the GWAS have been reported, PanScan I in 2009, PanScan II in 2010, and PanScan III in 2014.[28,60,61] The first 2 phases consisted of 12 case-control studies nested within prospective cohort studies and 8 case-control studies. The total number of subjects included 3851 patients diagnosed with pancreatic ductal adenocarcinoma (PDAC) and 3934 control subjects of European ancestry.[60,61] Combined analysis identified 4 genome-wide significant pancreatic cancer risk loci at chromosomes 9q34.2 (in the *ABO* blood group gene), 1q32.1 (*NR5A2*), 5p15.33 (*CLPTM1L-TERT* gene region), and 13q22.1 (nongenic). The third phase of PanScan (PanScan III) added 1582 newly genotyped pancreatic cancer cases and 5203 control subjects; 5 new cohort studies, 2 new case series, and 1 case-control study were included. Replication was mainly performed in samples from the Pancreatic Disease Research (PANDoRA) consortium[62] resulting in a grand total of 7683 cases and 14,397 control subjects.[28] **Fig. 3** depicts the current knowledge of the landscape of common and rare pancreatic risk variants identified through the GWAS approach as well as through linkage analysis of familial cancer syndromes and sequencing approaches.

The protective allele of the most significant single nucleotide polymorphism (SNP) on 9q34.2 in the *ABO* gene (rs505922, odds ratio [OR] = 1.20, $P = 5.4 \times 10^{-8}$) is in complete linkage disequilibrium (LD) with the O allele of the *ABO* locus ($r^2 = 1$). The *ABO* gene encodes a glycosyltransferase (histo-blood group ABO system transferase) that catalyzes the transfer of carbohydrates to the H antigen, thereby forming the A, B, and O blood group proteins as described initially by Karl Landsteiner in 1900. A set of small studies published more than 50 years ago reported an association between ABO blood type and gastrointestinal cancers.[63,64] The discovery of the ABO risk locus reawakened interest in the connection between blood groups and pancreatic cancer. Using PanScan GWAS data, individual ABO alleles were inferred and their association with pancreatic cancer risk determined, showing that individuals with inferred A (OR = 1.38), AB (OR = 1.47), and B (OR = 1.53) blood groups had an increased risk of pancreatic cancer as compared with the O group.[65] The fact that the A1 alleles conferred an increased risk of pancreatic cancer (OR = 1.38, 95% confidence interval 1.20–1.58) but A2 alleles did not furthermore indicated that increased glycosyltransferase activity of the former, either toward the H antigen or other proteins, might explain the risk.[66,67] Since the PanScan GWAS report linking ABO blood groups and risk of

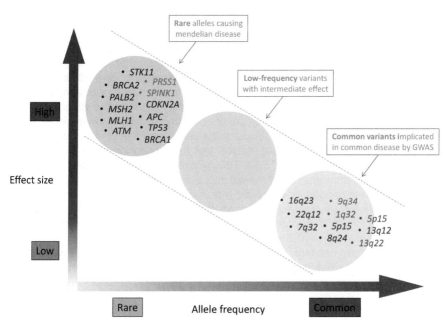

Fig. 3. The current landscape of inherited pancreatic cancer risk variants. Allele frequencies ranging from rare to common are shown on the x-axis, and effect sizes ranging from low to high on the y-axis. The clusters represent genes with germline mutations identified through linkage, candidate gene and sequencing approaches (*top left and middle*), and chromosomal band locations of common susceptibility loci identified through GWAS (*lower right*). Genes that are mutated as part of multicancer syndromes are listed in black; genes that influence hereditary pancreatitis are listed in green. Risk loci that are discussed in this article are shown in the lower right-hand part of the figure and colored according to PanScan GWAS phase they were identified: PanScan I (*blue*), PanScan II (*red*) and PanScan III (*purple*). GWAS loci from non-European populations were not included in the figure. (*From* Manolio TA, Collins FS, Cox NJ, et al. Finding the missing heritability of complex diseases. Nature 2009;461(7265):749; with permission.)

pancreatic cancer published in 2009, numerous studies have investigated the association of blood groups with cancer risk; the most consistently significant findings are for gastric and pancreatic cancer.[68–71]

The most significant SNP on chr1q32.1 (rs3790844, OR = 0.77, $P = 2.5 \times 10^{-10}$) maps to the first intron of the *NR5A2* gene. This gene encodes nuclear receptor subfamily 5 group A member 2 (NR5A2, also referred to as liver receptor homolog-1 or LRH-1), a transcription factor that plays an important role in early development, cholesterol synthesis, bile acid homeostasis, steroidogenesis, and regulating stemness.[72–74] NR5A2 is furthermore an important regulator of exocrine pancreatic function in the adult pancreas, where it cooperates with pancreas-specific transcription factor 1 to directly bind and activate a series of acinar-specific genes.[75] NR5A2 is required for early embryonic development, and mice that lack both copies of *Nr5a2* die at embryonic day 7.[76] Heterozygous *NR5A2* mice are viable but exhibit increased rates of pancreatic acinar to ductal metaplasia and impaired recovery after chemically induced acute pancreatitis.[77] Furthermore, *NR5A2* haploinsufficiency cooperates with pancreatitis in a pancreatic cancer mouse model driven by oncogenic *KRAS*, increasing the number of preneoplastic pancreatic intraepithelial neoplasia (PanIN) lesions and driving their progression toward PDAC.[77] Likewise, in mouse models, the induction of pancreatitis leads to a transient downregulation of multiple acinar and endocrine genes (including *NR5A2*, *HNF1A*, and *PDX1*) and increased acinar cell proliferation.[78] Thus, reduced expression of *NR5A2* and other acinar genes may contribute to increased proliferation and faster progression of PanINs in mouse pancreatic cancer models. Although the mechanism by which variants on chr1q32.1 mediate risk of pancreatic cancer is not clear, this may be related to effects on regulation of *NR5A2* gene expression and consequent effects on cell growth, especially in the presence of inflammatory conditions of the pancreas.

Two independent pancreatic cancer risk loci have been identified in the *TERT-CLPTM1L* gene region on chr5p15.33. This multicancer locus has been associated with lung, bladder, prostate, breast, melanoma, glioma, ovarian, melanoma, testicular, and basal cell skin cancers and chronic lymphocytic leukemia, intriguingly, with the same alleles showing increased risk for some cancers but decreased risk for other cancer types.[79–91] *TERT* encodes the catalytic subunit of telomerase, well known for its essential role in maintaining telomere ends and increased telomerase activity often seen in human cancers.[92–94] Telomerase also has telomere-independent functions, including in the regulation of gene expression, cell survival, epithelial to mesenchymal transition, and mitochondrial function.[95] The cleft lip and palate–associated transmembrane 1-like protein (CLPTM1L) seems to be a survival factor in lung cancer whereby it protects cells from apoptosis after treatment with DNA-damaging agents.[96,97] It has also been shown to induce cell growth and increase rates of aneuploidy in pancreatic cell lines, and it is overexpressed in pancreatic tumors.[98] The first pancreatic cancer signal (from PanScan II) was tagged by an intronic SNP (rs401681, OR = 1.19, $P = 3.7 \times 10^{-7}$) in *CLPTM1L*.[61] A second independent signal was identified in PanScan III, marked by a synonymous SNP in the second exon of *TERT* (rs2736098, OR = 0.80, $P = 9.8 \times 10^{-14}$).[28] Both SNPs were also identified in a subset-based meta-analysis of multiple cancer types in which pancreatic cancer contributed to risk in 6 independent loci[99] indicating that approaches leveling other cancer phenotypes can be useful to identify additional pancreatic cancer susceptibility variants in multicancer risk loci. The synonymous SNP in *TERT* and several correlated variants have been associated with telomere length in white blood cells and with *TERT* promoter activity in vitro.[85,100,101]

On chr13q22.1, the top-ranked GWAS SNP (rs9543325, OR = 1.26, $P = 3.27 \times 10^{-11}$) lies in a 600-kb nongenic region,[61] suggesting that the functional variant could affect gene expression at great distance through intrachromosomal or interchromosomal interactions. The chr13q22.1 risk locus is flanked by 2 genes encoding transcription factors of the Kruppel-like family: *KLF5* and *KLF12*; both encode proteins that regulate cell growth and transformation.[102–104] Furthermore, *KLF5* is upregulated in pancreatic cancer.[105] Additional genes, either nearby or at a greater distance could be functionally relevant to the mechanism by which the chr13q22.1 GWAS locus confers risk of PDAC.

A second independent signal was identified on chr13 in PanScan III, on 13q12.2 (rs9581943, OR = 1.15 $P = 2.4 \times 10^{-9}$). The top-ranked SNP is located in the promoter of the *PDX1* (pancreatic and duodenal homeobox1 protein 1) gene and is also intronic to *PDX1-AS1* (PDX1 antisense RNA 1), a noncoding RNA with unknown function. PDX1 plays a critical role in early pancreatic development, as well as the differentiation of exocrine pancreas, and regulates beta-cell function in the mature pancreas.[106,107] Mutations in this gene have been linked to agenesis of the pancreas[106] and MODY.[108] Furthermore, PDX1 has been implicated in glucose-dependent regulation of insulin gene transcription.[109]

The signal on 7q32.3 (rs6971499, OR = 0.79, P = 3.0 $\times$ 10^{-12}) lies in an intron of the *LINC-PINT* gene, a p53-induced long intergenic noncoding RNA. This SNP is also located between 2 additional plausible candidate genes, *MKLN1*, encoding muskelin 1, a mediator of cellular responses to the extracellular matrix, and *KLF14*, which encodes a member of the Kruppel-like family of transcription factors, which have been implicated as tumor suppressors.[110,111] KLF14 has also been identified as a regulator of several metabolic phenotypes, including type 2 diabetes.[112]

A synonymous SNP residing in the last exon of *BCAR1* (also known as p130Cas) was noted on 16q23.1 (rs7190458, OR = 1.46, P = 1.1 $\times$ 10^{-10}). BCAR1 functions as an adaptor protein that coordinates cell cycle control, cytoskeleton organization, and cell migration, and its aberrant expression has been linked to transformation and progression of multiple cancer types.[113,114] Two chymotrypsinogen genes, *CTRB1* and *CTRB2*, are also located close to this SNP (5 kb and 23 kb, respectively) and as important members of a family of serine proteases that are secreted by the pancreas into the gastrointestinal tract are plausible target genes for susceptibility variants at this locus.[115]

The most significant SNP at 22q12.1 (rs16986825, OR = 1.18 P = 1.2 $\times$ 10^{-8}), is intronic in the zinc and ring finger 3 (*ZNRF3*) gene, which encodes a transmembrane E3 ubiquitin protein ligase that negatively regulates the Wnt signaling pathway.[116] Although located 162 kb centromeric to the most notable SNP in this locus, *CHEK2* encodes a cell cycle checkpoint kinase that cooperates with p53, BRCA1, and ATM in response to DNA damage and may therefore represent a candidate gene worthy further follow-up.[117,118] Finally, a near-GWAS significant risk locus was identified in the well-known multicancer risk locus on 8q24.21 (rs1561927, OR = 0.87, P = 1.3 $\times$ 10^{-7}). The closest genes are located 400 to 800 kb centromeric to this SNP: *MIR1208*, *PVT1*, and *MYC*. Chromosome 8q24.21 is known to contain multiple cancer susceptibility loci that span over 2 Mb,[119,120] but most are located far away from this SNP, with low LD and are therefore not likely to represent the same signal. The highest LD is with an SNP that is 24 kb upstream and reported to be associated with ovarian cancer risk (rs10088218, r^2 = 0.37 in 1000G CEU (Utah residents with ancestry from northern and western europe) data).[121]

Common Pancreatic Cancer Risk Loci in Non-European Populations

In addition to PanScan, in which most subjects were of European ancestry, GWAS have now been performed in case-control studies from China and Japan. A Japanese GWAS of 991 advanced PDAC cases and 5209 control subjects reported 3 GWAS significant loci on chromosomes 6p25.3/*FOXQ1* (rs9502893, OR = 1.29, P = 3.30 $\times$ 10^{-7}), 7q36.2/*DPP6* (rs6464375, OR$_{Recessive}$ = 3.73, P = 4.4 $\times$ 10^{-7}), and 12p11.21/*BICD1* (rs708224, OR = 1.32, P = 3.3 $\times$ 10^{-7}).[122] Furthermore, a 2-phased GWAS with a combined set of 3584 pancreatic cancer cases and 4868 control subjects from China (ChinaPC) identified 5 risk loci on chr5p13.1/*DAB2* (rs2255280, OR = 0.81, P = 4.18 $\times$ 10^{-10}), chr10q26.11/*PRLHR* (rs12413624, OR = 1.23, P = 5.12 $\times$ 10^{-11}), chr21q21.3/*BACH1* (rs372883, OR = 0.79 P = 2.24 $\times$ 10^{-13}), chr21q22.3/*TFF1* (rs1547374, OR = 0.79, P = 3.71 $\times$ 10^{-13}), and chr22q13.32/*FAM19A5* (rs5768709, OR = 1.25, P = 1.41 $\times$ 10^{-10}).[123] Both the Chinese and Japanese GWAS scans replicated the chr13q22.1 locus initially discovered in PanScan and noted the risk locus on chr1q32.1, albeit with less significance. Chromosome chr5p15.33 was only noted in the Chinese scan (rs401681, P = 7.35 $\times$ 10^{-5}) and 9q34.2 (rs505922) only in the Japanese scan.

Assessment of the Chinese and Japanese pancreatic cancer risk loci in the European PANDoRA case-control consortium and in PanScan III did not replicate any of the pancreatic cancer susceptibility loci identified in Asians.[28,124]

Pathway Analyses of pancreatic Cancer Genome-Wide Association Studies Data Sets

Pathway-based analyses of GWAS data have been used to mine PanScan I and II data to identify genes, or groups of genes, enriched with variants whose individual effects may be too small to be detected in the GWAS.[60,61] These approaches have highlighted pancreatic development genes such as *HNF1A, HNF4G, HNF1B,* and *PDX1*,[26,27] which encode important components of the transcriptional networks that govern embryonic development of the pancreas and maintain homeostasis in adults.[29,30] In addition, mutations in *HNF1A, PDX1,* and *HNF1B* are responsible for MODY,[125–127] and common variants in *HNF1A* and *HNF1B* have been associated with risk of type 2 diabetes.[128–130] With the added numbers of cases and controls in the third phase of PanScan as compared with the first 2 phases, the significance of 2 of these genes *(PDX1* and *HNF1A)* improved markedly, indicating that pathway analysis can be a useful approach to tease out additional genes that influence risk of disease. These results furthermore suggest possible functional interrelationships between inherited variation in genes important for pancreatic development, diabetes, and cancer risk.

Functional Understanding of Common Pancreatic Cancer Risk Loci

Germline variants discovered in GWAS are usually non–protein coding and in most cases not the functional variants themselves. Much work is needed after GWAS to uncover the biological mechanism of the risk. Fine-mapping efforts followed by genomic and functional analysis of multiple highly correlated tag SNPs are the next steps after a GWAS identifies a risk locus for a specific disease or trait. These efforts involve genomic and functional approaches, such as investigating gene expression levels, splicing, promoter or enhancer strength, DNA methylation, protein to DNA binding, and chromosome conformation, to link risk genotypes to differences in specific molecular phenotypes to establish the underlying mechanism at each locus.

Future Gene Mapping Approaches

GWAS has already yielded valuable insights into the cause of pancreatic cancer. Although functional explanation of these loci is in its early stages, the results implicate genes that mediate diverse functions ranging from pancreatic development (*NR5A2, PDX1*), exocrine glandular function (*CTRB1/2*), and endocrine function (*PDX1, HNF1A*) to blood groups/glycosylation (*ABO*). As compared with more common cancers, the GWAS approach is still at an early stage for pancreatic cancer, and more findings can be expected as sample sets increase and additional populations are analyzed. For breast[131] and prostate cancers,[132] GWAS have already led to the identification of 67 and 100 risk loci, respectively. Altogether, these loci explain approximately 33% of the familial risk of prostate cancer and 28% for breast cancer in European populations. For pancreatic cancer, 18 risk loci have been identified to date through GWAS (in European and Asian populations) albeit with limited replication between European and Asian populations. Imputation and meta-analyses of existing and new GWAS data sets are bound to uncover even more loci. Efforts in pancreatic cancer GWAS outside of main effects are likely to expand by investigations of susceptibility variants for survival, pharmacologic responses, and gene-gene and gene-environmental interactions.[133–135] However, as for other diseases, susceptibility loci identified through GWAS may not explain most of the inherited risk for pancreatic cancer. With the emergence of next-generation sequencing, these efforts will grow in use for gene mapping. The identification of mutations in the *ATM* and *PALB2* genes in pancreatic cancer kindreds with unknown cause nicely demonstrated this use of next-generation sequencing.[136,137] Exome and whole-genome sequencing studies are likely to also be undertaken in sporadic cases and in cases with specific phenotypes such as an early age of onset and epidemiologic risk factors (eg, BMI, smoking, pancreatitis). As population-based sequencing studies have already shown, the number of uncommon and rare polymorphic variants in the human genome is high[138] and may explain a substantial portion of germline risk for disease. High-throughput sequencing approaches will furthermore enable the assessment of variants not captured on GWAS platforms, such as indels and copy number variants.

SUMMARY

Given the changing demographics of Western populations, the numbers of pancreatic cancer cases are projected to increase during the next decade.[6] Diabetes, recent cigarette smoking, and excess body weight are the most consistent risk factors for pancreatic cancer.[48] Diabetes associated with pancreatic cancer may have more heterogeneity than previously appreciated. In addition to type 2 diabetes, T3cDM related to exocrine pancreatic disease and common loci in genes related to MODY may contribute to the association between diabetes and pancreatic cancer.[23,24,26–28] Chronic pancreatitis is also associated with pancreatic cancer but accounts for a small proportion of the disease.[21,22] Coffee consumption is not associated with pancreatic cancer, whereas there is suggestive evidence for heavy alcohol use (>3 drinks per day) and high red meat, total fat and saturated fat, and fructose intake as risk factors.[48] Other nutrition-related factors and antidiabetic drugs are not consistently associated with pancreatic cancer.[9,31,32,48]

A small proportion of the familial aggregation of pancreatic cancer can be explained by hereditary cancer syndromes and inherited forms of pancreatitis, caused by rare high-risk inherited mutations.[136,139–146] However, the genetic basis for most familial aggregation of pancreatic cancer has yet to be explained. The search for common and rare germline variants that influence risk of pancreatic cancer through GWAS and high-throughput-sequencing–based studies is underway and holds promise of increasing the knowledge of variants and genes that play a role in inherited susceptibility of this devastating disease.

Although research gaps remain, the research reported in this review has advanced the understanding of pancreatic cancer. Understanding the etiology of pancreatic cancer and identifying modifiable factors may reduce the burden of this highly fatal disease. In addition, the need for translational research to improve prognostic and therapeutic modalities is urgent.

ACKNOWLEDGMENTS

The authors gratefully acknowledge Marina Piper for helping to collate some of the references used in this review.

REFERENCES

1. Ferlay J, Soerjomataram I, Dikshit R, et al. Cancer incidence and mortality worldwide: sources, methods and major patterns in GLOBOCAN 2012. Int J Cancer 2015;136(5):E359–86.
2. Edwards BK, Noone AM, Mariotto AB, et al. Annual Report to the Nation on the status of cancer, 1975–2010, featuring prevalence of comorbidity and impact on survival among persons with lung, colorectal, breast, or prostate cancer. Cancer 2014;120:1290–314.

3. SEER Stat fact sheets: pancreatic cancer. In: Surveillance, epidemiology, and end results program. 2014.

4. Anderson KE, Mack TM, Silverman DT. Cancer of the pancreas. In: Schottenfeld D, Fraumeni JF, editors. Cancer epidemiology and prevention. 3rd edition. New York: Oxford University Press; 2006. p. 721–63.

5. A snapshot of pancreatic cancer. 2014. Available at: www.cancer.gov/research/progress/snapshots/pancreatic.

6. Rahib L, Smith BD, Aizenberg R, et al. Projecting cancer incidence and deaths to 2030: the unexpected burden of thyroid, liver, and pancreas cancers in the United States. Cancer Res 2014;74:2913–21.

7. Ben Q, Xu M, Ning X, et al. Diabetes mellitus and risk of pancreatic cancer: a meta-analysis of cohort studies. Eur J Cancer 2011;47:1928–37.

8. Huxley R, Ansary-Moghaddam A, Berrington DG, et al. Type-II diabetes and pancreatic cancer: a meta-analysis of 36 studies. Br J Cancer 2005;92: 2076–83.

9. Bosetti C, Rosato V, Li D, et al. Diabetes, antidiabetic medications, and pancreatic cancer risk: an analysis from the International Pancreatic Cancer Case-Control Consortium. Ann Oncol 2014;25:2065–72.

10. Grote VA, Rohrmann S, Nieters A, et al. Diabetes mellitus, glycated haemoglobin and C-peptide levels in relation to pancreatic cancer risk: a study within the European Prospective Investigation into Cancer and Nutrition (EPIC) cohort. Diabetologia 2011;54:3037–46.

11. Wolpin BM, Bao Y, Qian ZR, et al. Hyperglycemia, insulin resistance, impaired pancreatic beta-cell function, and risk of pancreatic cancer. J Natl Cancer Inst 2013;105:1027–35.

12. Stolzenberg-Solomon RZ, Graubard BI, Chari S, et al. Insulin, glucose, insulin resistance, and pancreatic cancer in male smokers. JAMA 2005;294: 2872–8.

13. Douglas JB, Silverman DT, Pollak MN, et al. Serum IGF-I, IGF-II, IGFBP-3, and IGF-I/IGFBP-3 molar ratio and risk of pancreatic cancer in the prostate, lung, colorectal, and ovarian cancer screening trial. Cancer Epidemiol Biomarkers Prev 2010;19:2298–306.

14. Douglas JB, Silverman DT, Weinstein SJ, et al. Serum C-reactive protein and risk of pancreatic cancer in two nested, case-control studies. Cancer Epidemiol Biomarkers Prev 2011;20:359–69.

15. Jiao L, Weinstein SJ, Albanes D, et al. Evidence that serum levels of the soluble receptor for advanced glycation end products are inversely associated with pancreatic cancer risk: a prospective study. Cancer Res 2011;71: 3582–9.

16. Grote VA, Nieters A, Kaaks R, et al. The associations of advanced glycation end products and its soluble receptor with pancreatic cancer risk: a case-control study within the prospective EPIC Cohort. Cancer Epidemiol Biomarkers Prev 2012;21:619–28.

17. Grote VA, Rohrmann S, Dossus L, et al. The association of circulating adiponectin levels with pancreatic cancer risk: a study within the prospective EPIC cohort. Int J Cancer 2012;130:2428–37.

18. Kaaks R, Lukanova A. Energy balance and cancer: the role of insulin and insulin-like growth factor-I. Proc Nutr Soc 2001;60:91–106.

19. Mayers JR, Wu C, Clish CB, et al. Elevation of circulating branched-chain amino acids is an early event in human pancreatic adenocarcinoma development. Nat Med 2014;20:1193–8.

20. Newgard CB, An J, Bain JR, et al. A branched-chain amino acid-related metabolic signature that differentiates obese and lean humans and contributes to insulin resistance. Cell Metab 2009;9:311–26.

21. Duell EJ, Lucenteforte E, Olson SH, et al. Pancreatitis and pancreatic cancer risk: a pooled analysis in the International Pancreatic Cancer Case-Control Consortium (PanC4). Ann Oncol 2012;23:2964–70.

22. Lowenfels AB, Maisonneuve P, Cavallini G, et al. Pancreatitis and the risk of pancreatic cancer. International Pancreatitis Study Group. N Engl J Med 1993;328:1433–7.

23. Ewald N, Kaufmann C, Raspe A, et al. Prevalence of diabetes mellitus secondary to pancreatic diseases (type 3c). Diabetes Metab Res Rev 2012;28:338–42.

24. Andersen DK. The practical importance of recognizing pancreatogenic or type 3c diabetes. Diabetes Metab Res Rev 2012;28:326–8.

25. National Diabetes Information Clearinghouse. Monogenic forms of diabetes: neonatal diabetes mellitus and maturity-onset diabetes of the young. National Institute of Diabetes and Digestive and Kidney Diseases (NIDDK); National Institutes of Health, Department of Health and Human Services; 2014.

26. Pierce BL, Ahsan H. Genome-wide "pleiotropy scan" identifies HNF1A region as a novel pancreatic cancer susceptibility locus. Cancer Res 2011;71:4352–8.

27. Li D, Duell EJ, Yu K, et al. Pathway analysis of genome-wide association study data highlights pancreatic development genes as susceptibility factors for pancreatic cancer. Carcinogenesis 2012;33:1384–90.

28. Wolpin BM, Rizzato C, Kraft P, et al. Genome-wide association study identifies multiple susceptibility loci for pancreatic cancer. Nat Genet 2014;46:994–1000.

29. Maestro MA, Cardalda C, Boj SF, et al. Distinct roles of HNF1beta, HNF1alpha, and HNF4alpha in regulating pancreas development, beta-cell function and growth. Endocr Dev 2007;12:33–45.

30. Martin M, Hauer V, Messmer M, et al. Transcription factors in pancreatic development. Animal models. Endocr Dev 2007;12:24–32.

31. Bodmer M, Becker C, Meier C, et al. Use of antidiabetic agents and the risk of pancreatic cancer: a case-control analysis. Am J Gastroenterol 2012;107(4):620–6.

32. Gandini S, Puntoni M, Heckman-Stoddard BM, et al. Metformin and cancer risk and mortality: a systematic review and meta-analysis taking into account biases and confounders. Cancer Prev Res (Phila) 2014;7:867–85.

33. Lynch SM, Vrieling A, Lubin JH, et al. Cigarette smoking and pancreatic cancer: a pooled analysis from the Pancreatic Cancer Cohort Consortium. Am J Epidemiol 2009;170:403–13.

34. Bertuccio P, La VC, Silverman DT, et al. Cigar and pipe smoking, smokeless tobacco use and pancreatic cancer: an analysis from the International Pancreatic Cancer Case-Control Consortium (PanC4). Ann Oncol 2011;22:1420–6.

35. Maisonneuve P, Lowenfels AB. Risk factors for pancreatic cancer: a summary review of meta-analytical studies. Int J Epidemiol 2015;44(1):186–98.

36. Genkinger JM, Spiegelman D, Anderson KE, et al. A pooled analysis of 14 cohort studies of anthropometric factors and pancreatic cancer risk. Int J Cancer 2011;129:1708–17.

37. Aune D, Greenwood DC, Chan DS, et al. Body mass index, abdominal fatness and pancreatic cancer risk: a systematic review and non-linear dose-response meta-analysis of prospective studies. Ann Oncol 2012;23:843–52.

38. Eberle CA, Bracci PM, Holly EA. Anthropometric factors and pancreatic cancer in a population-based case-control study in the San Francisco Bay Area. Cancer Causes Control 2005;16:1235–44.

39. Fryzek JP, Schenk M, Kinnard M, et al. The association of body mass index and pancreatic cancer in residents of southeastern Michigan, 1996–1999. Am J Epidemiol 2005;162:222–8.

40. Li D, Morris JS, Liu J, et al. Body mass index and risk, age of onset, and survival in patients with pancreatic cancer. JAMA 2009;301:2553–62.

41. Ji BT, Hatch MC, Chow WH, et al. Anthropometric and reproductive factors and the risk of pancreatic cancer: a case-control study in Shanghai, China. Int J Cancer 1996;66:432–7.

42. Urayama KY, Holcatova I, Janout V, et al. Body mass index and body size in early adulthood and risk of pancreatic cancer in a central European multicenter case-control study. Int J Cancer 2011;129:2875–84.

43. Patel AV, Rodriguez C, Bernstein L, et al. Obesity, recreational physical activity, and risk of pancreatic cancer in a large U.S. cohort. Cancer Epidemiol Biomarkers Prev 2005;14:459–66.

44. Michaud DS, Giovannucci E, Willett WC, et al. Physical activity, obesity, height, and the risk of pancreatic cancer. JAMA 2001;286:921–9.

45. Levi Z, Kark JD, Afek A, et al. Measured body mass index in adolescence and the incidence of pancreatic cancer in a cohort of 720,000 Jewish men. Cancer Causes Control 2012;23:371–8.

46. Stolzenberg-Solomon RZ, Schairer C, Moore S, et al. Lifetime adiposity and risk of pancreatic cancer in the NIH-AARP Diet and Health Study cohort. Am J Clin Nutr 2013;98:1057–65.

47. World Cancer Research Fund and American Institute for Cancer Research. Continuous update project summary. Food, nutrition, physical activity, and the prevention of pancreatic cancer. 2012. Available at: www.dietandcancerreport.org.

48. Arem H, Reedy J, Sampson J, et al. The healthy eating index 2005 and risk of pancreatic cancer in the NIH-AARP Study. J Natl Cancer Inst 2013;105(17): 1298–305.

49. Jiao L, Mitrou PN, Reedy J, et al. A combined healthy lifestyle score and risk of pancreatic cancer in a large cohort study. Arch Invest Med 2009;169:764–70.

50. Bosetti C, Bravi F, Turati F, et al. Nutrient-based dietary patterns and pancreatic cancer risk. Ann Epidemiol 2013;23:124–8.

51. Chan JM, Gong Z, Holly EA, et al. Dietary patterns and risk of pancreatic cancer in a large population-based case-control study in the San Francisco Bay Area. Nutr Cancer 2013;65:157–64.

52. Jiao L, Silverman DT, Schairer C, et al. Alcohol use and risk of pancreatic cancer: the NIH-AARP Diet and Health Study. Am J Epidemiol 2009;169:1043–51.

53. Gapstur SM, Jacobs EJ, Deka A, et al. Association of alcohol intake with pancreatic cancer mortality in never smokers. Arch Invest Med 2011;171:444–51.

54. Lucenteforte E, La VC, Silverman D, et al. Alcohol consumption and pancreatic cancer: a pooled analysis in the International Pancreatic Cancer Case-Control Consortium (PanC4). Ann Oncol 2012;23:374–82.

55. Genkinger JM, Spiegelman D, Anderson KE, et al. Alcohol intake and pancreatic cancer risk: a pooled analysis of fourteen cohort studies. Cancer Epidemiol Biomarkers Prev 2009;18:765–76.

56. Stolzenberg-Solomon RZ, Vieth R, Azad A, et al. A prospective nested case-control study of vitamin D status and pancreatic cancer risk in male smokers. Cancer Res 2006;66:10213–9.

57. Stolzenberg-Solomon RZ, Hayes RB, Horst RL, et al. Serum vitamin D and risk of pancreatic cancer in the prostate, lung, colorectal, and ovarian screening trial. Cancer Res 2009;69:1439–47.

58. Stolzenberg-Solomon RZ, Jacobs EJ, Arslan AA, et al. Circulating 25-hydroxyvi-tamin D and risk of pancreatic cancer: Cohort Consortium Vitamin D Pooling Project of Rarer Cancers. Am J Epidemiol 2010;172:81–93.

59. Wolpin BM, Ng K, Bao Y, et al. Plasma 25-hydroxyvitamin D and risk of pancre-atic cancer. Cancer Epidemiol Biomarkers Prev 2012;21(1):82–91.

60. Amundadottir L, Kraft P, Stolzenberg-Solomon RZ, et al. Genome-wide associa-tion study identifies variants in the ABO locus associated with susceptibility to pancreatic cancer. Nat Genet 2009;41:986–90.

61. Petersen GM, Amundadottir L, Fuchs CS, et al. A genome-wide association study identifies pancreatic cancer susceptibility loci on chromosomes 13q22.1, 1q32.1 and 5p15.33. Nat Genet 2010;42:224–8.

62. Campa D, Rizzato C, Capurso G, et al. Genetic susceptibility to pancreatic can-cer and its functional characterisation: the PANcreatic Disease ReseArch (PANDoRA) consortium. Dig Liver Dis 2013;45:95–9.

63. Marcus DM. The ABO and Lewis blood-group system. Immunochemistry, ge-netics and relation to human disease. N Engl J Med 1969;280:994–1006.

64. Aird I, Bentall HH, Roberts JA. A relationship between cancer of stomach and the ABO blood groups. Br Med J 1953;1:799–801.

65. Wolpin BM, Kraft P, Gross M, et al. Pancreatic cancer risk and ABO blood group alleles: results from the Pancreatic Cancer Cohort Consortium. Cancer Res 2010;70:1015–23.

66. Wolpin BM, Kraft P, Xu M, et al. Variant ABO blood group alleles, secretor status, and risk of pancreatic cancer: results from the Pancreatic Cancer Cohort Con-sortium. Cancer Epidemiol Biomarkers Prev 2010;19:3140–9.

67. Yamamoto F, McNeill PD, Hakomori S. Human histo-blood group A2 transferase coded by A2 allele, one of the A subtypes, is characterized by a single base deletion in the coding sequence, which results in an additional domain at the carboxyl terminal. Biochem Biophys Res Commun 1992;187:366–74.

68. Zhang BL, He N, Huang YB, et al. ABO blood groups and risk of cancer: a systematic review and meta-analysis. Asian Pac J Cancer Prev 2014;15: 4643–50.

69. Franchini M, Liumbruno GM. ABO blood group: old dogma, new perspectives. Clin Chem Lab Med 2013;51:1545–53.

70. Khalili H, Wolpin BM, Huang ES, et al. ABO blood group and risk of colorectal cancer. Cancer Epidemiol Biomarkers Prev 2011;20:1017–20.

71. Gates MA, Wolpin BM, Cramer DW, et al. ABO blood group and incidence of epithelial ovarian cancer. Int J Cancer 2011;128:482–6.

72. Fayard E, Auwerx J, Schoonjans K. LRH-1: an orphan nuclear receptor involved in development, metabolism and steroidogenesis. Trends Cell Biol 2004;14: 250–60.

73. Kelly VR, Xu B, Kuick R, et al. Dax1 up-regulates Oct4 expression in mouse em-bryonic stem cells via LRH-1 and SRA. Mol Endocrinol 2010;24:2281–91.

74. Heng JC, Feng B, Han J, et al. The nuclear receptor Nr5a2 can replace Oct4 in the reprogramming of murine somatic cells to pluripotent cells. Cell Stem Cell 2010;6:167–74.

75. Holmstrom SR, Deering T, Swift GH, et al. LRH-1 and PTF1-L coregulate an exocrine pancreas-specific transcriptional network for digestive function. Genes Dev 2011;25:1674–9.

76. Pare JF, Malenfant D, Courtemanche C, et al. The fetoprotein transcription factor (FTF) gene is essential to embryogenesis and cholesterol homeostasis and is regulated by a DR4 element. J Biol Chem 2004;279:21206–16.

77. Flandez M, Cendrowski J, Canamero M, et al. Nr5a2 heterozygosity sensitises to, and cooperates with, inflammation in KRasG12V-driven pancreatic tumourigenesis. Gut 2014;63(4):647–55.

78. Molero X, Vaquero EC, Flandez M, et al. Gene expression dynamics after murine pancreatitis unveils novel roles for Hnf1alpha in acinar cell homeostasis. Gut 2012;61:1187–96.

79. Landi MT, Chatterjee N, Yu K, et al. A genome-wide association study of lung cancer identifies a region of chromosome 5p15 associated with risk for adenocarcinoma. Am J Hum Genet 2009;85:679–91.

80. McKay JD, Hung RJ, Gaborieau V, et al. Lung cancer susceptibility locus at 5p15.33. Nat Genet 2008;40:1404–6.

81. Amos CI, Wu X, Broderick P, et al. Genome-wide association scan of tag SNPs identifies a susceptibility locus for lung cancer at 15q25.1. Nat Genet 2008;40:616–22.

82. Broderick P, Wang Y, Vijayakrishnan J, et al. Deciphering the impact of common genetic variation on lung cancer risk: a genome-wide association study. Cancer Res 2009;69:6633–41.

83. Hsiung CA, Lan Q, Hong YC, et al. The 5p15.33 locus is associated with risk of lung adenocarcinoma in never-smoking females in Asia. PLoS Genet 2010;6 [pii: e1001051].

84. Kote-Jarai Z, Olama AA, Giles GG, et al. Seven prostate cancer susceptibility loci identified by a multi-stage genome-wide association study. Nat Genet 2011;43:785–91.

85. Rafnar T, Sulem P, Stacey SN, et al. Sequence variants at the TERT-CLPTM1L locus associate with many cancer types. Nat Genet 2009;41:221–7.

86. Chung CC, Ciampa J, Yeager M, et al. Fine mapping of a region of chromosome 11q13 reveals multiple independent loci associated with risk of prostate cancer. Hum Mol Genet 2011;20:2869–78.

87. Shete S, Hosking FJ, Robertson LB, et al. Genome-wide association study identifies five susceptibility loci for glioma. Nat Genet 2009;41:899–904.

88. Turnbull C, Rapley EA, Seal S, et al. Variants near DMRT1, TERT and ATF7IP are associated with testicular germ cell cancer. Nat Genet 2010;42:604–7.

89. Stacey SN, Sulem P, Masson G, et al. New common variants affecting susceptibility to basal cell carcinoma. Nat Genet 2009;41:909–14.

90. Barrett JH, Iles MM, Harland M, et al. Genome-wide association study identifies three new melanoma susceptibility loci. Nat Genet 2011;43:1108–13.

91. Berndt SI, Skibola CF, Joseph V, et al. Genome-wide association study identifies multiple risk loci for chronic lymphocytic leukemia. Nat Genet 2013;45:868–76.

92. Bodnar AG, Ouellette M, Frolkis M, et al. Extension of life-span by introduction of telomerase into normal human cells. Science 1998;279:349–52.

93. Hahn WC, Counter CM, Lundberg AS, et al. Creation of human tumour cells with defined genetic elements. Nature 1999;400:464–8.

94. Kim NW, Piatyszek MA, Prowse KR, et al. Specific association of human telomerase activity with immortal cells and cancer. Science 1994;266:2011–5.

95. Ding D, Zhou J, Wang M, et al. Implications of telomere-independent activities of telomerase reverse transcriptase in human cancer. FEBS J 2013;280:3205–11.

96. Yamamoto K, Okamoto A, Isonishi S, et al. A novel gene, CRR9, which was up-regulated in CDDP-resistant ovarian tumor cell line, was associated with apoptosis. Biochem Biophys Res Commun 2001;280:1148–54.

97. James MA, Wen W, Wang Y, et al. Functional characterization of CLPTM1L as a lung cancer risk candidate gene in the 5p15.33 locus. PLoS One 2012;7: e36116.

98. Jia J, Bosley AD, Thompson A, et al. CLPTM1L promotes growth and enhances aneuploidy in pancreatic cancer cells. Cancer Res 2014;74(10):2785–95.
99. Wang Z, Zhu B, Zhang M, et al. Imputation and subset based association analysis across different cancer types identifies multiple independent risk loci in the TERT-CLPTM1L region on chromosome 5p15.33. Hum Mol Genet 2014;23(24): 6616–33.
100. Bojesen SE, Pooley KA, Johnatty SE, et al. Multiple independent variants at the TERT locus are associated with telomere length and risks of breast and ovarian cancer. Nat Genet 2013;45:371–84.
101. Kote-Jarai Z, Saunders EJ, Leongamornlert DA, et al. Fine-mapping identifies multiple prostate cancer risk loci at 5p15, one of which associates with TERT expression. Hum Mol Genet 2013;22:2520–8.
102. McConnell BB, Yang VW. Mammalian Kruppel-like factors in health and diseases. Physiol Rev 2010;90:1337–81.
103. Dong JT, Chen C. Essential role of KLF5 transcription factor in cell proliferation and differentiation and its implications for human diseases. Cell Mol Life Sci 2009;66:2691–706.
104. Nakamura Y, Migita T, Hosoda F, et al. Kruppel-like factor 12 plays a significant role in poorly differentiated gastric cancer progression. Int J Cancer 2009;125: 1859–67.
105. Mori A, Moser C, Lang SA, et al. Up-regulation of Kruppel-like factor 5 in pancreatic cancer is promoted by interleukin-1beta signaling and hypoxia-inducible factor-1alpha. Mol Cancer Res 2009;7:1390–8.
106. Stoffers DA, Zinkin NT, Stanojevic V, et al. Pancreatic agenesis attributable to a single nucleotide deletion in the human IPF1 gene coding sequence. Nat Genet 1997;15:106–10.
107. MacDonald RJ, Swift GH, Real FX. Transcriptional control of acinar development and homeostasis. Prog Mol Biol Transl Sci 2010;97:1–40.
108. Vaxillaire M, Bonnefond A, Froguel P. The lessons of early-onset monogenic diabetes for the understanding of diabetes pathogenesis. Best Pract Res Clin Endocrinol Metab 2012;26:171–87.
109. Ohlsson H, Karlsson K, Edlund T. IPF1, a homeodomain-containing transactivator of the insulin gene. EMBO J 1993;12:4251–9.
110. Adams JC, Seed B, Lawler J. Muskelin, a novel intracellular mediator of cell adhesive and cytoskeletal responses to thrombospondin-1. EMBO J 1998;17: 4964–74.
111. Fernandez-Zapico ME, Lomberk GA, Tsuji S, et al. A functional family-wide screening of SP/KLF proteins identifies a subset of suppressors of KRAS-mediated cell growth. Biochem J 2011;435:529–37.
112. Small KS, Hedman AK, Grundberg E, et al. Identification of an imprinted master trans regulator at the KLF14 locus related to multiple metabolic phenotypes. Nat Genet 2011;43:561–4.
113. Barrett A, Pellet-Many C, Zachary IC, et al. p130Cas: a key signalling node in health and disease. Cell Signal 2013;25:766–77.
114. Cabodi S, del Pilar Camacho-Leal M, Di Stefano P, et al. Integrin signalling adaptors: not only figurants in the cancer story. Nat Rev Cancer 2010;10: 858–70.
115. Whitcomb DC, Lowe ME. Human pancreatic digestive enzymes. Dig Dis Sci 2007;52:1–17.
116. Hao HX, Xie Y, Zhang Y, et al. ZNRF3 promotes Wnt receptor turnover in an R-spondin-sensitive manner. Nature 2012;485:195–200.

117. Antoni L, Sodha N, Collins I, et al. CHK2 kinase: cancer susceptibility and cancer therapy - two sides of the same coin? Nat Rev Cancer 2007;7:925–36.
118. Gronwald J, Cybulski C, Piesiak W, et al. Cancer risks in first-degree relatives of CHEK2 mutation carriers: effects of mutation type and cancer site in proband. Br J Cancer 2009;100:1508–12.
119. Grisanzio C, Freedman ML. Chromosome 8q24-associated cancers and MYC. Genes Cancer 2010;1:555–9.
120. Huppi K, Pitt JJ, Wahlberg BM, et al. The 8q24 gene desert: an oasis of noncoding transcriptional activity. Front Genet 2012;3:69.
121. Pharoah PD, Tsai YY, Ramus SJ, et al. GWAS meta-analysis and replication identifies three new susceptibility loci for ovarian cancer. Nat Genet 2013;45:362–70, 370e1–2.
122. Low SK, Kuchiba A, Zembutsu H, et al. Genome-wide association study of pancreatic cancer in Japanese population. PLoS One 2010;5:e11824.
123. Wu C, Miao X, Huang L, et al. Genome-wide association study identifies five loci associated with susceptibility to pancreatic cancer in Chinese populations. Nat Genet 2012;44:62–6.
124. Campa D, Rizzato C, Bauer AS, et al. Lack of replication of seven pancreatic cancer susceptibility loci identified in two Asian populations. Cancer Epidemiol Biomarkers Prev 2013;22:320–3.
125. Glucksmann MA, Lehto M, Tayber O, et al. Novel mutations and a mutational hotspot in the MODY3 gene. Diabetes 1997;46:1081–6.
126. Carette C, Vaury C, Barthelemy A, et al. Exonic duplication of the hepatocyte nuclear factor-1beta gene (transcription factor 2, hepatic) as a cause of maturity onset diabetes of the young type 5. J Clin Endocrinol Metab 2007;92: 2844–7.
127. Yamagata K, Oda N, Kaisaki PJ, et al. Mutations in the hepatocyte nuclear factor-1alpha gene in maturity-onset diabetes of the young (MODY3). Nature 1996;384:455–8.
128. Voight BF, Scott LJ, Steinthorsdottir V, et al. Twelve type 2 diabetes susceptibility loci identified through large-scale association analysis. Nat Genet 2010;42: 579–89.
129. Furuta H, Furuta M, Sanke T, et al. Nonsense and missense mutations in the human hepatocyte nuclear factor-1 beta gene (TCF2) and their relation to type 2 diabetes in Japanese. J Clin Endocrinol Metab 2002;87:3859–63.
130. Holmkvist J, Cervin C, Lyssenko V, et al. Common variants in HNF-1 alpha and risk of type 2 diabetes. Diabetologia 2006;49:2882–91.
131. Garcia-Closas M, Couch FJ, Lindstrom S, et al. Genome-wide association studies identify four ER negative-specific breast cancer risk loci. Nat Genet 2013;45:392–8, 398e1–2.
132. Al Olama AA, Kote-Jarai Z, Berndt SI, et al. A meta-analysis of 87,040 individuals identifies 23 new susceptibility loci for prostate cancer. Nat Genet 2014; 46:1103–9.
133. Wu C, Kraft P, Stolzenberg-Solomon R, et al. Genome-wide association study of survival in patients with pancreatic adenocarcinoma. Gut 2014;63(1):152–60.
134. Willis JA, Olson SH, Orlow I, et al. A replication study and genome-wide scan of single-nucleotide polymorphisms associated with pancreatic cancer risk and overall survival. Clin Cancer Res 2012;18:3942–51.
135. Innocenti F, Owzar K, Cox NL, et al. A genome-wide association study of overall survival in pancreatic cancer patients treated with gemcitabine in CALGB 80303. Clin Cancer Res 2012;18:577–84.

136. Jones S, Hruban RH, Kamiyama M, et al. Exomic sequencing identifies PALB2 as a pancreatic cancer susceptibility gene. Science 2009;324:217.
137. Roberts NJ, Jiao Y, Yu J, et al. ATM mutations in patients with hereditary pancreatic cancer. Cancer Discov 2012;2:41–6.
138. Marth GT, Yu F, Indap AR, et al. The functional spectrum of low-frequency coding variation. Genome Biol 2011;12:R84.
139. Goldstein AM, Chan M, Harland M, et al. High-risk melanoma susceptibility genes and pancreatic cancer, neural system tumors, and uveal melanoma across GenoMEL. Cancer Res 2006;66:9818–28.
140. Lynch HT, Fusaro RM, Lynch JF, et al. Pancreatic cancer and the FAMMM syndrome. Fam Cancer 2008;7:103–12.
141. van Lier MG, Wagner A, Mathus-Vliegen EM, et al. High cancer risk in Peutz-Jeghers syndrome: a systematic review and surveillance recommendations. Am J Gastroenterol 2010;105:1258–64 [author reply: 1265].
142. Kastrinos F, Mukherjee B, Tayob N, et al. Risk of pancreatic cancer in families with Lynch syndrome. JAMA 2009;302:1790–5.
143. Breast Cancer Linkage Consortium. Cancer risks in BRCA2 mutation carriers. J Natl Cancer Inst 1999;91:1310–6.
144. Lowenfels AB, Maisonneuve P, DiMagno EP, et al. Hereditary pancreatitis and the risk of pancreatic cancer. International Hereditary Pancreatitis Study Group. J Natl Cancer Inst 1997;89:442–6.
145. Howes N, Lerch MM, Greenhalf W, et al. Clinical and genetic characteristics of hereditary pancreatitis in Europe. Clin Gastroenterol Hepatol 2004;2:252–61.
146. Witt H, Luck W, Hennies HC, et al. Mutations in the gene encoding the serine protease inhibitor, Kazal type 1 are associated with chronic pancreatitis. Nat Genet 2000;25:213–6.
147. Michaud DS, Wolpin B, Giovannucci E, et al. Prediagnostic plasma C-peptide and pancreatic cancer risk in men and women. Cancer Epidemiol Biomarkers Prev 2007;16:2101–9.
148. Stolzenberg-Solomon RZ, Weinstein S, Pollak M, et al. Prediagnostic adiponectin concentrations and pancreatic cancer risk in male smokers. Am J Epidemiol 2008;168:1047–55.
149. Bao Y, Giovannucci EL, Kraft P, et al. A prospective study of plasma adiponectin and pancreatic cancer risk in five US cohorts. J Natl Cancer Inst 2013;105:95–103.
150. Stolzenberg-Solomon RZ, Limburg P, Pollak M, et al. Insulin-like growth factor (IGF)-1, IGF-binding protein-3, and pancreatic cancer in male smokers. Cancer Epidemiol Biomarkers Prev 2004;13:438–44.
151. Rohrmann S, Grote VA, Becker S, et al. Concentrations of IGF-I and IGFBP-3 and pancreatic cancer risk in the European Prospective Investigation into Cancer and Nutrition. Br J Cancer 2012;106:1004–10.
152. Wolpin BM, Michaud DS, Giovannucci EL, et al. Circulating insulin-like growth factor axis and the risk of pancreatic cancer in four prospective cohorts. Br J Cancer 2007;97:98–104.
153. Wolpin BM, Michaud DS, Giovannucci EL, et al. Circulating insulin-like growth factor binding protein-1 and the risk of pancreatic cancer. Cancer Res 2007;67:7923–8.
154. Grote VA, Kaaks R, Nieters A, et al. Inflammation marker and risk of pancreatic cancer: a nested case-control study within the EPIC cohort. Br J Cancer 2012;106:1866–74.

155. Bao Y, Giovannucci EL, Kraft P, et al. Inflammatory plasma markers and pancreatic cancer risk: a prospective study of five U.S. cohorts. Cancer Epidemiol Biomarkers Prev 2013;22:855–61.
156. Jacobs EJ, Newton CC, Silverman DT, et al. Serum transforming growth factor-beta1 and risk of pancreatic cancer in three prospective cohort studies. Cancer Causes Control 2014;25:1083–91.

Familial Pancreatic Adenocarcinoma

Gloria M. Petersen, PhD

KEYWORDS

- Genetic susceptibility • Familial risk • Genetic testing
- Risk assessment and management

KEY POINTS

- Familial pancreatic cancer (FPC) kindreds have 2 or more first-degree relatives ever diagnosed with pancreatic ductal adenocarcinoma.
- Patients with FPC constitute 8% to 10% of all patients with pancreatic cancer. Positive family history of pancreatic cancer is a consistent risk factor, with twofold increased risk to first-degree relatives.
- Although novel genes that predispose to FPC remain to be discovered, increased risk of pancreatic cancer is now known to be associated with half a dozen inherited syndromes with known germline mutations, including *BRCA1, BRCA2, CDKN2A, PALB2*, ataxia telangiectasia mutated (*ATM*), mismatch repair genes, as well as *PRSS1* and *SPINK2* of hereditary pancreatitis.
- Predisposition genetic testing for individuals in FPC kindreds is feasible and typically consists of sequencing a panel of multiple genes. Cancer risk assessment is less precise, and research into prevention and screening is nascent.
- Guidelines for management of family members at risk for FPC are being developed or disseminated. Owing to limited experience worldwide, guidance is often based on expert opinion. It is agreed that more research is needed to improve the shaping of options.

INTRODUCTION

Pancreatic cancer is a devastating diagnosis for patients and their families, and it is the fourth leading cause of cancer death. Among the major cancers, pancreatic cancer has the worst survival and historically, has been the least studied. Approximately 95% of pancreatic neoplasms are ductal adenocarcinomas. The rapid mortality of patients with pancreatic adenocarcinoma makes this cancer challenging for research into basic, translational, and epidemiologic studies. For genetic or molecular

Disclosures: The author has no conflicts.
Supported in part by National Cancer Institute grants R01 CA97075 and P50 CA102701.
Department of Health Sciences Research, Mayo Clinic Cancer Center, Mayo Clinic, Charlton 6-243, Rochester, MN 55905, USA
E-mail address: Petersen.gloria@mayo.edu

investigations that require biospecimens for DNA studies, involving patients who are often too ill to participate and whose disease precludes surgical resection (with consequent lack of tumor tissue) has posed difficulties.

This longstanding dearth of knowledge has resulted in only minimal inroads to improve risk reduction or survival. In the United States, the incidence and mortality rates have remained largely unchanged since 1973. During 2005–2009, the incidence rate for whites and African Americans was 11.6 of 105 and 15.2 of 105, respectively. Mortality rates were 10.7 of 105 for whites and 13.8 of 105 for African Americans.[1] The 5-year survival has been 4% to 6% for decades.[2] The low survival from pancreatic cancer is primarily due to the advanced stage at diagnosis in most cases: by the time of diagnosis, 80% of pancreatic carcinomas are no longer localized to the pancreas. To date, no reliable screening tests or effective cures for pancreatic cancer are available; there are few long-term survivors.

It is crucial to advance the knowledge of etiology to enable evidence-based strategies to decrease incidence and mortality. For years, pancreatic cancer was thought to be a sporadic disease, due in part to the lack of systematic studies and the inherent challenges as described earlier. Over the past 2 decades, however, there has been sustained effort to elucidate its genetics. As demonstrated for a variety of cancers, genetic epidemiology and family-based approaches have led to important breakthroughs in a variety of diseases, and particularly cancer.[3–5] Discerning familial patterns of cancer incidence, combined with detailed studies of clinical and DNA variation, has defined a variety of inherited cancer syndromes and their causal genes. This article reviews the evidence for a genetic component of pancreatic cancer, studies of hereditary syndromes that feature increased risk of pancreatic cancer, and the current status of clinical translation of the findings.

EVIDENCE FOR GENETIC BASIS OF PANCREATIC CANCER
Familial Clustering

Early reports of familial clusters of pancreatic cancer provided the first suggestion that at least a hereditary, but rare form of pancreatic cancer might exist. Reports of clusters included families in which multiple siblings were affected (but not the parents)[6–9] or 1 family in which 3 generations contained an affected member each.[10]

Familial Aggregation Studies and Analysis of Families

More formal study designs that apply epidemiologic and genetic segregation analysis methods are widely accepted standards to uncover existence of genetic basis for a cancer. One conventional approach to investigating potential host susceptibility is to perform case-control comparisons of family history of pancreatic cancer. A comprehensive summary of these studies and estimated risks are listed in **Table 1**. Seven case-control studies, 2 cohort studies, 1 population-based genealogic analysis, and 1 case series that estimated the incidence of pancreatic cancer in relatives have found that first-degree relatives have at least a 2-fold increased risk of developing pancreatic cancer. These findings are remarkably consistent, given that case ascertainment and data collection spanned 30 or more years, multiple countries and cultures, and different methods for estimating risk. A systematic review and meta-analysis by Permuth-Wey and Egan[22] of 1 cohort study and 7 case-control studies totaling 6568 pancreatic cancer cases calculated an overall relative risk of 1.80 (95% confidence interval [CI], 1.48–2.12). The investigators also found that 1.3% of pancreatic cancers in the population is attributable to family history. The risk was consistent for both males and females, and did not differ by early or late

Table 1
Family history and estimated risks of pancreatic cancer in case-control and cohort studies

Location, Years of Study	Cases, N	Controls, N	Risk of Pancreatic Cancer in Family Members		Reference
			Risk	95% CI	
Louisiana, 1979–1983	362	1408	5.25	2.1–13.2	Falk et al,[11] 1988
Canada, 1984–1988	174	136	5.0	1.2–24.5	Ghadirian et al,[12] 2002
Italy, 1983–1992	363	1234	2.8	1.3–6.3	Fernandez et al,[13] 1994
United States, 1986–1989	484	2099	3.2	1.8–5.6	Silverman et al,[14] 1999
Japan, cohort, 1988–1999	200	2200	2.09	1.01–4.33	Inoue et al,[15] 2003
United States, 1996–1999	247	420	2.49	1.3–4.7	Schenk et al,[16] 2001
Texas, 2000–2006	888	888	3.3	1.8–6.1	Hassan et al,[17] 2007
United States, 2005–2009	654	697	2.79	1.44–4.08	Austin et al,[18] 2013
International, PanScan Cohort Consortium (1 case-control and 10 cohort studies), 1985–2001	1183	1205	1.76	1.19–2.61	Jacobs et al,[19] 2010
Utah, genealogy database, 1966–2010	1411	—	RR = 1.84	1.47–2.29	Shirts et al,[20] 2010
Minnesota, case series, 2000–2004	426	—	SIR = 1.88	1.27–2.68	McWilliams et al,[21] 2005

Case-control study designs reported unless otherwise specified.
Abbreviations: CI, confidence interval; RR, relative risk; SIR, standardized incidence ratio.
Data from Axilbund J, Wiley E. Genetic testing by cancer site: pancreas. Cancer J 2012;18(4):350–4; and Klein AP. Genetic susceptibility to pancreatic cancer. Mol Carcinog 2012;51(1):14–24.

age at diagnosis. With respect to risk for second-degree relatives (aunts, uncles, grandparents, grandchildren), both Hassan and colleagues[17] and Shirts and colleagues[20] reported risks comparable to those of first-degree relatives (relative risks of 2.9 [95% CI, 1.3–6.3] and 1.59 [95% CI, 1.31–2.91], respectively). In addition, a large multicenter cohort study examined risk by number of affected individuals and showed high risk associated with having 2 or more first-degree relatives with pancreatic cancer with odds ratio (OR) of 4.26 (95% CI, 0.48–37.79).[19]

The authors' experience and those of the others has shown that 8% to 10% of patients with pancreatic adenocarcinoma report having had a first-degree relative (parent, sibling, or child) with pancreatic cancer.[23,24] This proportion is congruent with family history patterns observed in series of patients with colorectal cancer, breast cancer, lung cancer, and prostate cancer. In addition, a population-based twin study of cancer in Sweden by Lichtenstein and colleagues[25] estimated pancreatic cancer heritability to be 36%, similar to that of colorectal cancer (35%), higher than that of breast cancer (27%), and slightly lower than that of prostate cancer (42%). Taken together, this implies that pancreatic adenocarcinoma susceptibility patterns would be consistent with those seen for the more common cancers and it could be likewise expected that predisposition genes exist.

Segregation analysis is a statistical method that determines if a gene consistent with a mendelian inheritance pattern could cause the observed familial aggregation of a trait. Klein and colleagues[26] analyzed family histories of 287 patients with pancreatic cancer seen from 1994–1999 at Johns Hopkins Hospital in Baltimore, MD, USA. The analysis rejected nongenetic transmission models. The data best fit a major gene model that was predicted to follow an autosomal dominant pattern of a rare allele; 0.7% of the population would carry a high risk of developing pancreatic cancer because of this putative gene. A smaller study of 70 families by Banke and colleagues[27] arrived at a similar conclusion.

Familial Pancreatic Cancer Defined to Advance Research

Increased attention on the genetic analysis of pancreatic cancer required that a standard definition be applied so that research on risk factors and gene discovery in the familial setting would be consistent. In 1998, Hruban and colleagues[28] proposed that FPC would be defined as kindreds containing at least a pair of individuals who were affected with pancreatic adenocarcinoma and who were first-degree relatives. This definition was simple, yet provided a sufficient boundary and is now widely used and facilitates a variety of studies. In particular, the multicenter Pancreatic Cancer Genetic Epidemiology (PACGENE) Consortium was formed to systematically collect risk factor and family history data plus germline DNA from blood or saliva from members of FPC kindreds. The resources would be used for gene discovery and genetic epidemiologic characterization.[23] Many of the advances described here were enabled by the ongoing activities of the PACGENE Consortium members. To date, 44,183 patients at 7 sites have been screened for family history, of whom 3190 (7.2%) with positive family history have been enrolled, along with 7012 adult (99% unaffected) relatives of these patients.

Characteristics of familial pancreatic cancer: sex, incident risk, age at onset, smoking, other cancers

Based on the PACGENE data, approximately half of the patients with FPC are males, which is consistent with the proportion observed in sporadic pancreatic cancer. With respect to incident risk, family history studies described earlier clearly document the risk. Klein and colleagues[29] analyzed 5179 individuals in 838 Johns Hopkins FPC kindreds and quantified risk using standardized incidence ratios (SIRs) that compared the number of incident pancreatic cancers observed with those expected using Surveillance, Epidemiology, and End Results (SEER)[30] rates. During the follow-up period from the time of enrollment, 19 pancreatic cancers developed among the relatives. The observed-to-expected rate of pancreatic cancer was 9.0 (95% CI, 4.5–16.1), significantly increased compared with members of sporadic kindreds. It was also noted that with increasing number of affected individuals in the pedigree, the risk increased: 3 affected first-degree relatives in the kindred had an SIR of 32.0 (95% CI, 10.2–74.7), 2 affected had an SIR of 6.4 (95% CI, 1.8–16.4), and 1 affected had an SIR of 4.6 (95% CI, 0.5–16.4). Compared with the general population incidence of 9 per 100,000, relatives with FPC with 3 affected individuals in the pedigree have an estimated incidence of 288 per 100,000, relatives with 2 affected individuals in the kindred have an incidence of 57.6 per 100,000, and those with 1 affected individual in the kindred have an incidence of 41.1 per 100,000.

Risk of developing pancreatic cancer in the FPC setting was higher in smokers than in nonsmokers. Individuals with a strong family history of pancreatic cancer have a significantly increased risk of developing pancreatic cancer. Unlike hereditary breast cancer or hereditary colorectal cancer syndromes, where the age of onset can be much less by 10 to 20 years compared with sporadic cases, the difference in median age at diagnosis in FPC is approximately 5 years. Compared with the general pancreatic cancer population (from SEER data) in which the mean age at diagnosis was 70.0 ± 12.1 years, the mean age among FPC cases was 65.4 ± 11.6 years. Among the PACGENE kindreds, mean ages at diagnosis did not significantly differ when stratified by number of affected individuals in the pedigree. With respect to smoking history, 37% are never smokers, 47.1% are ever smokers, and smoking status is unknown in 14.9%. In an Australian sample of 68 patients with FPC, 60.3% were never smokers.[24] The authors and other investigators have observed increased risk of other cancers in FPC kindreds, particularly breast cancer, melanoma, and colorectal cancer. However, these risks have not been systematically disentangled from analyses that also include germline mutations in cancer susceptibility genes. In addition, much of the focus is on cancer among at-risk relatives.

GENETIC STUDIES OF FAMILIAL PANCREATIC CANCER
Hereditary Syndromes with Increased Risk of Pancreatic Cancer

In 1996, Lynch and colleagues[31] asserted that genetic factors were estimated to play a significant role in 5% of the total pancreatic cancer burden. Much research has been accomplished in the intervening time. Although novel genes that predispose to FPC remain to be discovered, increased risk of pancreatic cancer is now known to be associated with half a dozen inherited syndromes with known germline mutations, including *BRCA1, BRCA2, CDKN2A, PALB2, ATM,* mismatch repair genes, and *PRSS1* and *SPINK1* of hereditary pancreatitis.[32] These syndromes are summarized in **Table 2**, along with associated malignancies and estimates of pancreatic risk in these syndromic settings. The most prominent syndromes are hereditary breast-ovarian cancer syndrome, particularly due to germline mutations in *BRCA2*, and familial atypical mole and melanoma syndrome, due to mutations in *CDKN2A*.

It is also important to note that this review does not discuss low-penetrance common genetic polymorphisms that confer modest risk of pancreatic cancer (OR<1.3). The susceptibility variants were identified by genome-wide association studies involving large samples of sporadic pancreatic cancer cases and healthy controls. The variants offer opportunities to study gene pathways and gene-environment interactions.[32] However, translation of these findings to the clinic is unlikely for some time.

Gene Discovery Studies in Familial Pancreatic Cancer

Family-based gene discovery studies focused on linkage studies and candidate gene approaches. Genetic linkage analysis requires a panel of hundreds to thousands of genetic markers spaced across the genome, which are then used in conjunction with the family structure and cancer phenotypes to assess the probability that an allele in a specific marker is cotransmitted through the pedigree with the cancer phenotype. A lod score (log of the odds that the allele is transmitted with the phenotype vs independently of the phenotype) is calculated for each family and examined in aggregate. To date, no formal linkage analysis of a large number of families has been published. The only linkage analysis of a single FPC kindred in the literature examined a linkage region on chromosome 4p[38] and erroneously concluded that the *PALLD* gene encoding the palladin protein was the predisposition gene.[39] *PALLD* mutation analysis of 48 patients with FPC was unable to support the original linkage finding.[40]

An alternative approach to FPC gene discovery is candidate gene analysis. Studies that use this approach are based on a plausible biological or clinical rationale for examining a candidate gene in patients with pancreatic cancer. For example, van

Table 2
Genes and syndromes associated and estimates of risk of developing pancreatic adenocarcinoma

Gene	Chromosome	Predisposition Syndrome	Associated Malignancies	Risk of Pancreatic Cancer	Patients with FPC Deleterious Mutations		
					Proportion	%	Reference
ATM	11q23	Familial breast cancer	Breast	Increased risk: not well defined	2/168	1.2	Roberts et al,[33] 2012
					1/39	2.6	Grant et al,[34] 2014
BRCA1	17q21.31	Hereditary breast and ovarian cancer	Breast (particularly premenopausal), ovary, male breast, prostate	No effect up to OR = 2.26 (95% CI, 1.26–4.06); SIR = 2.55 (95% CI, 1.03–5.31)[35]	6/516	1.2	Zhen et al,[36] 2014
BRCA2	13q13.1		Breast (particularly premenopausal), ovary, male breast, prostate, melanoma	OR = 3.5 (95% CI, 1.87–6.58); SIR = 2.13 (95% CI, 0.36–7.03)[35]	19/516	3.7	Zhen et al,[36] 2014
CDKN2A	9p21.3	Familial atypical mole and melanoma	Melanoma	SIR = 13–38	14/519	2.7	Zhen et al,[36] 2014
Mismatch repair:		Hereditary nonpolyposis colorectal cancer (Lynch syndrome)	Colorectum, endometrium, ovary, stomach, small bowel, urinary tract (ureter, renal pelvis) biliary, glioblastoma, skin (sebaceous)	No effect up to SIR = 8.6 (95% CI, 4.7–15.7)	—	—	—
MLH1	3p22.2						
MSH2	2p21						
MSH6	2p16.3						
PMS2	7p22.1						
PALB2	16p12.2	Familial breast cancer	Fanconi anemia, breast, esophagus, prostate, stomach	Increased risk: not well defined	3/96	3.1	Jones et al,[37] 2009
					3/521	0.6	Zhen et al,[36] 2014
PRSS1	7q34	Hereditary pancreatitis	—	SIR = 67 (95% CI, 8–80)	—	—	—
SPINK1	5q32						
STK11 (LKB1)	19p13.3	Peutz-Jeghers syndrome	Colorectum, small bowel, stomach, breast, gynecologic	SIR = 132	—	—	—

The probabilities of detecting a deleterious mutation in the predisposition genes shown were based on studies that sequenced the entire gene in a series of patients with FPC.

Abbreviations: CI, confidence interval; OR, odds ratio; SIR, standardized incidence ratio.

Adapted from Axilbund J, Wiley E. Genetic testing by cancer site: pancreas. Cancer J 2012;18(4):350–4; and Klein AP. Genetic susceptibility to pancreatic cancer. Mol Carcinog 2012;51(1):14–24.

der Heijden and colleagues[41] identified mutations in *FANCC* and *FANCG* gene in Fanconi anemia among patients with young-onset pancreatic cancer. Rogers and colleagues[42] examined 38 FPC kindreds for mutations but was not able to attribute mutations to FPC. Couch and colleagues[43] performed a mutation screen of the *FANCC* and *FANCG* genes in 421 unselected Mayo Clinic cases and found 2 mutations of *FANCC* in sporadic young-onset patients, but none in *FANCG*.

In another candidate gene study, McWilliams and colleagues[44] analyzed 39 mutations in the cystic fibrosis transmembrane regulator (*CFTR*) gene in 949 unselected white Mayo Clinic pancreatic cancer cases and used data on 13,340 white controls from a clinical laboratory database. The investigators found that 5.3% carried a common *CFTR* mutation versus 3.8% of controls, giving an OR of 1.40 (95% CI, 1.04–1.89). Among patients who were younger when their disease was diagnosed (<60 years), the carrier frequency was higher than in controls (OR, 1.82; 95% CI, 1.14–2.94).

Analogously, Murphy and colleagues[45] reported 17% prevalence of *BRCA2* mutations among affected individuals from 26 European FPC kindreds containing 3 or more affected members with pancreatic cancer. Subsequent studies of individuals with pancreatic cancer from families meeting FPC criteria estimated *BRCA2* prevalence ranging between 6% and 10%.[46] Among Ashkenazi Jews, similar mutation prevalences were observed for both *BRCA1* and *BRCA2*.[47]

Novel gene discovery in patients with familial pancreatic cancer using next-generation sequencing

Advances in sequencing technology, bioinformatics, and computing capacity have moved genomic researchers considerably forward in the discovery of susceptibility genes for FPC. High-throughput sequencing of FPC kindreds has resulted in the discovery of 2 genes that were not previously known to increase the risk of pancreatic cancer: *PALB2* and *ATM*. In both cases, functional roles were supported by the loss of heterozygosity of the wild-type allele in the pancreatic tumor of the patients. In the course of complete exome sequencing of unselected patients with pancreatic cancer, Jones and colleagues[37] identified a germline truncating mutation in *PALB2* that cosegregated in a patient with FPC. This finding led to screening of the DNA of 96 more patients with FPC specifically for *PALB2* mutations. Truncating mutations were detected in 3 additional patients; however, no difference was observed in the age at diagnosis of the mutation carriers. No *PALB2* mutations were found in 1084 normal controls. Similarly, mutations in the *ATM* gene were discovered to segregate with the pancreatic cancer phenotype in 2 FPC kindreds by Roberts and colleagues[33] The investigators screened the *ATM* gene for mutations in 166 patients with FPC and identified 4 carriers of deleterious mutations. No similar mutations were seen in 190 controls.

Taken together, the candidate gene approach and the unbiased genomic sequencing approach are revealing, gene by gene, the extensive genetic heterogeneity of the FPC phenotype (**Fig. 1**). In addition to adding to the catalog of genes, they provide an opportunity to study the potential effect of genetic mutations on age at diagnosis and risk of developing other cancers.

Genetic analysis of cancer syndrome genes

With the identification of susceptibility genes, particularly in the context of hereditary cancer syndromes, genetic testing for multiple susceptibility genes is readily feasible. The approach used with this opportunity is to characterize the genetic variation in patients with FPC, tested across genes. In the PACGENE Consortium study, Zhen and colleagues[36] collected and performed mutation analysis of germline DNA samples from 727 unrelated probands with positive family history (521 met criteria for FPC).

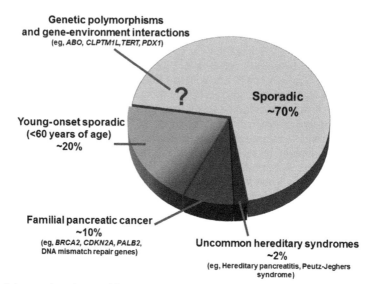

Fig. 1. Subsets of patients with pancreatic adenocarcinoma who carry gene mutations or variants that increase susceptibility. Most cases of pancreatic adenocarcinoma are considered sporadic without any known associated genetic or hereditary factor. Low-penetrance genetic polymorphisms, which confer modest risks (odds ratio<1.3), were identified in genome-wide association studies. A modest proportion of patients with young-onset sporadic pancreatic cancer carry deleterious germline mutations in known cancer genes or polymorphisms associated with pancreatic cancer risk. The genetic basis of FPC is only partly explained by known cancer genes. Uncommon hereditary syndromes confer increased risk of pancreatic cancer.

All patient samples were tested for mutations in *BRCA1, BRCA2, PALB2*, and *CDKN2A*. Prevalence of mutations among FPC probands was estimated. The prevalence of deleterious mutations among FPC probands was as follows: *BRCA1*, 1.2%; *BRCA2*, 3.7%; *PALB2*, 0.6%; and *CDKN2A*, 2.5%. The probability of testing positive for deleterious mutations in any of the 4 genes ranges up to 10.4%, depending on family history of cancers. *BRCA2* and *CDKN2A* account for most mutations in FPC. These results are summarized in **Table 2**.

In the Ontario Pancreas Cancer Registry study,[34] the prevalence of germline mutations was investigated in a panel of 13 genes (*APC, ATM, BRCA1, BRCA2, CDKN2A, MLH1, MSH2, MSH6, PALB2, PMS2, PRSS1, STK11*, and *TP53*) in 290 patients with varying degrees of family history. Although a total of 11 deleterious mutations were found (3 in *ATM*, 1 in *BRCA1*, 2 in *BRCA2*, 1 in *MLH1*, 2 in *MSH2*, 1 in *MSH6,* and 1 in *TP53*), the only mutation detected among 39 patients with FPC was one in *ATM*. Owing to the variation in family history and FPC status, the aggregate probability of having a positive result of gene test is 3.8% in the Ontario study compared with over 10% in familial subsets in the PACGENE study.

The emerging trend of multiple genetic testing of patients regardless of family history indications is a concern. Commercial testing is already offered through genetic testing companies, but recommendations regarding who is appropriate for genetic testing are nascent. Although there is a need for more genetic epidemiologic evidence, the aggregate prevalence of mutations in current genetic panels is such that useful information may be learned. Several whole genome and whole exome sequencing studies of large numbers of patients with pancreatic cancer and FPC series are ongoing. These studies are expected to inform risk assessment and genetic testing using multigene panels.

CLINICAL TRANSLATION OF FAMILIAL PANCREATIC CANCER RESEARCH

As with other cancer genes, the transfer of discoveries to the clinical laboratory and bedside is occurring rapidly. Regrettably, there still remain gaps in knowledge so that strategies cannot be fully shaped to guide patients and their families. Multiple fronts have been opened: personalized therapy, risk assessment and genetic testing, as well as screening and surveillance.

Personalized Therapy

When a novel germline mutation is identified, its relevance and contribution to the cancer phenotype is investigated. As described for *PALB2* and *ATM*, a functional role is sought, such as examining the matched tumor for additional mutations and loss of heterozygosity. Work then proceeds to identify mechanisms to establish whether existing therapies could be redirected to address effect of the genetic alteration. In particular, several investigations of poly (ADP-ribose) polymerase inhibitor in patients with *BRCA1* or *BRCA2* mutations in germline and/or tumor have been initiated,[48,49] and several pancreatic-cancer-specific trials are enrolling.[50] It is still too early to know whether the clinical trial outcomes will lend credence to personalized therapy for mutation carriers.

Genetic Testing and Cancer Risk Assessment

By far, the most rapid translational activity after discovery of a susceptibility gene is determining the gene/mutation utility and suitability for genetic testing, risk assessment, and counseling. Family history alone may trigger a referral to a cancer genetic counselor. With the array of genetic tests available, it is unclear whether health care providers or patients will seek to take up these new options. Genetic testing of at-risk individuals, particularly in high-risk cancer clinics, may be routinely offered. As discussed earlier, the cancer multigene testing panels are a double-edged sword. Genetic testing can provide more information than was previously available and the yield may be higher, but interpretation may be hampered for lack of evidence on which to develop the next steps.[51–53]

Screening Options for High-Risk Individuals

Clinicians are being pushed by the pace of genetic discoveries and testing for FPC. It has been a challenge to develop commensurate screening, surveillance, and management guidelines for genetically high-risk individuals. Clinical experiences of 49 experts were shared in the Cancer of the Pancreas Screening (CAPS) Consortium to develop consensus on several clinical scenarios.[54,55] There was excellent agreement on goals of a screening program (should detect and treat T1N0M0 margin-negative PC and high-grade dysplastic precursor lesions). Candidates for screening include first-degree relatives of an affected patient in an FPC kindred, patients with Peutz-Jeghers syndrome, and mutation carriers of FPC hereditary cancer syndrome genes with an affected first-degree relative. Although initial screening should include endoscopic ultrasonography (EUS) and/or MRI/magnetic resonance cholangiopancreatography, the CAPS Consortium could not reach consensus on ages to initiate or stop surveillance and on longer-term management of problematic scenarios.[54]

The American College of Gastroenterology (ACG) has published its clinical guidelines on genetic testing and management of hereditary gastrointestinal cancer syndromes, including hereditary pancreatic cancer.[52] Agreeing with the CAPS Consortium, the ACG states that surveillance of genetically high-risk individuals should be performed at experienced centers with a multidisciplinary approach. The ACG guidelines include a conditional recommendation with low quality of evidence that surveillance for pancreatic cancer should be with EUS and/or MRI annually starting at the age of 50 years, or 10 years less than the earliest age of pancreatic cancer in the family. The quality of the supporting data for the guidelines is low, and, combined with the experience and caution of others,[56,57] it is important to maintain perspective when counseling high-risk relatives. Taken together, experts most familiar with screening and surveillance of at-risk individuals in the setting of FPC are taking careful steps forward, but the challenges to achieve consensus underscore the need for more research and collaboration.

SUMMARY

FPC kindreds contain at least 2 first-degree relatives with pancreatic ductal adenocarcinoma. Genetic studies of FPC have uncovered important new genes and insights about the genetics of pancreatic cancer. Over a decade of research reveals that a half dozen known hereditary syndromes or genes are associated with increased risk of developing pancreatic cancer, the most prominent of which are *BRCA2* and *CDKN2A*. Next-generation sequencing technologies successfully identified new FPC genes, *PALB2* and *ATM*. At the same time, with rapid dissemination of the knowledge to the clinical setting, many challenges have been generated. Genetic testing, risk assessment, and management of those at risk have proved the need for effective, evidence-based criteria. Guidelines are based on expert opinion, although all agree that research is needed to improve management.

REFERENCES

1. American Cancer Society. Cancer facts & figures. Atlanta (GA): American Cancer Society; 2013. Available at: http://www.cancer.org/acs/groups/content/@epidemiologysurveilance/documents/document/acspc-036845.pdf.
2. American Cancer Society. Cancer facts & figures. Atlanta (GA): American Cancer Society; 2015. Available at: http://www.cancer.org/acs/groups/content/@editorial/documents/document/acspc-044552.pdf.
3. de la Chapelle A. Genetic predisposition to colorectal cancer. Nat Rev Cancer 2004;4(10):769–80.
4. Hemminki K, Rawal R, Chen B, et al. Genetic epidemiology of cancer: from families to heritable genes. Int J Cancer 2004;111(6):944–50.
5. Antoniou AC, Easton DF. Models of genetic susceptibility to breast cancer. Oncogene 2006;25(43):5898–905.
6. Ghadirian P, Simard A, Baillargeon J. Cancer of the pancreas in two brothers and one sister. Int J Pancreatol 1987;2(5–6):383–91.
7. Dat NM, Sontag SJ. Pancreatic carcinoma in brothers. Ann Intern Med 1982; 97(2):282.
8. MacDermott RP, Kramer P. Adenocarcinoma of the pancreas in four siblings. Gastroenterology 1973;65(1):137–9.
9. Friedman JM, Fialkow PJ. Familial carcinoma of the pancreas. Clin Genet 1976; 9(5):463–9.
10. Ehrenthal D, Haeger L, Griffin T, et al. Familial pancreatic adenocarcinoma in three generations. A case report and a review of the literature. Cancer 1987;59(9):1661–4.

11. Falk RT, Pickle LW, Fontham ET, et al. Life-style risk factors for pancreatic cancer in Louisiana: a case–control study. Am J Epidemiol 1988;128(2):324–36.
12. Ghadirian P, Liu G, Gallinger S, et al. Risk of pancreatic cancer among individuals with a family history of cancer of the pancreas. Int J Cancer 2002;97(6):807–10.
13. Fernandez E, La Vecchia C, D'Avanzo B, et al. Family history and the risk of liver, gallbladder, and pancreatic cancer. Cancer Epidemiol Biomarkers Prev 1994; 3(3):209–12.
14. Silverman DT, Schiffman M, Everhart J, et al. Diabetes mellitus, other medical conditions and familial history of cancer as risk factors for pancreatic cancer. Br J Cancer 1999;80(11):1830–7.
15. Inoue M, Tajima K, Takezaki T, et al. Epidemiology of pancreatic cancer in Japan: a nested case-control study from the Hospital-based Epidemiologic Research Program at Aichi Cancer Center (HERPACC). Int J Epidemiol 2003;32(2):257–62.
16. Schenk M, Schwartz AG, O'Neal E, et al. Familial risk of pancreatic cancer. J Natl Cancer Inst 2001;93(8):640–4.
17. Hassan MM, Bondy ML, Wolff RA, et al. Risk factors for pancreatic cancer: case-control stud. Am J Gastroenterol 2007;102(12):2696–707.
18. Austin MA, Kuo E, Van Den Eeden SK, et al. Family history of diabetes and pancreatic cancer as risk factors for pancreatic cancer: the PACIFIC study. Cancer Epidemiol Biomarkers Prev 2013;22(10):1913–7.
19. Jacobs EJ, Chanock SJ, Fuchs CS, et al. Family history of cancer and risk of pancreatic cancer: a pooled analysis from the Pancreatic Cancer Cohort Consortium (PanScan). Int J Cancer 2010;127(6):1421–8.
20. Shirts BH, Burt RW, Mulvihill SJ, et al. A population-based description of familial clustering of pancreatic cancer. Clin Gastroenterol Hepatol 2010;8(9):812–6.
21. McWilliams RR, Rabe KG, Olswold C, et al. Risk of malignancy in first-degree relatives of patients with pancreatic carcinoma. Cancer 2005;104(2):388–94.
22. Permuth-Wey J, Egan KM. Family history is a significant risk factor for pancreatic cancer: results from a systematic review and meta-analysis. Fam Cancer 2009; 8(2):109–17.
23. Petersen GM, de Andrade M, Goggins M, et al. Pancreatic cancer genetic epidemiology consortium. Cancer Epidemiol Biomarkers Prev 2006;15(4):704–10.
24. Humphris JL, Johns AL, Simpson SH, et al, Australian Pancreatic Cancer Genome Initiative. Clinical and pathologic features of familial pancreatic cancer. Cancer 2014;120(23):3669–75.
25. Lichtenstein P, Holm NV, Verkasalo PK, et al. Environmental and heritable factors in the causation of cancer–analyses of cohorts of twins from Sweden, Denmark, and Finland. N Engl J Med 2000;343(2):78–85.
26. Klein AP, Beaty TH, Bailey-Wilson JE, et al. Evidence for a major gene influencing risk of pancreatic cancer. Genet Epidemiol 2002;23(2):133–49.
27. Banke MG, Mulvihill JJ, Aston CE. Inheritance of pancreatic cancer in pancreatic cancer-prone families. Med Clin North Am 2000;84(3):677–90, x–xi.
28. Hruban RH, Petersen GM, Kern S, et al. Genetics of cancer of the pancreas: from genes to families. In: Pitt HA, editor. Surgical oncology clinics of North America, vol. 7, No. 1, pancreatic cancer. New York: W. B. Saunders; 1998. p. 1–23.
29. Klein AP, Brune KA, Petersen GM, et al. Prospective risk of pancreatic cancer in familial pancreatic cancer kindreds. Cancer Res 2004;64(7):2634–8.
30. National Cancer Institute Surveillance, Epidemiology, and End Results Program. Available at: http://seer.cancer.gov/. Accessed May 22, 2015.
31. Lynch HT, Smyrk T, Kern SE, et al. Familial pancreatic cancer: a review. Semin Oncol 1996;23(2):251–75.

32. Klein AP. Genetic susceptibility to pancreatic cancer. Mol Carcinog 2012;51(1): 14–24.

33. Roberts NJ, Jiao Y, Yu J, et al. ATM mutations in patients with hereditary pancreatic cancer. Cancer Discov 2012;2(1):41–6.

34. Grant RC, Selander I, Connor AA, et al. Prevalence of germline mutations in cancer predisposition genes in patients with pancreatic cancer. Gastroenterology 2014;148(3):556–64.

35. Iqbal J, Ragone A, Lubinski J, et al, Hereditary Breast Cancer Study Group. The incidence of pancreatic cancer in BRCA1 and BRCA2 mutation carriers. Br J Cancer 2012;107(12):2005–9.

36. Zhen DB, Rabe KG, Gallinger S, et al. BRCA1, BRCA2, PALB2, and CDKN2A mutations in familial pancreatic cancer (FPC): a PACGENE study. Genet Med 2014. http://dx.doi.org/10.1038/gim.2014.153.

37. Jones S, Hruban RH, Kamiyama M, et al. Exomic sequencing identifies PALB2 as a pancreatic cancer susceptibility gene. Science 2009;324(5924):217.

38. Eberle MA, Pfutzer R, Pogue-Geile KL, et al. A new susceptibility locus for autosomal dominant pancreatic cancer maps to chromosome 4q32-34. Am J Hum Genet 2002;70:1044–8.

39. Pogue-Geile KL, Chen R, Bronner MP, et al. Palladin mutation causes familial pancreatic cancer and suggests a new cancer mechanism. PLoS Med 2006; 3:e516.

40. Klein AP, Borges M, Griffith M, et al. Absence of deleterious palladin mutations in patients with familial pancreatic cancer. Cancer Epidemiol Biomarkers Prev 2009; 18(4):1328–30.

41. van der Heijden MS, Yeo CJ, Hruban RH, et al. Fanconi anemia gene mutations in young-onset pancreatic cancer. Cancer Res 2003;63(10):2585–8.

42. Rogers CD, van der Heijden MS, Brune K, et al. The genetics of FANCC and FANCG in familial pancreatic cancer. Cancer Biol Ther 2004;3(2):167–9.

43. Couch FJ, Johnson MR, Rabe K, et al. Germ line Fanconi anemia complementation group C mutations and pancreatic cancer. Cancer Res 2005;65(2):383–6.

44. McWilliams RR, Petersen GM, Rabe KG, et al. Cystic fibrosis transmembrane conductance regulator (CFTR) gene mutations and risk for pancreatic adenocarcinoma. Cancer 2010;116(1):203–9.

45. Murphy KM, Brune KA, Griffin C, et al. Evaluation of candidate genes MAP2K4, MADH4, ACVR1B, and BRCA2 in familial pancreatic cancer: deleterious BRCA2 mutations in 17%. Cancer Res 2002;62(13):3789–93.

46. Couch FJ, Johnson MR, Rabe KG, et al. The prevalence of BRCA2 mutations in familial pancreatic cancer. Cancer Epidemiol Biomarkers Prev 2007;16(2):342–6.

47. Stadler ZK, Salo-Mullen E, Patil SM, et al. Prevalence of BRCA1 and BRCA2 mutations in Ashkenazi Jewish families with breast and pancreatic cancer. Cancer 2012;118(2):493–9.

48. Lowery MA, Kelsen DP, Stadler ZK, et al. An emerging entity: pancreatic adenocarcinoma associated with a known BRCA mutation: clinical descriptors, treatment implications, and future directions. Oncologist 2011;16(10):1397–402.

49. Vyas O, Leung K, Ledbetter L, et al. Clinical outcomes in pancreatic adenocarcinoma associated with BRCA-2 mutation. Anticancer Drugs 2015;26(2):224–6.

50. National Institutes of Health. Available at: http://ClinicalTrials.gov. Accessed May 22, 2015.

51. Verna EC, Hwang C, Stevens PD, et al. Pancreatic cancer screening in a prospective cohort of high-risk patients: a comprehensive strategy of imaging and genetics. Clin Cancer Res 2010;16(20):5028–37.

52. Syngal S, Brand RE, Church JM, et al. ACG clinical guideline: genetic testing and management of hereditary gastrointestinal cancer syndromes. Am J Gastroenterol 2015;110(2):223–62.
53. Fendrich V, Langer P, Bartsch DK. Familial pancreatic cancer–status quo. Int J Colorectal Dis 2014;29(2):139–45.
54. Canto MI, Harinck F, Hruban RH, et al, International Cancer of Pancreas Screening (CAPS) Consortium. International Cancer of the Pancreas Screening (CAPS) Consortium summit on the management of patients with increased risk for familial pancreatic cancer. Gut 2013;62(3):339–47.
55. Bartsch DK, Gress TM, Langer P. Familial pancreatic cancer–current knowledge. Nat Rev Gastroenterol Hepatol 2012;9(8):445–53.
56. Langer P, Kann PH, Fendrich V, et al. Five years of prospective screening of high-risk individuals from families with familial pancreatic cancer. Gut 2009;58(10):1410–8.
57. Templeton AW, Brentnall TA. Screening and surgical outcomes of familial pancreatic cancer. Surg Clin North Am 2013;93(3):629–45.

Diagnosis and Management of Pancreatic Cystic Neoplasms

Teresa S. Kim, MD[a], Carlos Fernandez-del Castillo, MD[b],*

KEYWORDS

- Pancreatic cyst • Intraductal papillary mucinous neoplasm (IPMN)
- Mucinous cystic neoplasm (MCN) • Serous cystadenoma (SCA)
- Endoscopic ultrasound (EUS)

KEY POINTS

- Pancreatic cystic neoplasms are becoming increasingly prevalent due to increased awareness and increased utilization of high-resolution cross-sectional imaging.
- Different types of pancreatic cystic neoplasms vary in risk of current and future malignancy. Accurate diagnosis is, therefore, key to selecting optimal management, which involves either surgical resection or clinical and radiologic surveillance.
- Intraductal papillary mucinous neoplasms (IPMNs) present as 1 of 2 variants, main duct (MD-IPMNs) or branch duct (BD-IPMNs), with differing malignant potential and, hence, management. MD-IPMNs have a higher risk of malignancy and should be referred for surgical resection. BD-IPMNs are more likely to be benign and, particularly in older patients without high-risk features, such as mural nodules, can be observed.
- Mucinous cystic neoplasms (MCNs) represent another type of mucinous tumor with malignant potential. MCNs most often present in middle-aged women, in the body or tail of the pancreas, and should be referred for surgical resection.
- Serous cystadenomas (SCAs) are nonmucinous, benign lesions that often occur in older women and can be observed unless symptomatic or growing.
- Cystic pancreatic endocrine neoplasms (CPENs) are rare, potentially malignant tumors, with characteristic arterially enhancing walls on CT. CPENs should be referred for surgical resection.
- Solid pseudopapillary neoplasms (SPNs) are rare, potentially malignant tumors almost exclusively seen in young women. SPNs should be referred for surgical resection.

Disclosure of Potential Conflicts of Interest: The authors have no conflicts of interest to disclose.
[a] Department of Surgery, Massachusetts General Hospital, 55 Fruit Street, GRB-425, Boston, MA 02114, USA; [b] Department of Surgery, Massachusetts General Hospital, 55 Fruit Street, WAC-460, Boston, MA 02114, USA
* Corresponding author.
E-mail address: cfernandez@partners.org

Hematol Oncol Clin N Am 29 (2015) 655–674
http://dx.doi.org/10.1016/j.hoc.2015.04.002
0889-8588/15/$ – see front matter © 2015 Elsevier Inc. All rights reserved.

hemonc.theclinics.com

INTRODUCTION

Cystic lesions of the pancreas pose a growing diagnostic and management challenge. Incidental pancreatic cysts are now detected in 2.6% to 13.5% of adults undergoing CT or MRI, with an even higher prevalence, up to 10% to 40%, in those above the age of 80.[1–3] A vast majority of such cystic lesions do not contain invasive cancer, but many subtypes—IPMNs, MCNs, CPENs, and SPNs—carry a risk of current or future malignancy and, therefore, may require surgical resection.[4] The morbidity and mortality of pancreatic resection, however, mandate careful risk/benefit analysis of surgery versus surveillance for each individual patient and lesion. The current challenge for oncologists, gastroenterologists, and surgeons is 2-fold. The malignant behavior of pancreatic cysts must be predicted more accurately and then this information used to better stratify patients into surgical versus nonoperative management.

To provide clinical context to this question, this article reviews the most common types of pancreatic cystic neoplasms, detailing each disease's characteristic clinical and radiologic features and recommended management, followed by a generalized approach to diagnosis and treatment. International consensus guidelines[5] are included where relevant. Attention is paid to controversial diagnostic and treatment questions requiring further investigation.

DISEASE ENTITIES

In light of increased use of high-resolution cross-sectional imaging and heightened awareness of pancreatic cystic neoplasms, pancreatic cysts are diagnosed with increasing frequency, at a smaller size (median diameter 1.6 cm vs 2.4 cm in the most recent vs prior decades), and, increasingly incidentally, now in more than two-thirds of cases.[6,7] The most common types of resected pancreatic cystic neoplasms include IPMNs (27%–48%), MCNs (11%–23%), SCAs (13%–23%), CPENs (4%–7%), SPNs (2%–5%), and, infrequently, cystic degeneration of pancreatic ductal adenocarcinomas (PDACs) (1%–2%) (**Fig. 1**).[6–8] Over the past several decades, MCNs and SCAs have decreased in frequency, whereas IPMN has become the most common pathologic diagnosis.[6,8] Current knowledge about each disease entity's presentation, diagnosis, and management is discussed.

Intraductal Papillary Mucinous Neoplasm

IPMNs have markedly increased in incidence over the past 20 years and are now the most commonly diagnosed and resected type of pancreatic cystic neoplasm.[4,6,8] From a histologic standpoint, IPMNs are cystic, intraductal, mucin-producing tumors whose dysplastic cells range from benign adenoma to invasive carcinoma (**Fig. 2**).[4] IPMNs are suspected to represent a different disease entity than PDACs but are thought to progress through a similar pathway of benign to dysplastic to invasive disease.[9,10] Two variants, MD-IPMNs and BD-IPMNs, are distinguished based on main pancreatic duct involvement, which, in the absence of histology, is defined as ductal dilatation on imaging.[5] Mixed or combined IPMNs involving both the main pancreatic duct and side branches behave similarly to MD-IPMNs and are often grouped with MD-IPMNs for simplicity.[11,12] Because MD-IPMNs carry a higher risk of malignancy at presentation and require immediate surgical resection, whereas the more commonly encountered BD-IPMNs are more likely benign lesions that can be managed nonoperatively, it is important to discern the variant of IPMN at the time of diagnosis to help guide management and determine prognosis.[5]

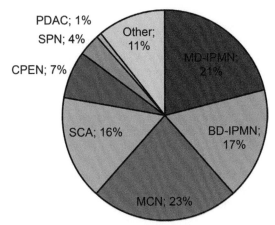

Fig. 1. Mucinous neoplasms are the most frequent type of resected pancreatic cystic neoplasm based on 851 resected pancreatic cysts over 33 years at a tertiary-care center. "Other" includes pancreatic pseudocyst, benign epithelial cyst, acinar cell cystadenoma or cystadenocarcinoma, lymphoepithelial cyst, choledochal cyst, lymphangioma, hemangioma, and other unclassified epithelial cyst. (*Adapted from* Valsangkar NP, Morales-Oyarvide V, Thayer SP, et al. 851 Resected cystic tumors of the pancreas: a 33-year experience at the Massachusetts General Hospital. Surgery 2012;152(3 Suppl 1):S6; with permission.)

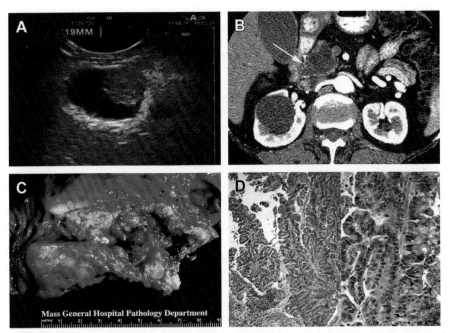

Fig. 2. BD-IPMN of the head and uncinate process of the pancreas. This patient presented with weight loss. EUS demonstrated a large nodule (*A*), which was not as apparent within the large cystic lesion on CT (*B*) (*arrow*). The patient underwent a Whipple procedure. (*C*) Macroscopic appearance of the tumor. (*D*) Histology by hematoxylin and eosin staining revealed extensive high-grade dysplasia (carcinoma in situ), 10 × and 40 × magnification (*left, right*).

Prevalence

BD-IPMNs are thought to represent the majority of small pancreatic cysts discovered incidentally on cross-sectional imaging.[4] In several large surgical series, IPMNs are also the most commonly resected pancreatic cystic lesions, comprising 30% to 40% of all specimens, with slight predominance of MD-IPMNs over BD-IPMNs.[6,8]

Demographics

IPMNs have an equal gender distribution and present at a median age of 65 to 67 years.[9,10,12,13] Based on case series dating from the 1980s onward, a majority of patients with IPMN (60%–88%) present with symptoms, most often abdominal pain and, less frequently, weight loss, obstructive jaundice, or pancreatitis.[9,10,12,13] Jaundice, in particular, occurs more frequently in patients with invasive versus noninvasive disease.[10,12] More recently, however, IPMNs, in particular BD-IPMNs, are increasingly presenting as incidental radiologic findings.[7,12]

Radiologic features

IPMNs are best characterized by 1 of 2 imaging modalities: (1) pancreas protocol CT, which uses multidetector acquisition of images with thin cuts through the pancreas and dual arterial and portal venous phases of intravenous contrast enhancement, or (2) MRI/magnetic resonance cholangiopancreatography (MRCP), which combines routine contrast-enhanced MRI with special fast spin-echo sequences plus optional 3-D imaging of the pancreatic and biliary ducts.[14,15] MRCP is more accurate than CT at detecting ductal communication, involvement of the main pancreatic duct, extent of disease throughout the pancreas, and high-risk cyst characteristics, such as mural nodules, and is, therefore, the imaging modality of choice for initial evaluation of a suspected IPMNs.[5,14,15]

On either MRCP or CT, MD-IPMNs appear as a cystic and tortuous dilatation of the main pancreatic duct, with two-thirds of cases involving the head of the pancreas, 8% involving the entire duct, and a variable appearance of the associated pancreatic parenchyma, ranging from atrophic to enlarged and inflamed.[11] BD-IPMNs, on the other hand, appear as solitary or multifocal cysts that communicate with the pancreatic ductal system but do not involve the main duct (ie, are associated with a normal-sized pancreatic duct; see **Fig. 2**B).[13]

Management

When clinical and imaging characteristics are insufficient to establish a diagnosis of MD-IPMNs or BD-IPMNs (eg, in the setting of a solitary cyst with normal-sized pancreatic duct), further evaluation with endoscopic ultrasound (EUS) and EUS-guided fine-needle aspiration (FNA) of cyst fluid can aid diagnosis and management decisions.[5,15] Endoscopically, one-third of MD-IPMNs present with pathognomonic bulging of the papilla and mucus extrusion.[11] EUS can additionally confirm the presence or absence of main duct involvement and better characterize solid components that raise the concern for malignancy (see **Fig. 2**A).[11,16,17] Cyst fluid analysis can also differentiate between mucinous and nonmucinous lesions, such as inflammatory pseudocysts or benign SCAs, but results are imperfect. Viscous, mucin-positive fluid is not always identified from mucinous lesions. Chemical fluid analysis demonstrating an elevated carcinoembryonic antigen (CEA) level above an optimal cutoff of 192 to 200 ng/mL is only approximately 80% accurate in distinguishing mucinous versus nonmucinous cysts and can neither differentiate IPMN from MCN nor predict malignancy.[5,18,19] Cyst fluid results, therefore, serve only as an adjunct to diagnostic evaluation and must be interpreted within the context of a patient's overall clinical and radiologic presentation.

Regarding definitive management, MD-IPMNs more frequently harbor malignancy than BD-IPMNs, with approximately 43% of MD-IPMNs containing invasive carcinoma at the time of resection and an additional 19% harboring high-grade dysplasia (synonymous with carcinoma in situ).[5,9,10,12] Current consensus guidelines from the 2010 meeting of the International Association of Pancreatology in Fukuoka, Japan (published in 2012,[5] updated from the 2006 Sendai guidelines[20]), therefore, recommend surgical resection for all MD-IPMNs, as determined radiologically by either main pancreatic duct dilatation of 10 mm or greater on CT or MRI or borderline ductal dilatation of 5 to 9 mm with subsequent EUS confirmation of main duct involvement (ie, thickened walls or intraductal mucin or nodules).[5]

BD-IPMNs, on the other hand, are much less likely to be malignant, with only up to 18% of cases containing invasive cancer and 8% containing high-grade dysplasia (reviewed by Tanaka and colleagues[5] and Al-Haddad and colleagues[21]), frequencies that may be overestimated given the lack of specification between invasive carcinoma arising from an IPMN and concomitant PDAC arising in a separate site of the pancreas.[4,22] Given the lower risk of malignancy with BD-IPMNs, and older age at presentation, current management has moved away from unconditional operation.[5,11,20] The current 2012 Fukuoka guidelines recommend the following:

- Selective surgical resection of only high-risk BD-IPMNs, as determined by either of the following: (1) high-risk stigmata of malignancy (clinical: obstructive jaundice; CT/MRCP: enhancing solid component or main duct greater than or equal to 10 mm); or (2) worrisome features (clinical: pancreatitis; CT/MRCP: main duct 5–9 mm, nonenhancing mural nodule, thickened/enhancing cyst wall, abrupt change in duct caliber with distal atrophy, lymphadenopathy, or cyst size greater than or equal to 3 cm) plus EUS confirmation of either main duct involvement (as discussed previously), mural nodule (as opposed to a ball of mucin) (see **Fig. 2**A), or cyst fluid cytology suspicious or positive for malignancy.[5]
- Nonoperative surveillance for all other BD-IPMNs without high-risk or worrisome features.[5] Frequency and type of surveillance is stratified by cyst size: (1) 2–3 cm: EUS in 3–6 months, then alternating EUS and MRCP (can lengthen interval if stable; consider surgery in young, fit patients who would otherwise require prolonged surveillance); (2) 1–2 cm: yearly MRCP or CT (can lengthen interval after 2 years of stability); or (3) less than 1 cm: 1-time follow-up MRCP or CT in 2 to 3 years.[5]

Cyst size may be a weaker predictor of malignancy than other radiologic features, such as mural nodules,[23] so it is allowable within the 2012 Fukuoka guidelines to observe BD-IPMNs larger than 3 cm, as long as no other high-risk or worrisome features are present and close surveillance with alternating EUS and MRCP is maintained every 3 to 6 months.[5] In 1 series of 82 patients with BD-IPMN and no mural nodules (including 10 with cysts larger than 3 cm), all patients were managed nonoperatively, and only 5% developed new nodules over a median follow-up of 5 years, with only 1 of 4 cases containing high-grade dysplasia, and zero containing invasive carcinoma at the time of resection.[24] A larger multicenter Japanese series of 349 BD-IPMN patients without mural nodules yielded similar results, with only 3% developing mural nodules or ductal dilatation and subsequent malignancy on surgical pathology.[25]

A population that requires special consideration is patients with hereditary pancreatic cancer, defined by at least 2 other first-degree relatives with PDAC. These patients are at increased risk of PDAC and, if presenting with BD-IPMN, should be offered surgical resection at a lower threshold (ie, if they present with any worrisome features on MRCP or CT).[5,26] If not immediately operated on, such patients should be managed with close endoscopic and radiologic surveillance.[5]

Of historical note, the 2006 consensus Sendai guidelines had recommended surgery for all BD-IPMNs with either symptoms, main pancreatic ductal dilation greater than 6 mm, mural nodules, or cyst size greater than or equal to 3 cm.[20] Subsequent studies found these guidelines to be nonspecific, with a positive predictive value of only 22% for malignancy (high-grade dysplasia or invasive carcinoma),[13,27] thereby providing the impetus for the updated 2012 guidelines,[5] discussed previously.

Outcomes

For both MD-IPMNs and BD-IPMNs, noninvasive disease is associated with excellent long-term survival, whereas invasive IPMN portends worse prognosis, albeit better than standard PDAC.[5,20] After resection, 5-year disease-specific survival for noninvasive IPMN (including adenoma, borderline, and high-grade dysplasia) compared with invasive IPMN (carcinoma) is estimated to be 95% to 100% compared with 46% to 63%.[5,9,13,28] Recurrence, either locally or with distant metastases, occurs more frequently in patients with invasive IPMN, with variable frequency and timing reported in the literature, in up to 41% to 44% of invasive cases, at a mean duration of 21 to 28 months after initial resection.[5,12,28]

The histologic subtype of IPMN also has an impact on prognosis.[11,29–31] A majority of MD-IPMNs demonstrate intestinal-type histology and frequently progress to colloid carcinoma, which is invasive but more indolent than standard PDACs.[29,30] A minority of MD-IPMNs are of the oncocytic subtype, which can progress to an indolent form of oncocytic carcinoma, or the pancreaticobiliary subtype, which rarely can progress to tubular carcinoma, an aggressive histology that behaves similarly to PDACs.[29,30] Alternatively, most BD-IPMNs are of the gastric subtype, which only infrequently progresses to the aggressive form of tubular carcinoma.[29,30] Five-year overall survival was found 89%, 84%, 52%, and 94% for the intestinal, oncocytic, pancreaticobiliary, and gastric subtypes, respectively.[29] Likewise, in a series of resected MD-IPMNs and BD-IPMNs, 5-year overall survival for patients with invasive disease was significantly better for those with colloid versus tubular carcinoma (83% vs 24%).[10]

Current controversies and future directions

More accurate diagnosis and prediction of malignancy represent major challenges in current IPMN management as well as management of pancreatic cysts in general. Few studies report predictors of malignancy in MD-IPMNs, except to say that main duct involvement, itself, is associated with invasive disease in IPMNs.[5,32] Based on multivariate analysis of a cohort of 219 patients with resected MD-IPMNs or BD-IPMNs, Correa-Gallego and colleagues[33] developed a preoperative nomogram to better predict high-grade dysplasia or invasive carcinoma in IPMNs prior to surgical resection. Weight loss, history of prior malignancy, male gender, and solid component were significantly associated with malignant MD-IPMNs, whereas solid component, weight loss, and cyst size were significantly associated with malignant BD-IPMNs.[33] The nomograms require prospective validation and are limited by lack of inclusion of EUS/FNA features.

The exact role of EUS/FNA in risk-stratifying IPMN lesions remains to be determined. EUS, in particular contrast-enhanced EUS, may be able to better characterize mural nodules and thus predict which lesions warrant resection.[16,17] EUS-guided FNA of cyst fluid with subsequent cytologic analysis for high-grade atypical epithelial cells or obviously malignant cells is approximately 80% accurate at predicting malignant disease in IPMNs and MCNs.[34,35] Cell yield from cyst fluid, however, can be low. Chemical analysis of cyst fluid, in particular CEA level, was suggested by some groups to predict malignancy[36,37] but has not been reproducible.[19,38] Molecular assessment of cyst fluid (eg, DNA analysis for oncogenic *KRAS* or *GNAS* mutations and/or amplifications),[38,39] microRNA (miRNA) profiling,[40] cytokine measurement (eg, of interleukin [IL]-1β[41] and prostaglandin E_2 [PGE_2]),[42] and mucin proteomic profiling[43] may each improve prediction of malignancy but require further investigation. Overall, EUS/FNA is promising but prone to interobserver variability and operator dependency, should be performed in centers with expertise in these techniques, and requires further validation prior to widespread use.[44] Ultimately, predicting current and future malignancy within an IPMN lesion likely requires incorporation of clinical, imaging, and multiple EUS/FNA features.

An additional question pertains to the frequency of surveillance after resection of IPMNs. In the setting of invasive disease, the 2012 Fukuoka guidelines recommend similar surveillance as recommended for PDACs.[5] Even with noninvasive IPMNs, however, there is an estimated 1% annual risk of developing concomitant PDAC, supporting the hypothesis of a field defect wherein the entire pancreas is predisposed to malignancy and leading some groups to maintain twice-yearly clinical and imaging surveillance even after resection of benign IPMNs.[5,25,45,46]

Mucinous Cystic Neoplasm

MCNs represent a different type of mucinous cystic tumor of the pancreas, more often premalignant than frankly malignant and distinguished from IPMNs based on the presence of a pathognomonic ovarian-like stroma surrounding the cyst's inner epithelial layer as well as an absence of communication with the pancreatic duct (**Fig. 3**).[5]

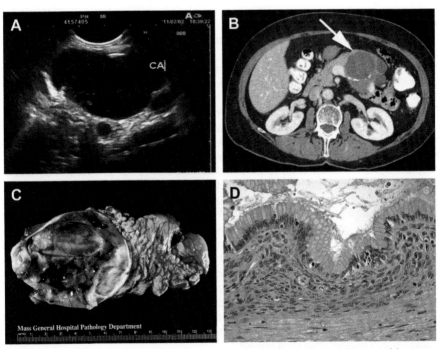

Fig. 3. MCN involving the body and tail of the pancreas. The patient, a 55-year-old woman, presented with nonspecific upper abdominal pain. (*A*) EUS demonstrated a large complex cyst; fluid was aspirated and showed thick mucus. (*B*) CT likewise revealed a multiloculated cyst (*arrow*) and rim calcification. The patient underwent a distal pancreatectomy with splenic preservation. Surgical pathology revealed typical (*C*) macroscopic and (*D*) microscopic appearance, with mucinous epithelium and ovarian-like stroma on hematoxylin and eosin staining, 40 × magnification.

Despite a low risk of malignancy at presentation, MCNs harbor a risk of progressing to invasive carcinoma and, therefore, warrant surgical resection in young and healthy patients who would otherwise require years of radiologic surveillance.[5] Presentation and management are discussed.

Prevalence
MCNs have decreased in prevalence but still comprise 25% of all resected pancreatic cystic neoplasms.[8]

Demographics
MCNs almost exclusively present in middle-aged women at an average age of 40 to 50 years.[47–49] In several large series, approximately 60% to 70% of patients presented with symptoms, most often abdominal pain, whereas the remainder were diagnosed incidentally on imaging.[47,48]

Radiologic features
Initial diagnostic evaluation should include pancreas protocol CT or MRCP, as for IPMN evaluation. MCNs nearly always present as a solitary cyst in the body or tail of the pancreas (see **Fig. 3**B).[47–49] These lesions lack communication with the pancreatic duct and can have thickened walls or septae in more than half of cases.[4,50] Mural nodules are predictive of malignancy, as is the case with IPMNs.[47,49,50]

Management
A solitary cyst in the body or tail of the pancreas, in a middle-aged woman, without ductal communication strongly suggests a diagnosis of MCN and eliminates the need for further evaluation prior to treatment.[5] If clinical and imaging features are indeterminate, however, EUS can be performed to better characterize the relationship of the lesion to the pancreatic duct (ie, to help distinguish MCNs from IPMNs [see **Fig. 3**A]).[4,5] EUS-guided FNA of cyst fluid also allows for molecular analysis (eg, cyst fluid CEA level, which, if greater than 192–200 ng/mL, favors a diagnosis of mucinous over serous lesions, and DNA sequencing, which, in the setting of a *KRAS* mutation without *GNAS* mutation, favors a diagnosis of MCN over other cystic neoplasms).[18,39,44] Such tests require further validation prior to widespread use in diagnosis of MCNs and other pancreatic cystic lesions.[44]

Regarding definitive management, the current 2012 Fukuoka consensus guidelines recommend surgical resection for all MCN.[5] Rationale includes the 17% to 18% risk of malignancy (high-grade dysplasia or invasive cystadenocarcinoma), the risk of future progression even in benign disease, current inability to predict which lesions contain or will progress to malignancy, and the characteristic presentation of a distal lesion in an otherwise young and healthy patient, allowing for a less morbid operation (ie, distal pancreatectomy with possible splenic preservation as opposed to pancreaticoduodenectomy) in patients with relatively low perioperative risk.[5,47–49,51] Alternative management, with nonoperative clinical and radiologic surveillance, would entail years of repeated cross-sectional imaging and, in the patient population described previously, would involve greater cost than benefit.[5]

On surgical pathology, diagnosis of MCN is confirmed by the presence of ovarian-type stroma (see **Fig. 3**D).[5] If invasive cystadenocarcinoma is noted, postoperative surveillance, as for PDAC, is recommended but has not been shown to improve prognosis.[5] If there is no invasion noted on pathology, the patient is considered cured, with zero risk of recurrence based on several large case series,[47,48] and no special oncologic surveillance is required.[5]

Outcomes

Prognosis is excellent after resection of noninvasive cystadenoma or in situ carcinoma but is variably poor for invasive cystadenocarcinoma. Five-year overall survival in 1 series was estimated to be 89% versus 17% for patients with noninvasive versus invasive disease, and 5 of the 6 invasive patients recurred and died within 5 years of surgery.[48] More recent series describe slightly less dismal prognosis, with 5-year disease-specific survival rates of 95% to 100% and 57% to 83% for noninvasive and invasive MCNs, respectively, and an estimated recurrence rate of 40% at a mean duration of 33 months after surgery for those with invasive disease.[47,49] Zero recurrences were detected after resection of noninvasive MCNs at an average follow-up of at least 5 years after surgery.[47–49]

Current controversies and future directions

As for IPMNs, more accurate prediction of malignant behavior in MCNs will help identify which lesions require up-front resection and which, if any, can be observed. Cyst size greater than 4 cm or presence of mural nodules predicts malignancy with 100% sensitivity but lacks specificity and does not help identify those noninvasive lesions that will or will not progress to invasive carcinoma.[47,49,50] Cyst fluid cytology from EUS/FNA, conversely, is specific but not sufficiently sensitive to predict invasive disease prior to surgical resection.[34,35] Further molecular assessment of cyst fluid, as for IPMNs, may ultimately aid with risk stratification of MCN lesions.

A final question pertains to disease mechanisms and systemic therapy. Use of adjuvant chemotherapy after resection of invasive cystadenocarcinoma has not been rigorously studied and remains questionable in its impact on survival. Recent studies identifying activation of the Wnt/β-catenin signaling pathway within the ovarian-like stroma of human MCNs and an analogous transgenic mouse model highlight novel potential therapeutic targets, but much remains to be elucidated about the molecular mechanisms of MCN progression.[52]

Serous Cystadenoma

SCAs are nonmucinous, benign cystic neoplasms of the pancreas, which can be observed rather than resected and, therefore, stand apart from most other types of pancreatic cystic neoplasms.[4] Cyst lining is composed of cuboidal epithelial cells rich in glycogen (**Fig. 4D**).[4] The more common microcystic variant is composed of numerous small cysts grouped together in a honeycomb appearance (see **Fig. 4A–C**), whereas the less common oligo- or macrocystic variant appears as a solitary cyst that is difficult to distinguish from pseudocysts, MCNs, or unifocal BD-IPMNs. Management requires careful diagnosis (detailed later).

Prevalence

SCAs have decreased in prevalence and comprise approximately 16% of resected pancreatic cystic neoplasms.[8]

Demographics

SCAs frequently affect older women, with 75% to 85% female predominance, and an average age at presentation ranging from mid-50s to mid-60s.[53–56] Approximately one-half to two-thirds of patients present with symptoms, most commonly abdominal pain, less commonly a palpable abdominal mass or jaundice.[53–56] SCAs occur sporadically or, in approximately 2% of cases, in the setting of von Hippel-Lindau (VHL) disease, an autosomal dominant genetic disease arising from germline loss of the *VHL* tumor suppressor gene.[55,56]

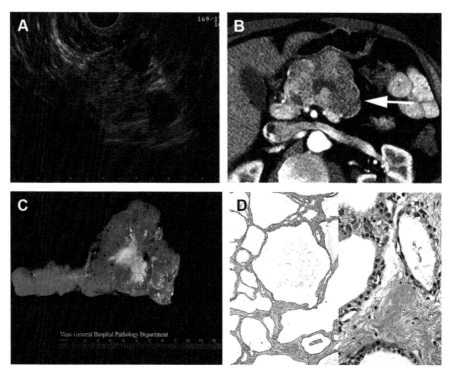

Fig. 4. Radiologic and histologic features of SCA. Multiple small cysts create the spongy appearance of the microcystic variant of SCA, as seen on (*A*) EUS and CT (*B*) (*arrow*). (*C*) Macroscopic appearance is similar and typically includes a central scar. (*D*) Histology by hematoxylin and eosin staining demonstrates characteristic cuboidal epithelium, 10 × and 40 × magnification (*left, right*).

Radiologic features

Initial evaluation with pancreas protocol CT or MRCP is recommended. SCAs are distributed evenly throughout the pancreas.[55,56] Microcystic SCAs present as a unifocal, multilobulated lesion with many tiny cysts together creating a classic honeycomb or spongelike appearance, often with central calcifications (see **Fig.** 4B–C).[4,55,56] The less common oligocystic variant appears as a solitary cyst, which can mimic MCNs, BD-IPMNs, or pancreatic pseudocysts (discussed previously).

Management

Particularly for oligocystic lesions, when clinical and imaging features are insufficient to establish a diagnosis of SCA, EUS/FNA is recommended for further cyst characterization. EUS-guided FNA of cyst fluid allows for biochemical and cytologic analysis, which has the same limitations noted previously but can identify serous lesions in the setting of characteristic cytology, very low CEA (less than 5 ng/mL),[55] or, potentially, wild-type *KRAS* and *GNAS*.[39]

Unlike mucinous neoplasms, such as IPMNs or MCNs, serous cystic neoplasms have an extremely low risk of malignancy, with fewer than 1% of cases in the literature designated as invasive serous cystadenocarcinomas.[4,8,54,56] Management has, therefore, moved away from unconditional operation to serial surveillance for asymptomatic lesions.[4] Compared with smaller SCAs less then 4 cm in diameter, however, larger SCAs are 3-fold more likely to cause symptoms and, in 1 series, demonstrated a significantly faster growth rate of 2 cm versus 0.1 cm per year.[56] Additional reports suggest that age, number of years after diagnosis, oligocystic morphology, and history of other malignancies correlate with faster growth.[57] Consideration should, therefore, be given to surgical resection in these cases.

Outcomes
Survival after surgical resection has been reported to be approximately 100% at an average follow-up period of 3 to 4 years after surgery, with isolated reports of recurrence in less than 1% of patients.[53–55] Nonoperative surveillance of asymptomatic or stable to slow-growing lesions is a viable treatment option. Zero of 26 cases in 1 series required an operation after a median follow-up of 38 months,[55] and only 23 of 145 cases (16%) required surgery at a median duration of 4 years after initial diagnosis.[57]

Current controversies and future directions
Because management for SCAs differs drastically from MCNs, MD-IPMNs, and other malignant pancreatic cystic neoplasms, accurate diagnosis is paramount. Clinical, radiologic, and cyst fluid characteristics are often adequate to establish a diagnosis of SCA, but for indeterminate cases, additional cyst markers, such as *VHL* mutation or chromosomal loss (as is found in VHL disease), or elevated fluid levels of vascular endothelial growth factor (VEGF), a cytokine regulated by VHL and critical to vascular maintenance and angiogenesis, may serve as diagnostic aides, pending prospective validation.[58,59]

Finally, despite approximate predictors of growth rate (described previously), conflicting results about the impact of cyst size on growth rate remain to be resolved.[56,57] Ultimately, more accurate prediction of SCA growth will better guide management with respect to the need and timing of surgery and, alternatively, the optimal frequency of nonoperative surveillance.

Cystic Pancreatic Endocrine Neoplasm

CPENs are a rare cystic variant of pancreatic neuroendocrine tumors (PNETs) that carry a risk of malignancy and, therefore, require surgical resection (**Fig. 5**). Presentation and management are described.

Prevalence
CPENs comprise 5% to 7% of all resected pancreatic cystic neoplasms and 10% to 17% of resected PNETs.[8,60–62]

Demographics
CPENs have an equal gender distribution and present at an average age of 50 to 60 years.[60–62] Although older case series noted symptoms in a majority of patients, more recent studies suggest that most CPENs now present incidentally.[61,62] More so than solid PNETs, a majority (greater than 80%) of CPENs are nonfunctioning (ie, without clinical manifestation of hormone overproduction).[60] Compared with solid PNETs, CPENs may also have a higher association with the genetic syndrome multiple endocrine neoplasia type 1 (MEN-1), which involves germline mutation of the *MEN1* tumor suppressor gene and predisposes to endocrine tumors of the pituitary, parathyroid, and pancreas.[60]

Radiologic features
At least 45% up to a majority of CPENs present with an arterially enhancing cyst wall on pancreas protocol CT (see **Fig. 5B**).[60–62] Solid components and septae are also present in approximately one-quarter of cases.[62]

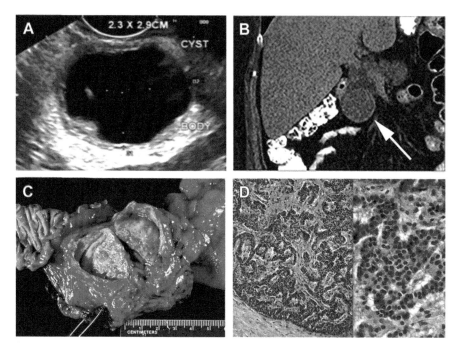

Fig. 5. CPEN of the head of the pancreas. This was an incidental finding. (*A*) EUS revealed a thick, irregular wall, which was enhancing (*B*) (*arrow*) on CT. Surgical resection revealed the pictured (*C*) macroscopic and (*D*) microscopic appearance. Hematoxylin and eosin staining is shown at 10 × and 40 × magnification (*left, right*).

Management

If clinical and radiologic findings are insufficient to establish a diagnosis of CPEN, EUS/FNA can provide further cyst characterization. Hypervascular or thickened walls can be seen on EUS (see **Fig. 5A**).[61,63] Additionally, positive or suspicious cytology and confirmatory immunostaining of chromogranin A and synaptophysin can establish a diagnosis of CPEN in 73% to 78% of cases.[62–64] On final surgical pathology, most specimens demonstrate positive immunostaining for synaptophysin (100%) and chromogranin (82%).[60]

Once a diagnosis of CPEN has been established, the recommended treatment is surgical resection. Although some series suggest that CPENs have a lower Ki67 proliferative index and risk of carcinoma than solid PNETs, CPENs still harbor an 11% to 14% risk of malignancy and 8% to 14% risk of nodal or distant metastases, necessitating surgical resection as the only potential curative treatment.[8,61]

Outcomes

Patients with resected CPENs have an excellent prognosis, with an estimated 5-year overall survival of 87% to 100% and disease-free survival of 94% to 96%, similar to those with solid PNETs.[60–62]

Current controversies and future directions

Given the low risk of invasive disease, some groups advocate for nonanatomic resection of CPENs, but others maintain that anatomic resection with lymphadenectomy aids in detecting nodal disease and establishing prognosis.[62] Optimal extent of resection remains to be determined.

Recurrence is infrequent but can occur late (ie, 5–10 years after initial resection). Some groups perform postoperative clinical and radiologic surveillance every 6 months for 5 years, then yearly if stable.[61] Optimal frequency of postoperative surveillance remains to be determined.

From a broader disease perspective, it remains unclear whether CPENs represent necrotic or cystic degeneration of solid PNETs, as suggested in 1 series by the larger presenting size of CPENs,[60] or whether CPENs represent de novo cyst formation or a unique disease process, as suggested by lack of necrosis in most resected CPEN specimens and differing clinical features, including lower rate of malignancy and possible disproportionate association with MEN-1.[60–62] Better understanding of the relationship between cystic and solid PNETs will dictate whether changes in the management of solid PNETs (ie, nonoperative surveillance of small, nonfunctioning solid PNETs)[65] can be applied to CPENs.

Finally, as with other pancreatic cystic neoplasms, more accurate prediction of malignancy will help stratify CPENs into those that require immediate resection and those that can safely be observed. Based on multivariate analysis of 21 CPENs and 161 solid PNETs, Boninsegna and colleagues[61] suggest that cystic versus solid morphology, symptoms at presentation, and increasing size (continuous variable) correlate with malignancy. Such factors require prospective validation.

Solid Pseudopapillary Neoplasm

SPNs are rare, heterogeneous tumors that most commonly afflict young women and harbor a risk of malignancy, therefore necessitating surgical resection. Presentation and management are detailed.

Prevalence
SPNs comprise 3% of resected pancreatic cystic neoplasms.[8]

Demographics
SPNs almost exclusively affect young women, presenting at an average age of 30 to 38 years.[66,67] A majority (up to 84%–87%) of patients with SPNs present with symptoms, most often abdominal pain and less frequently pancreatitis, jaundice, or palpable mass.[66,67]

Radiologic features
On CT, SPNs present as heterogeneous masses with mixed solid and cystic components, anywhere throughout the pancreas.[66] Additional less common features include an arterially enhancing wall[67] and calcifications (16% in 1 series).[66]

Management
Percutaneous or endoscopic biopsy can sometimes aid diagnosis, with a 56% to 62% diagnostic yield reported in 2 series.[66,67] Definitive management with surgical resection is currently recommended for all SPNs, because 10% to 20% of cases demonstrate malignant behavior (ie, local invasion, nodal metastases, distant liver metastases, or local or distant recurrence after resection).[4,66,67] On surgical pathology, SPNs contain loosely cohesive cells that form delicate pseudopapillae supported by capillary-sized fibrovascular cores.[66,67] Histopathologic diagnosis is confirmed with immunostaining of characteristic markers, including CD56, CD10, vimentin, and nuclear labeling of β-catenin.[66,68]

Outcomes
Overall, greater than 80% of SPN patients experience long-term survival after surgery.[66]

Current controversies and future directions

As with other pancreatic cystic neoplasms, more accurate prediction of malignancy could help stratify SPNs into those that require immediate resection and those that can be observed.

After surgery, recurrence is infrequent but can occur late, in 1 case 8 years after initial resection.[67] Optimal frequency of postoperative surveillance remains to be determined.

Regarding management of metastatic disease, anecdotal data suggest that resection of synchronous or metachronous liver metastases can be associated with long-term survival, although only a small number of cases are reported in the literature. Further investigation is required to better predict which patients will benefit from such radical resection and, either alternatively or in conjunction with surgery, which chemotherapy may be effective for metastatic SPN. Recent gene expression profiling studies have demonstrated overactivation of the Wnt/β-catenin, hedgehog, and epithelial-to-mesenchymal transition signaling pathways in SPNs and may highlight new potential therapeutic targets for systemic disease.[69]

GENERAL APPROACH TO DIAGNOSIS AND MANAGEMENT

Having reviewed the most clinically relevant types of pancreatic cystic neoplasms, a generalized approach to diagnosis and management is provided, summarizing key points discussed previously (**Fig. 6**).

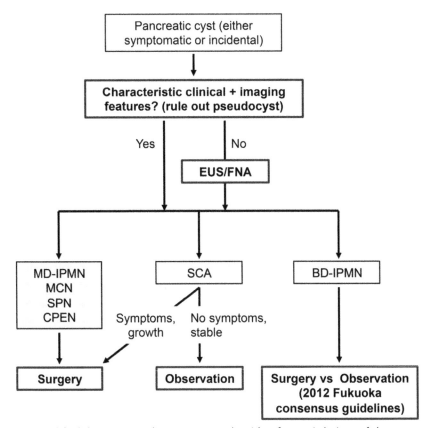

Fig. 6. Simplified diagnostic and management algorithm for cystic lesions of the pancreas.

Initial Evaluation

Any patient presenting with a pancreatic cyst should first undergo standard clinical evaluation, with attention paid to patient demographics (ie, age and gender), pertinent symptoms (eg, abdominal pain, jaundice, pancreatitis, or weight loss), notable family history of PDAC or heritable genetic syndromes, and any notable physical examination findings (eg, palpable mass or jaundice). Importantly, a recent episode of acute pancreatitis makes a diagnosis of inflammatory pseudocyst more likely but does not rule out neoplasm. Demographics can often contribute significantly to the preoperative diagnosis (eg, with SCAs predominantly arising in older women, MCNs almost exclusively affecting middle-aged women, and SPNs almost always occurring in younger women). A family history of MEN-1 suggests CPENs, whereas VHL disease suggests a possible diagnosis of SCAs. In general, other symptoms and signs are nonspecific but may help predict risk of malignancy and, in cases of suspected benign lesions, may help direct management (ie, surgery for symptomatic lesions).

Subsequent radiologic evaluation with MRCP or pancreas protocol CT should be performed, with attention paid to the number of cysts, appearance, location within the pancreas, and any identifying features, including pancreatic ductal dilatation (MD-IPMNs), ductal communication (MD-IPMNs or BD-IPMNs), thickened walls or septae (MCNs and others), honeycomb appearance and central calcifications (microcystic SCAs), arterially enhancing wall (CPENs or sometimes SPNs), and mixed solid and cystic components (SPNs). Multiple cysts almost always represent multifocal BD-IPMNs and may be observed without high-risk features. A solitary cyst in the body or tail of the pancreas in a middle-aged woman with no history of prior pancreatitis is most likely an MCN. Other solitary cystic lesions, however, have a larger differential diagnosis, including mucinous tumors, such MCNs and solitary BD-IPMNs; serous tumors, such as oligocystic SCAs; and benign pseudocysts. Neither CT nor MRI/MRCP can distinguish mucinous from nonmucinous lesions[70,71] or predict malignancy[10,14] with sufficient accuracy. Such indeterminate lesions, therefore, require further diagnostic evaluation.

Further Investigation

To aid diagnosis, EUS/FNA is an invasive but generally safe technique that better characterizes pancreatic cysts.[4] EUS can confirm communication with the pancreatic duct (IPMNs or pseudocysts) and specific neoplastic involvement of the main duct, manifesting as ductal dilation or intraductal mucin, wall thickening, or nodules (MD-IPMNs).[5] Cyst fluid analysis is fraught with limitations but in the appropriate clinical and radiologic context can facilitate diagnosis. For example, mucin, elevated CEA (above 200 ng/mL), and *KRAS* mutation favor a mucinous diagnosis, whereas *GNAS* mutation additionally favors a diagnosis of IPMNs over MCNs.[44] Alternatively, very low CEA (less than 5 ng/mL)[55] and possibly elevated fluid VEGF[58] favor a diagnosis of SCA. Characteristic cytology is not sensitive but can improve diagnosis in some cases (mucinous tumors, SCAs, CPENs, SPNs). In the appropriate clinical context, low amylase (less than 250 U/L) renders a diagnosis of pseudocyst unlikely.[72]

Specifically for BD-IPMNs, EUS/FNA can also help risk stratify lesions into those at risk of harboring malignancy and those that are likely benign and safe to observe. Mural nodules or suspicious cytology warrants resection in the 2012 Fukuoka guidelines.[5] In the future, a panel of molecular tests in the cyst fluid, including *KRAS* amplification, miRNA profiling, elevated cytokine levels of IL-1β and PGE$_2$, and mucin subtype profiling, may ultimately improve assessment of malignant behavior within IPMNs.[44]

Management: Resection versus Surveillance

Generally, all pancreatic cystic neoplasms have malignant potential and require surgical resection except for SCAs and a subset of BD-IPMNs. Therefore, MD-IPMNs, MCNs, CPENs, SPNs, and indeterminate lesions that raise concern for any of these diagnoses should be referred for surgical resection, with postoperative surveillance based on degree of invasion detected on surgical pathology. SCA, the major nonmucinous tumor, is benign and can be observed; surgical resection is reserved for only those lesions that are symptomatic or large and/or growing. BD-IPMNs represent a spectrum of benign to malignant disease and must be stratified based on clinical and radiologic risk features into low-risk lesions that can be watched and high-risk lesions that require resection, per the 2012 Fukuoka guidelines.[5]

OUTCOMES

For patients with pancreatic cystic neoplasms, overall prognosis is excellent, but more accurate diagnosis and selection of surgical versus nonoperative management are needed.[7,73] Perioperative morbidity (18%–38%) and mortality (0%–2%) are approximately comparable to rates after pancreatectomy for all patients, including those with PDAC.[7–10] Management of pancreatic cystic neoplasms should ideally avoid unnecessary surgery for benign lesions while also considering the personal and financial costs of prolonged radiologic surveillance in young otherwise healthy patients with premalignant lesions. Long-term (5-year) survival after surgery is disease dependent but is nearly 100% for patients with noninvasive lesions and variably poor, ranging from approximately 20% to 80%, for those with invasive disease on surgical pathology.

SUMMARY AND DISCUSSION

Pancreatic cysts are becoming increasingly common, incidental diagnoses. The most common types, including MD-IPMNs and BD-IPMNs, MCNs, and SCAs represent a spectrum from malignant disease warranting surgical resection to benign lesions that can be watched safely. Understanding of these diagnoses has markedly improved over the past 20 years, but many questions remain, notably how to improve diagnosis with the adjunct of cyst fluid biomarkers and how to better predict malignant behavior to best direct patients to surgical resection or nonoperative surveillance. Evaluation within a multidisciplinary setting is ideal.[74]

REFERENCES

1. Laffan TA, Horton KM, Klein AP, et al. Prevalence of unsuspected pancreatic cysts on MDCT. AJR Am J Roentgenol 2008;191(3):802–7.
2. Lee KS, Sekhar A, Rofsky NM, et al. Prevalence of incidental pancreatic cysts in the adult population on MR imaging. Am J Gastroenterol 2010;105(9):2079–84.
3. Kimura W, Nagai H, Kuroda A, et al. Analysis of small cystic lesions of the pancreas. Int J Pancreatol 1995;18(3):197–206.
4. Farrell JJ, Fernandez-del Castillo C. Pancreatic cystic neoplasms: management and unanswered questions. Gastroenterology 2013;144(6):1303–15.
5. Tanaka M, Fernandez-del Castillo C, Adsay V, et al. International consensus guidelines 2012 for the management of IPMN and MCN of the pancreas. Pancreatology 2012;12(3):183–97.
6. Gaujoux S, Brennan MF, Gonen M, et al. Cystic lesions of the pancreas: changes in the presentation and management of 1,424 patients at a single institution over a 15-year time period. J Am Coll Surg 2011;212(4):590–600 [discussion: 600–3].

7. Ferrone CR, Correa-Gallego C, Warshaw AL, et al. Current trends in pancreatic cystic neoplasms. Arch Surg 2009;144(5):448–54.
8. Valsangkar NP, Morales-Oyarvide V, Thayer SP, et al. 851 resected cystic tumors of the pancreas: a 33-year experience at the Massachusetts General Hospital. Surgery 2012;152(3 Suppl 1):S4–12.
9. Salvia R, Fernandez-del Castillo C, Bassi C, et al. Main-duct intraductal papillary mucinous neoplasms of the pancreas: clinical predictors of malignancy and long-term survival following resection. Ann Surg 2004;239(5):678–85 [discussion: 685–7].
10. Sohn TA, Yeo CJ, Cameron JL, et al. Intraductal papillary mucinous neoplasms of the pancreas: an updated experience. Ann Surg 2004;239(6):788–97 [discussion: 797–9].
11. Fernandez-del Castillo C, Adsay NV. Intraductal papillary mucinous neoplasms of the pancreas. Gastroenterology 2010;139(3):708–13, 713.e1–2.
12. Crippa S, Fernandez-Del Castillo C, Salvia R, et al. Mucin-producing neoplasms of the pancreas: an analysis of distinguishing clinical and epidemiologic characteristics. Clin Gastroenterol Hepatol 2010;8(2):213–9.
13. Rodriguez JR, Salvia R, Crippa S, et al. Branch-duct intraductal papillary mucinous neoplasms: observations in 145 patients who underwent resection. Gastroenterology 2007;133(1):72–9 [quiz: 309–10].
14. Waters JA, Schmidt CM, Pinchot JW, et al. CT vs MRCP: optimal classification of IPMN type and extent. J Gastrointest Surg 2008;12(1):101–9.
15. Berland LL, Silverman SG, Gore RM, et al. Managing incidental findings on abdominal CT: white paper of the ACR incidental findings committee. J Am Coll Radiol 2010;7(10):754–73.
16. Kurihara N, Kawamoto H, Kobayashi Y, et al. Vascular patterns in nodules of intraductal papillary mucinous neoplasms depicted under contrast-enhanced ultrasonography are helpful for evaluating malignant potential. Eur J Radiol 2012;81(1): 66–70.
17. Ohno E, Hirooka Y, Itoh A, et al. Intraductal papillary mucinous neoplasms of the pancreas: differentiation of malignant and benign tumors by endoscopic ultrasound findings of mural nodules. Ann Surg 2009;249(4):628–34.
18. Brugge WR, Lewandrowski K, Lee-Lewandrowski E, et al. Diagnosis of pancreatic cystic neoplasms: a report of the cooperative pancreatic cyst study. Gastroenterology 2004;126(5):1330–6.
19. Correa-Gallego C, Warshaw AL, Fernandez-del Castillo C. Fluid CEA in IPMNs: a useful test or the flip of a coin? Am J Gastroenterol 2009;104(3):796–7.
20. Tanaka M, Chari S, Adsay V, et al. International consensus guidelines for management of intraductal papillary mucinous neoplasms and mucinous cystic neoplasms of the pancreas. Pancreatology 2006;6(1–2):17–32.
21. Al-Haddad M, Schmidt MC, Sandrasegaran K, et al. Diagnosis and treatment of cystic pancreatic tumors. Clin Gastroenterol Hepatol 2011;9(8):635–48.
22. Yamaguchi K, Kanemitsu S, Hatori T, et al. Pancreatic ductal adenocarcinoma derived from IPMN and pancreatic ductal adenocarcinoma concomitant with IPMN. Pancreas 2011;40(4):571–80.
23. Schmidt CM, White PB, Waters JA, et al. Intraductal papillary mucinous neoplasms: predictors of malignant and invasive pathology. Ann Surg 2007;246(4): 644–51 [discussion: 651–4].
24. Tanno S, Nakano Y, Nishikawa T, et al. Natural history of branch duct intraductal papillary-mucinous neoplasms of the pancreas without mural nodules: long-term follow-up results. Gut 2008;57(3):339–43.

25. Maguchi H, Tanno S, Mizuno N, et al. Natural history of branch duct intraductal papillary mucinous neoplasms of the pancreas: a multicenter study in Japan. Pancreas 2011;40(3):364–70.

26. Shi C, Klein AP, Goggins M, et al. Increased prevalence of precursor lesions in familial pancreatic cancer patients. Clin Cancer Res 2009;15(24):7737–43.

27. Tang RS, Weinberg B, Dawson DW, et al. Evaluation of the guidelines for management of pancreatic branch-duct intraductal papillary mucinous neoplasm. Clin Gastroenterol Hepatol 2008;6(7):815–9 [quiz: 719].

28. Wada K, Kozarek RA, Traverso LW. Outcomes following resection of invasive and noninvasive intraductal papillary mucinous neoplasms of the pancreas. Am J Surg 2005;189(5):632–6 [discussion: 637].

29. Furukawa T, Hatori T, Fujita I, et al. Prognostic relevance of morphological types of intraductal papillary mucinous neoplasms of the pancreas. Gut 2011;60(4):509–16.

30. Mino-Kenudson M, Fernandez-del Castillo C, Baba Y, et al. Prognosis of invasive intraductal papillary mucinous neoplasm depends on histological and precursor epithelial subtypes. Gut 2011;60(12):1712–20.

31. Freeny PC, Saunders MD. Moving beyond morphology: new insights into the characterization and management of cystic pancreatic lesions. Radiology 2014;272(2):345–63.

32. Hwang DW, Jang JY, Lee SE, et al. High-grade atypical epithelial cells in pancreatic mucinous cysts are a more accurate predictor of malignancy than "positive" cytology. Langenbecks Arch Surg 2012;397(1):93–102.

33. Correa-Gallego C, Do R, Lafemina J, et al. Predicting dysplasia and invasive carcinoma in intraductal papillary mucinous neoplasms of the pancreas: development of a preoperative nomogram. Ann Surg Oncol 2013;20(13):4348–55.

34. Genevay M, Mino-Kenudson M, Yaeger K, et al. Cytology adds value to imaging studies for risk assessment of malignancy in pancreatic mucinous cysts. Ann Surg 2011;254(6):977–83.

35. Pitman MB, Genevay M, Yaeger K, et al. High-grade atypical epithelial cells in pancreatic mucinous cysts are a more accurate predictor of malignancy than "positive" cytology. Cancer Cytopathol 2010;118(6):434–40.

36. Hirono S, Tani M, Kawai M, et al. The carcinoembryonic antigen level in pancreatic juice and mural nodule size are predictors of malignancy for branch duct type intraductal papillary mucinous neoplasms of the pancreas. Ann Surg 2012;255(3):517–22.

37. Maire F, Voitot H, Aubert A, et al. Intraductal papillary mucinous neoplasms of the pancreas: performance of pancreatic fluid analysis for positive diagnosis and the prediction of malignancy. Am J Gastroenterol 2008;103(11):2871–7.

38. Khalid A, Zahid M, Finkelstein SD, et al. Pancreatic cyst fluid DNA analysis in evaluating pancreatic cysts: a report of the PANDA study. Gastrointest Endosc 2009;69(6):1095–102.

39. Wu J, Matthaei H, Maitra A, et al. Recurrent GNAS mutations define an unexpected pathway for pancreatic cyst development. Sci Transl Med 2011;3(92):92ra66.

40. Matthaei H, Wylie D, Lloyd MB, et al. miRNA biomarkers in cyst fluid augment the diagnosis and management of pancreatic cysts. Clin Cancer Res 2012;18(17):4713–24.

41. Maker AV, Katabi N, Qin LX, et al. Cyst fluid interleukin-1beta (IL1beta) levels predict the risk of carcinoma in intraductal papillary mucinous neoplasms of the pancreas. Clin Cancer Res 2011;17(6):1502–8.

42. Schmidt CM, Yip-Schneider MT, Ralstin MC, et al. PGE(2) in pancreatic cyst fluid helps differentiate IPMN from MCN and predict IPMN dysplasia. J Gastrointest Surg 2008;12(2):243–9.

43. Jabbar KS, Verbeke C, Hyltander AG, et al. Proteomic mucin profiling for the identification of cystic precursors of pancreatic cancer. J Natl Cancer Inst 2014;106(2):djt439.

44. Maker AV, Carrara S, Jamieson NB, et al. Cyst fluid biomarkers for intraductal papillary mucinous neoplasms of the pancreas: a critical review from the international expert meeting on pancreatic branch-duct-intraductal papillary mucinous neoplasms. J Am Coll Surg 2015;220(2):243–53.

45. Ohtsuka T, Kono H, Tanabe R, et al. Follow-up study after resection of intraductal papillary mucinous neoplasm of the pancreas; special references to the multifocal lesions and development of ductal carcinoma in the remnant pancreas. Am J Surg 2012;204(1):44–8.

46. Uehara H, Nakaizumi A, Ishikawa O, et al. Development of ductal carcinoma of the pancreas during follow-up of branch duct intraductal papillary mucinous neoplasm of the pancreas. Gut 2008;57(11):1561–5.

47. Crippa S, Salvia R, Warshaw AL, et al. Mucinous cystic neoplasm of the pancreas is not an aggressive entity: lessons from 163 resected patients. Ann Surg 2008; 247(4):571–9.

48. Sarr MG, Carpenter HA, Prabhakar LP, et al. Clinical and pathologic correlation of 84 mucinous cystic neoplasms of the pancreas: can one reliably differentiate benign from malignant (or premalignant) neoplasms? Ann Surg 2000;231(2): 205–12.

49. Yamao K, Yanagisawa A, Takahashi K, et al. Clinicopathological features and prognosis of mucinous cystic neoplasm with ovarian-type stroma: a multiinstitutional study of the Japan pancreas society. Pancreas 2011;40(1): 67–71.

50. Le Baleur Y, Couvelard A, Vullierme MP, et al. Mucinous cystic neoplasms of the pancreas: definition of preoperative imaging criteria for high-risk lesions. Pancreatology 2011;11(5):495–9.

51. Rodriguez JR, Madanat MG, Healy BC, et al. Distal pancreatectomy with splenic preservation revisited. Surgery 2007;141(5):619–25.

52. Sano M, Driscoll DR, De Jesus-Monge WE, et al. Activated wnt signaling in stroma contributes to development of pancreatic mucinous cystic neoplasms. Gastroenterology 2014;146(1):257–67.

53. Bassi C, Salvia R, Molinari E, et al. Management of 100 consecutive cases of pancreatic serous cystadenoma: wait for symptoms and see at imaging or vice versa? World J Surg 2003;27(3):319–23.

54. Galanis C, Zamani A, Cameron JL, et al. Resected serous cystic neoplasms of the pancreas: a review of 158 patients with recommendations for treatment. J Gastrointest Surg 2007;11(7):820–6.

55. Le Borgne J, de Calan L, Partensky C. Cystadenomas and cystadenocarcinomas of the pancreas: a multiinstitutional retrospective study of 398 cases. French Surgical Association. Ann Surg 1999;230(2):152–61.

56. Tseng JF, Warshaw AL, Sahani DV, et al. Serous cystadenoma of the pancreas: tumor growth rates and recommendations for treatment. Ann Surg 2005;242(3): 413–9 [discussion: 419–21].

57. Malleo G, Bassi C, Rossini R, et al. Growth pattern of serous cystic neoplasms of the pancreas: observational study with long-term magnetic resonance surveillance and recommendations for treatment. Gut 2012;61(5):746–51.

58. Yip-Schneider MT, Wu H, Dumas RP, et al. Vascular endothelial growth factor, a novel and highly accurate pancreatic fluid biomarker for serous pancreatic cysts. J Am Coll Surg 2014;218(4):608–17.

59. Moore PS, Zamboni G, Brighenti A, et al. Molecular characterization of pancreatic serous microcystic adenomas: evidence for a tumor suppressor gene on chromosome 10q. Am J Pathol 2001;158(1):317–21.

60. Bordeianou L, Vagefi PA, Sahani D, et al. Cystic pancreatic endocrine neoplasms: a distinct tumor type? J Am Coll Surg 2008;206(3):1154–8.

61. Boninsegna L, Partelli S, D'Innocenzio MM, et al. Pancreatic cystic endocrine tumors: a different morphological entity associated with a less aggressive behavior. Neuroendocrinology 2010;92(4):246–51.

62. Gaujoux S, Tang L, Klimstra D, et al. The outcome of resected cystic pancreatic endocrine neoplasms: a case-matched analysis. Surgery 2012;151(4):518–25.

63. Yoon WJ, Daglilar ES, Pitman MB, et al. Cystic pancreatic neuroendocrine tumors: endoscopic ultrasound and fine-needle aspiration characteristics. Endoscopy 2013;45(3):189–94.

64. Morales-Oyarvide V, Yoon WJ, Ingkakul T, et al. Cystic pancreatic neuroendocrine tumors: the value of cytology in preoperative diagnosis. Cancer Cytopathol 2014; 122(6):435–44.

65. Lee LC, Grant CS, Salomao DR, et al. Small, nonfunctioning, asymptomatic pancreatic neuroendocrine tumors (PNETs): role for nonoperative management. Surgery 2012;152(6):965–74.

66. Butte JM, Brennan MF, Gonen M, et al. Solid pseudopapillary tumors of the pancreas. Clinical features, surgical outcomes, and long-term survival in 45 consecutive patients from a single center. J Gastrointest Surg 2011;15(2):350–7.

67. Reddy S, Cameron JL, Scudiere J, et al. Surgical management of solid-pseudopapillary neoplasms of the pancreas (Franz or Hamoudi tumors): a large single-institutional series. J Am Coll Surg 2009;208(5):950–7 [discussion: 957–9].

68. Abraham SC, Klimstra DS, Wilentz RE, et al. Solid-pseudopapillary tumors of the pancreas are genetically distinct from pancreatic ductal adenocarcinomas and almost always harbor beta-catenin mutations. Am J Pathol 2002;160(4):1361–9.

69. Park M, Kim M, Hwang D, et al. Characterization of gene expression and activated signaling pathways in solid-pseudopapillary neoplasm of pancreas. Mod Pathol 2014;27(4):580–93.

70. Chaudhari VV, Raman SS, Vuong NL, et al. Pancreatic cystic lesions: discrimination accuracy based on clinical data and high resolution CT features. J Comput Assist Tomogr 2007;31(6):860–7.

71. de Jong K, Nio CY, Mearadji B, et al. Disappointing interobserver agreement among radiologists for a classifying diagnosis of pancreatic cysts using magnetic resonance imaging. Pancreas 2012;41(2):278–82.

72. van der Waaij LA, van Dullemen HM, Porte RJ. Cyst fluid analysis in the differential diagnosis of pancreatic cystic lesions: a pooled analysis. Gastrointest Endosc 2005;62(3):383–9.

73. Del Chiaro M, Segersvard R, Pozzi Mucelli R, et al. Comparison of preoperative conference-based diagnosis with histology of cystic tumors of the pancreas. Ann Surg Oncol 2014;21(5):1539–44.

74. Sahani DV, Lin DJ, Venkatesan AM, et al. Multidisciplinary approach to diagnosis and management of intraductal papillary mucinous neoplasms of the pancreas. Clin Gastroenterol Hepatol 2009;7(3):259–69.

Imaging and Endoscopic Approaches to Pancreatic Cancer

Michael H. Rosenthal, MD, PhD[a,b,c,]*, Alexander Lee, MD[c,d],
Kunal Jajoo, MD[c,d]

KEYWORDS

- Imaging • Endoscopy • Pancreatic adenocarcinoma • Cancer diagnosis
- Cancer staging

KEY POINTS

- Imaging and endoscopy have complementary strengths that should be used as part of a multidisciplinary oncology care plan.
- Computed tomography (CT) is the primary imaging modality for routine diagnosis, staging, and monitoring of patients with cancer, but MRI and PET with fludeoxyglucose F 18 (FDG-PET) can be useful in certain problem-solving situations.
- Endoscopy provides accurate local and regional nodal staging via endoscopic ultrasonography (EUS) and can provide immediate diagnostic tissue sampling and supportive interventions.

INTRODUCTION

Noninvasive imaging and endoscopy play important and complementary roles in the diagnosis and management of patients with pancreatic cancer. Imaging, primarily in the form of ultrasonography (US) and CT, is often the first line of investigation for the symptoms of pancreatic cancer. Imaging is widely available and can provide noninvasive diagnostic and staging information, while endoscopy offers complementary diagnostic and therapeutic tools throughout the spectrum of care. The following sections examine the roles and importance of each of these modalities for pancreatic cancer.

[a] Department of Imaging, Dana-Farber Cancer Institute, 450 Brookline Avenue, Boston, MA 02215, USA; [b] Department of Radiology, Brigham and Women's Hospital, 75 Francis Street, Boston, MA 02115, USA; [c] Harvard Medical School, 25 Shattuck Street, Boston, MA 02115, USA; [d] Division of Gastroenterology, Department of Medicine, Brigham and Women's Hospital, 75 Francis Street, Boston, MA 02115, USA
* Corresponding author. Department of Imaging, Dana-Farber Cancer Institute, 450 Brookline Avenue, Boston 02215, MA.
E-mail address: Michael_Rosenthal@dfci.harvard.edu

Hematol Oncol Clin N Am 29 (2015) 675–699
http://dx.doi.org/10.1016/j.hoc.2015.04.008
0889-8588/15/$ – see front matter © 2015 Elsevier Inc. All rights reserved.

hemonc.theclinics.com

NONINVASIVE IMAGING IN PANCREATIC CANCER
Image-Based Anatomy of the Pancreas

As shown in **Fig. 1**, the pancreas is conceptually divided into 4 parts based on adjacent landmarks, as follows:

- Head: The head is the rightmost portion of the pancreas. All parenchyma to the right of the superior mesenteric vein (SMV) is included in the pancreatic head. The head contains the common bile duct and central portion of the pancreatic duct.
- Neck: The pancreatic neck is a narrow band of tissue that is located anterior to the SMV. This part is defined medially by the right edge of the portal vein and laterally by the left edge of the portal vein-SMV confluence.
- Body: The body of the pancreas is located lateral to the left edge of the portal vein-SMV confluence. While the American Joint Committee on Cancer (AJCC) manual states that the left edge of the aorta is the dividing line between the body and tail, this often results in little or no parenchyma in the body and is not uniformly accepted.[1] The empirical division is often chosen to be 2 to 3 cm to the left of the aorta.
- Tail: The tail of the pancreas is the most lateral component and all pancreatic tissue lateral to the pancreatic body. The tail is typically located near the splenic hilum.

In addition, the uncinate process is a small, variable projection of the pancreatic head that extends posterior to the SMV.

Ductal anatomy
There are 2 ductal systems that traverse the pancreas: the pancreatic ducts and the common bile duct. **Fig. 2** shows the typical configuration of these ductal systems within the pancreas.

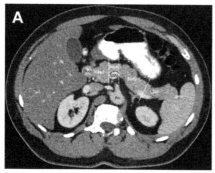
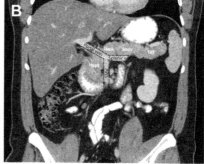

Fig. 1. CT anatomy of the pancreas. Axial (*A*) and coronal (*B*) curved reformats from a portal venous phase CT of the pancreas demonstrate the normal appearance of pancreatic parenchyma and the surrounding landmarks. The head of the pancreas lies to the right of the superior mesenteric vein (SMV) and the neck is immediately anterior to the SMV and confluence. The parenchyma to the left of the portal confluence is divided into the body and tail. While the American Joint Committee on Cancer manual identifies the left border of the aorta as the landmark that divides the body and tail, this is not widely used because it frequently results in a small or absent pancreatic body. The empirical division is often chosen to be 2 to 3 cm to the left of the aorta. The splenic vein extends along the posterior margin of the body and tail, and the portal vein extends superiorly and to the right from the portal confluence. The duodenum travels along the right and inferior margins of the pancreatic head.

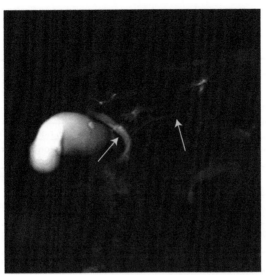

Fig. 2. Biliary anatomy on magnetic resonance cholangiopancreatography (MRCP). The common bile duct (CBD) (*left arrow*) and pancreatic duct (*right arrow*) are clearly defined and not dilated in this normal-appearing MRCP. Dilatation of the pancreatic duct is a common finding in pancreatic cancer.

The common bile duct is formed from the fusion of the proper hepatic duct and the cystic duct, which occurs superior to the pancreas in most people. In standard anatomy, the common bile duct traverses the pancreatic head and merges with the pancreatic duct before draining through the sphincter of Oddi at the ampulla of Vater.

The main pancreatic duct begins in the tail of the pancreas and extends through the body and neck of the pancreas (see **Fig. 2**). The main pancreatic duct typically extends inferomedially through the pancreatic head as the ventral duct of Wirsung. The dorsal duct of Santorini fuses with and drains into the main duct during typical embryologic development. Common variants of this configuration are described by Yu and colleagues.[2]

Vascular anatomy
Correct identification of the vessels in and around the pancreas is critical to assessing the feasibility of surgery for pancreatic cancer. There is substantial variability in the arterial anatomy in this region, so the radiologist plays a key role in delineating each patient's anatomy for the surgical oncology team.

Table 1 describes the arterial segments that are most important in pancreatic cancer. As shown by Winston and colleagues,[3] up to 49% of patients have variations in one of the important arteries that can be involved in a pancreatic resection. **Fig. 3** shows the typical arterial anatomy on CT angiograms. Detailed and accurate reporting of these variations is crucial for preoperative planning studies.

The detailed venous anatomy around the pancreas is less crucial for surgical planning, but 3 major veins must be assessed to determine resectability (**Fig. 4**). The SMV drains the small bowel and colon. The SMV is located at the lateral border of the pancreatic head and is immediately posterior to the pancreatic neck. The SMV merges with the splenic vein, which travels along the posterior margin of the tail, body, and neck of the pancreas, to form the portal vein. The portal vein then travels superiorly and to the right to the hepatic hilum.

Table 1		
Important arterial anatomy for pancreatic surgery		
Artery	**Standard Origin**	**Variants**
Celiac axis	Aorta	Common trunk with SMA (<1%)
Left gastric	Celiac axis	Aortic origin (3%)
Splenic	Celiac axis	—
Common hepatic	Celiac axis	SMA origin (2%), aortic origin (2%)
GDA	Common hepatic	SMA origin (<1%), right hepatic origin (<1%)
Proper hepatic	Common hepatic (at origin of GDA)	Immediate trifurcation of common hepatic (4%)
Left hepatic	Proper hepatic	Left gastric origin (13%), common hepatic (<1%), celiac axis (<1%)
Right hepatic	Proper hepatic	SMA origin (15%), celiac axis (4%), GDA origin (1%), aorta (<1%)
Accessory hepatic	Not typically present	Numerous, primarily from contralateral hepatic (5%) and left gastric (4%)
SMA	Aorta	Common trunk with celiac (<1%)

Abbreviations: GDA, gastroduodenal artery; SMA, superior mesenteric artery.

Data from Winston CB, Lee NA, Jarnagin WR, et al. CT angiography for delineation of celiac and superior mesenteric artery variants in patients undergoing hepatobiliary and pancreatic surgery. AJR Am J Roentgenol 2007;189(1):W18.

Adjacent structures

The anterior and superior margins of the pancreas are covered by the peritoneum of the lesser sac, so lesions that extend anteriorly or superiorly may involve the peritoneal cavity and metastasize through that pathway. A narrow fold of the transverse mesocolon extends anteriorly and inferiorly from the lower anterior margin of the pancreas and forms the inferior boundary of the lesser sac; this can be a direct retroperitoneal pathway of spread of cancer and is the mechanism through which the colon obstruction sign is observed on kidney-ureter-bladder (KUB) films in patients with pancreatic pathology.[4]

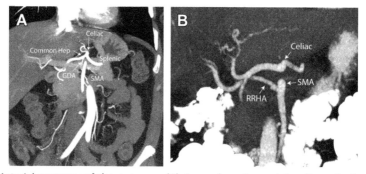

Fig. 3. Arterial anatomy of the pancreas. (*A*) Coronal maximum-intensity projection image from an arterial phase CT shows the normal trifurcation of the celiac axis into the left gastric, splenic, and common hepatic (Common hep) arteries. The gastroduodenal artery (GDA) extends inferior from the common hepatic artery. The superior mesenteric artery (SMA) arises from the aorta inferior to the celiac axis. (*B*) A maximum-intensity projection image from an arterial phase CT scan shows a replaced right hepatic artery (RRHA) arising from the SMA.

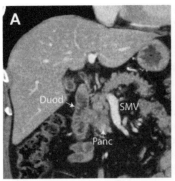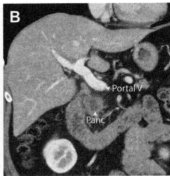

Fig. 4. Important veins near the pancreas (Panc) on coronal CT images. (*A*) The SMV drains the bowel and courses along the left border of the pancreatic head. (*B*) The SMV and splenic vein join at the portal confluence to form the portal vein (Portal v), which travels superiorly and rightward to the hepatic hilum. Duod, duodenum.

The anterior, inferior margin of the uncinate process, body, and tail of the pancreas are in close proximity to the greater sac of the peritoneum as well as the root of the mesentery. Tumor that extends anteriorly and inferiorly from this area can spread along the mesentery around the superior mesenteric artery (SMA) and SMV (as in **Fig. 12**D) or may directly invade into the peritoneum.

The inferior margin of the pancreas is retroperitoneal and is bordered by the duodenum. The posterior margin is also retroperitoneal and is bordered by the inferior vena cava, aorta, left adrenal gland, and left kidney. Lesions arising from the uncinate process or posterior body and tail may extend along these planes and sometimes metastasize into the left perirenal space.

Imaging Techniques

The following noninvasive imaging techniques are typically used in the evaluation of pancreatic cancer:

- CT
  - CT is the primary method of abdominal imaging
  - This technique uses X-rays to create images of thin sections of the body
  - CT is typically performed using intravenous iodinated contrast
  - Standard studies are performed with a single scan acquired in the portal venous phase, approximately 70 seconds after the start of contrast injection
  - Specialized pancreatic cancer protocols typically involve the following 3 scans after contrast injection:
    - Early arterial phase scan for assessment of arterial anatomy for surgery (25 seconds after injection)
    - Late arterial/pancreatic parenchymal phase scan for detection of pancreatic lesions and venous anatomy (at 40–45 seconds)
    - Portal venous phase scan for assessment of regional and metastatic disease, particularly in the liver (at 70 seconds)
- MRI
  - This technique uses a combination of strong magnetic fields and nonionizing radiowaves to produce images of the body
  - MRI is a problem-solving modality; it can detect and characterize lesions that may be occult or indeterminate on other modalities

○ Each MRI sequence exploits a different combination of physical characteristics to produce contrast between tissue types
○ MRI of the pancreas is typically performed with intravenous gadolinium contrast
   ■ Oral contrast such as water or milk can be used to improve visualization of the gastric and duodenal margins near the pancreas
○ A typical MRI of the pancreas includes T2-weighted sequence, heavily T2-weighted magnetic resonance cholangiopancreatography (MRCP), T1 precontrast sequence, multiphase postcontrast sequence, and diffusion-weighted sequence; views should be acquired in at least 2 planes
○ Secretin injection can be used to augment ductal dilatation in MRCP when strictures or main duct communication are questioned[5]
○ The typical appearance of the pancreas on MRI is demonstrated in **Fig. 5**
● US
○ This method uses high-frequency sound waves to image the structure of tissues of interest
○ US is often used to assess for biliary or gallbladder pathology during initial evaluation of symptoms
○ Transabdominal US of the pancreas can be limited by gastric and duodenal air
○ US is a relatively low-cost and accessible technique, but performance and interpretation depend highly on the skill of the sonographer and radiologist
○ The typical appearance of the pancreas on US is demonstrated in **Fig. 6**

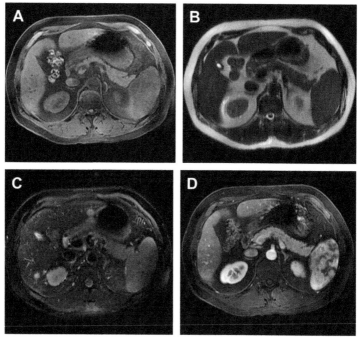

Fig. 5. Normal appearance of the pancreas on MRI. The normal pancreas is hyperintense on precontrast T1-weighted images (*A*) and mildly hypointense on T2-weighted images (*B*) without fat saturation, and (*C*) with fat saturation. Normal parenchyma shows increased signal on postcontrast images (*D*); appearance of spleen is due to phase contrast.

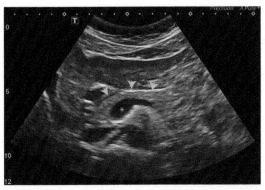

Fig. 6. Normal appearance of the pancreas on US. This transverse US image shows the typical homogeneously echogenic appearance of the pancreatic head, neck, and proximal body (*arrowheads*). The anechoic portal confluence is visible centrally (*asterisk*), and a portion of the splenic vein extends leftward from the confluence along the posterior margin of the pancreas.

- PET
  - PET produces images of positrons that are created by radioactive decay
  - PET uses radiotracers, which are compounds labeled with a radioactive atom, that localize to a process or structure of interest
    - FDG, an analog of glucose and a marker of energy metabolism, is the most commonly used radiotracer
  - PET is often coupled with low-dose CT for correction of attenuation within the body
  - This technique is highly sensitive to sites of disease throughout the body and is often used for systemic staging in cancer care
- Radiography and fluoroscopy
  - These methods use X-rays to create projection images of the body
  - These techniques are of limited use in modern pancreatic cancer diagnosis and treatment
  - Historically, abdominal radiographs and barium enemas could show transverse colon obstruction from spread of pancreatic cancer along the transverse mesocolon

Imaging Across the Spectrum of Care

Initial diagnosis
The initial assessment of the symptoms of pancreatic cancer often begins with a diagnostic CT or US examination. The initial diagnostic use of these modalities is as follows:

- CT is the preferred diagnostic modality because it can be used to assess for the local, regional, and systemic signs of disease and has utility for a wide range of alternative diagnoses.[6]
- US is often used as an initial study in patients who present with right upper quadrant pain or jaundice because of its sensitivity for biliary tract obstruction and for the alternative diagnosis of choledocholithiasis.
- MRI is used as a problem-solving tool when the initial diagnosis is uncertain because of the modality's superior soft tissue contrast and ability to characterize the structure and composition of unknown lesions.[7,8]

- PET-CT is not typically part of the initial diagnostic strategy but may rarely be used for detection of an occult primary tumor when a patient has systemic signs of malignancy (eg, cachexia) without localizing symptoms.

When a pancreatic lesion is detected on the initial diagnostic workup, there are a variety of benign and malignant differential considerations that should be entertained. The most common considerations and their diagnostic features are as follows:

- Adenocarcinoma (see **Fig. 12**)
  - Ill-defined, hypodense, infiltrative mass on CT
  - Solid (except carcinomas arising from cystic pancreatic lesions)
  - Hypoechoic, nonshadowing mass on US
  - T1-hypointense and minimally T2-hyperintense appearance of the primary mass on MRI
  - Hypoenhancing on postcontrast pancreatic and portal venous phases
  - Mildly restricted diffusion on diffusion-weighted imaging
  - Significant FDG avidity
  - Hepatic and peritoneal metastases are common
- Neuroendocrine tumors, including carcinoids (**Fig. 7**)
  - Arterial and pancreatic phase hyperenhancement on CT and MRI
  - Washout of contrast on delayed imaging
  - T1 hypointensity or isointensity of the mass to pancreas and T2 hyperintensity on MRI
  - Typically solid, but rare complex cystic variants are seen
  - Restricted diffusion on diffusion-weighted MRI
  - Variation of FDG uptake by grade
  - Hepatic metastases are common
- Cystic pancreatic neoplasms
  - Mixture of solid and fluid density components on CT
  - May have a capsule or calcifications
  - MRI shows T2-hyperintense cystic components with enhancing mural nodules or septations
  - MRCP can be used to show relationship to pancreatic duct
  - Entities include mucinous cystic tumors, serous cystadenomas (most commonly microcystic), solid pseudopapillary epithelial neoplasms,

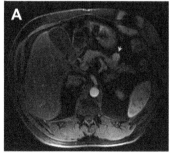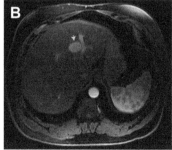

Fig. 7. Multiple gastrinomas in a patient with multiple endocrine neoplasia type 1. MRI of the pancreas demonstrates a representative example of several well-circumscribed hypervascular lesions (*arrow*) that were seen throughout the pancreas (*A*). A hypervascular liver metastasis was also identified (*B*) (*arrow*). The serum gastrin level was elevated to 20,140 pg/mL (normal < 100 pg/mL). Hyperparathyroidism was also present.

intraductal papillary mucinous neoplasms (IPMN; main duct or sidebranch varieties; **Fig. 8**), and rare cystic neuroendocrine tumors

- Metastases
  - Uncommon overall, but most commonly associated with renal cell carcinoma, melanoma, as well as lung and breast cancers. **Fig. 9** shows a rare solitary pancreatic metastasis from a colorectal adenocarcinoma.
  - Variable appearance on CT, MRI, and PET-CT depending on the primary source
  - Synchronous metastases are typically present elsewhere in the body
- Pancreatitis
  - CT shows ill-defined, homogeneous hypodensity with loss of internal paren-chymal architecture (**Fig. 10**)
  - Adjacent inflammatory fat stranding, necrosis, or pseudocyst formation may be present depending on the severity
  - Calcifications and CT hypodensity without stranding are markers of chronic pancreatitis (**Fig. 11**)
  - US shows loss of parenchymal architecture and hypoechoic parenchyma
  - MRI of acute pancreatitis shows T1 hypointensity, T2 hyperintensity, and post-contrast hypoenhancement throughout the affected area
  - Autoimmune pancreatitis appears similar to other forms of acute pancreatitis but may have a sausagelike configuration of homogeneous inflammation with restricted diffusion on MRI[7]

There are many other uncommon entities that are included within the radiologic differential diagnosis but are beyond the scope of this discussion.

The combination of imaging features, nodal involvement, and signs of systemic metastasis can be used to produce a narrow differential diagnosis, as is often the case with sidebranch IPMNs and serous microcystic adenomas. Certain entities can only be definitively distinguished by tissue biopsy, such as metastasis versus primary pancreatic adenocarcinoma in a patient with a resected stage II lung cancer. Endoscopy and final-needle aspiration (FNA) are crucial in such determinations.

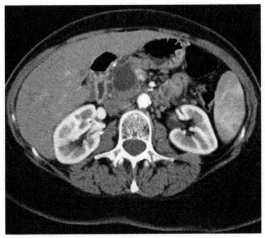

Fig. 8. IPMN of the head of the pancreas. Pancreatic phase CT demonstrates a 2.7-cm cystic mass in the head of the pancreas that is confluent with the main pancreatic duct. This lesion was resected and found to contain areas of moderate dysplasia.

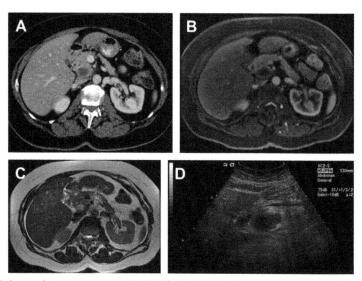

Fig. 9. Colorectal cancer metastasis mimicking pancreatic adenocarcinoma. Portal venous phase CT (*A*) demonstrates a 3.7-cm hypodense solid mass in the head of the pancreas. MRI of the pancreas shows a hypoenhancing mass (*B*) that is hyperintense on T2-weighted images (*C*). A previous US (*D*) demonstrated a hypoechoic, nonshadowing mass at this location.

Initial staging

CT is the preferred modality for the initial staging of pancreatic cancer.[6] The staging of pancreatic cancer is currently performed using the seventh edition of the AJCC's *Cancer Staging Manual*.[1] Radiology plays a key role in classifying each patient's extent of disease using the 3-part TNM staging system described below.

Primary tumor T stage As shown in **Fig. 12**, the T staging of pancreatic cancer is based on both the size and the degree of involvement of surrounding tissues and vascular structures. The current T staging system is as follows[1]:

- T1: Limited to the pancreas, 2 cm or less in greatest dimension
- T2: Limited to the pancreas, more than 2 cm in greatest dimension

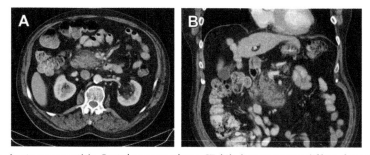

Fig. 10. Acute pancreatitis. Portal venous phase CT (*A*) demonstrates diffuse fat stranding around the head and uncinate process of the pancreas. No distinct mass is seen. A coronal view from the same CT (*B*) shows that the parenchymal architecture of the pancreas is preserved, which suggests an inflammatory process rather than an invasive adenocarcinoma.

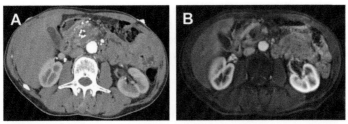

Fig. 11. Chronic pancreatitis mimicking pancreatic adenocarcinoma. Pancreatic phase CT (*A*) demonstrates an ill-defined region of hypodensity in the head of the pancreas. The distal pancreatic duct was dilated up to a transition point in this area. Multiple small calcifications in this area suggested chronic pancreatitis. MRI (*B*) also shows an ill-defined area of hypo-enhancement in the pancreatic head. No restricted diffusion was present, and the area was isointense on T2-weighted images (not shown). Whipple resection confirmed chronic pancreatitis and showed no evidence of cancer.

- T3: Extends beyond the pancreas but does not involve the celiac axis or SMA; involvement of the portal vein and/or SMV is included in this category
- T4: Involves celiac axis or SMA; also termed locally advanced in the absence of metastases

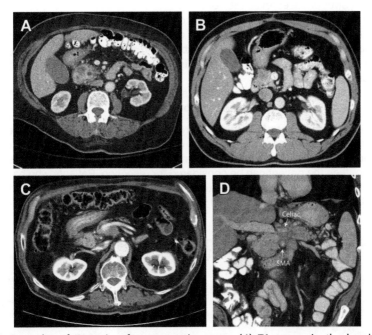

Fig. 12. Examples of T staging for pancreatic cancer. (*A*) T1 cancer in the head of the pancreas measures less than 2 cm and does not involve adjacent structures or vessels. (*B*) T2 cancer in the head of the pancreas measures more than 2 cm and does not involve adjacent structures or vessels. (*C*) T3 cancer involves the portal confluence. There is a fat plane between the mass and the SMA. (*D*) Coronal view of a T4 tumor in the pancreatic body that encases the celiac axis and SMA.

Regional nodes The regional lymph nodes for the pancreas include the portal, peripancreatic, celiac, SMV, and splenic hilar stations. Any involved lymph node below the renal veins or above the diaphragm is considered to represent distant metastasis. The N staging system is a simple binary system[1] and is as follows:

- N0: No regional nodal involvement
- N1: Regional nodal involvement

Metastatic disease Pancreatic adenocarcinoma frequently metastasizes, with 55% of patients presenting with metastatic disease at initial diagnosis.[9] The most common sites of metastasis are the liver, peritoneum, and lungs, with less-frequent metastases occurring to the bones and brain. Metastases can occur nearly anywhere in the body in advanced disease. **Fig. 13** demonstrates several examples of such metastases.

M staging for pancreatic cancer is also a simple binary system[1] and is as follows:

- M0: No metastasis
- M1: Any metastasis

Resectability For patients who have no evidence of metastatic disease on their initial staging studies and who do not have contraindications to surgery, the resectability of the primary tumor is primarily determined by the extent of vascular involvement by the tumor. The current criteria for resectability are widely debated, and the details of this debate are beyond the scope of this article.[10–14] The following factors are considered in most of the proposed standards:

- Is the SMA encased over 180° or more?
- Is the celiac axis abutted or encased over 180° or more?
- Is the portal vein or SMV involved to a degree that would preclude resection with reconstruction (the criteria for resectability of tumors that involve the major veins are particularly disputed and may include abutment, invasion, stenosis, or occlusion)?
- Are other critical vascular structures, such as the common hepatic artery, aorta, or vena cava, involved in a way that precludes resection?

With allowances for the aforementioned resectability debate, if the answer to any of these questions is yes, then the patient is considered to have nonresectable locally advanced disease and is referred for systemic therapy. If the answer to all these questions is no, then the patient can be considered for resection. Patients who have some degree of vascular contact by tumor but do not meet the above-mentioned criteria for locally advanced disease are labeled as having borderline resectable disease and

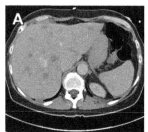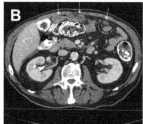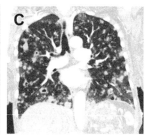

Fig. 13. Examples of metastases from pancreatic adenocarcinoma. The most common sites of metastasis include the liver (*A*), peritoneum (*B*) (*arrows*), and lungs (*C*), with less-frequent metastases seen in the bones and brain.

typically undergo neoadjuvant therapy to improve their odds of achieving a disease-free resection.

Treatment monitoring

After neoadjuvant therapy For patients who undergo neoadjuvant therapy, a pancreatic protocol CT scan is typically used to reassess the disease burden to ensure that the patient's tumor remains resectable. This study should include assessments of the primary tumor extent, degree of vascular involvement, and surveillance of potential sites of nodal and metastatic disease in the chest, abdomen, and pelvis.

The significance of residual radiographic vascular abutment after neoadjuvant therapy remains uncertain. Cassinotto and colleagues[15] recently reported that in a cohort of 47 patients with borderline resectable pancreatic head adenocarcinoma, postneoadjuvant chemoradiotherapy CT scans that showed regression of tumor size and decrease in venous contact were all positive predictors of R0 resection. Larger tumor sizes, elevated postneoadjuvant cancer antigen 19-9 (CA19-9) levels, and residual SMA contact were negative predictors of R0 resection. Importantly, the presence of residual venous contact was not a predictor of R0 outcome. However, Katz and colleagues[16] found that most patients who had radiographically stable disease after neoadjuvant therapy were able to achieve R0 resections at surgery.

After surgery For patients who undergo surgical resection, imaging is used in the immediate postoperative period to detect complications such as anastomotic leaks, enteric and biliary strictures, hemorrhage, abscess formation, and pancreatitis. A new baseline CT scan is typically performed before the start of any adjuvant chemotherapy to provide a reliable reference for detection of new lesions during treatment.

During adjuvant and palliative chemotherapy The primary purposes of imaging during adjuvant or palliative chemotherapy are as follows:

1. To detect any signs of treatment resistance, such as new metastases or unequivocal growth of existing lesions
2. To assess for any lesions that may cause significant morbidity or mortality, particularly those that are amenable to palliative interventions
3. To detect any complications of treatment, such as drug-related pneumonitis or colitis

There is no consensus on the optimal type and timing of imaging during treatment, but a common approach is to acquire CT scans of the chest, abdomen, and pelvis every 8 to 12 weeks or if new symptoms develop.

Surveillance

Patients who have no evidence of disease after resection and any adjuvant therapy typically undergo surveillance through a combination of clinical assessments, biomarker testing, and imaging surveillance. The National Comprehensive Cancer Network guidelines currently recommend CT imaging every 3 to 6 months for the first 2 years and annually thereafter.[17]

Future Considerations

Dual-energy computed tomography imaging

Dual-energy CT uses 2 different X-ray spectra, either by changing the spectrum of a single source or by using 2 different sources, to estimate the local material composition of a volume of interest.[18,19] This technology can be used to improve the contrast between enhancing and nonenhancing tissues, which has the potential to improve the assessment of pancreatic cancers. This technique is not currently in widespread use.

Stromal transport characterization

Koay and colleagues[20] recently reported that metrics based on preoperative CT contrast enhancement characteristics strongly correlated with the extent of gemcitabine incorporation into tumor DNA after intraoperative gemcitabine infusion. These metrics also correlated with the stromal characteristics of the tumor on histology. These findings suggest that contrast kinetics could be useful in treatment optimization, but further work is needed to validate this methodology.

ENDOSCOPY IN PANCREATIC CANCER

Introduction

Endoscopy plays a central role in the management of pancreatic cancer.

Imaging techniques such as US, CT, or MRI are typically the first to identify a pancreatic mass. Subsequent endoscopy is often needed to confirm the diagnosis of pancreatic cancer, to stage disease, and/or to render therapy.[21]

This section examines the role and performance characteristics of endoscopy in the management of pancreatic cancer.

Diagnosis

Endoscopic retrograde cholangiopancreatography

During endoscopic retrograde cholangiopancreatography (ERCP), cholangiography and/or pancreatography can detect physical impingement upon the ductal systems by malignancy or lymphadenopathy, visualized as ductal strictures or irregularity.

More than 60% of exocrine pancreatic neoplasms occur in the pancreatic head, and ERCP is particularly effective in detecting lesions at that location due its proximity to the bile duct (**Fig. 14**). An early meta-analysis demonstrated greater than 90% sensitivity and specificity of ERCP for pancreatic cancer.[22]

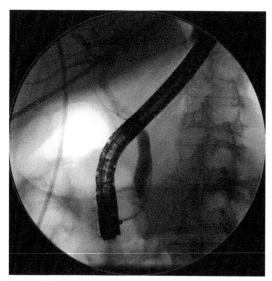

Fig. 14. Cholangiogram during ERCP consistent with pancreatic cancer. Narrowing at the distal common bile duct is secondary to malignant stricture from malignancy in the pancreatic head.

Complications of ERCP are shown in **Table 2**. Although certainly safe in experienced hands, ERCP is recognized as one of the most high-risk endoscopic procedures; the overall mortality rate is 0.2%.[23] Thus, ERCP has evolved into a primarily therapeutic tool (ie, for biliary obstruction) rather than a diagnostic one.[24] In settings in which the diagnosis of pancreatic cancer is still uncertain after imaging, ERCP can provide tissue diagnosis.

Biliary aspirate During ERCP, bile or pancreatic juice can be obtained for cytology proximal to a suspected malignant ductal stricture. However, sensitivity for malignancy is very low, ranging from 6% to 32%. At present, this technique is used only in combination with other techniques.[30]

Brushing Sensitivity for detection of malignancy by brushing of ductal strictures during ERCP (**Fig. 15**) is weak, ranging from 35% to 70% in the literature; the specificity does exceed 90%.[31] Recent advances in brush instruments and technique have demonstrated sensitivity and specificity exceeding 90% in some studies.[32]

Biopsy Forceps may be deployed through the scope during ERCP to obtain biopsies of a stricture. Sensitivity is wide ranging in the literature at approximately 40% to 80%, with specificity comparable to brush cytology. Some experts promote use of both biopsy and brush cytology in combination; increases in sensitivity with combination technique versus brushing alone have ranged from 8% to 25%.[33]

Ductoscopy A miniature endoscope (ductoscope) can be passed through the ERCP scope into the bile duct or pancreatic duct to interrogate a stricture, and this facilitates endoscopically targeted biopsies.[34] Sensitivity for malignancy as high as 96% has been reported, but this technique is largely limited to specialized centers.[35] Novel ductoscopes have recently been developed that directly access the desired duct and do not require passage through the ERCP scope (**Fig. 16**).

Endoscopic ultrasonography

EUS provides excellent visualization of pancreatic lesions, because of the pancreas' location adjacent to the stomach and duodenum (**Fig. 17**). Resolution is also much higher than that of transabdominal US. Multiple studies have demonstrated excellent sensitivity of EUS for detection of pancreatic tumors, ranging from 90% to 99%, even in small lesions.[36]

Table 2
Complications from endoscopic procedures

Complication	EGD	ERCP	EUS/EUS-FNA	Enteral Stent[a]	EUS-CPN[b]
Pancreatitis (%)	0	3.50	0.04–2.00	<0.01	0
Bleeding (%)	0.50	1.30	0.13	5.00	0.13
Bowel perforation (%)	0.03	0.60	0.03–0.06	0.70	0.03–0.06
Infection (%)	<0.01	1.00	0.40–1.00	<0.01	<0.01
Tumor seeding (%)	0	0	<0.01	0	0

Abbreviations: CPN, celiac plexus neurolysis; EGD, esophagogastroduodenoscopy; EUS, endoscopic ultrasound.
   [a] Additional complications include distal migration (5%) and restenosis (18%).
   [b] Additional complications include diarrhea (7%), hypotension (4%), and neurologic sequelae (<0.01%).
   Data from Refs.[23,25–29]

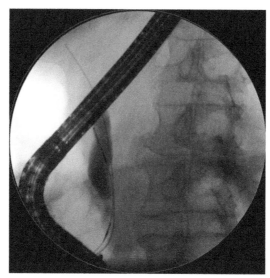

Fig. 15. Cytologic brushings obtained during ERCP. The brush instrument has been deployed into the bile duct and is across the stricture.

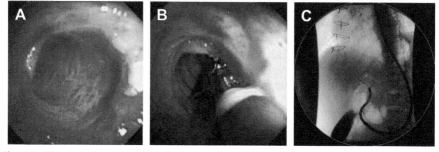

Fig. 16. Biliary ductoscopy (choledochoscopy). Stricture and associated abnormal mucosa are seen (*A*) with directed biopsy (*B*). Fluoroscopy demonstrates the ductoscope in the bile duct (*C*).

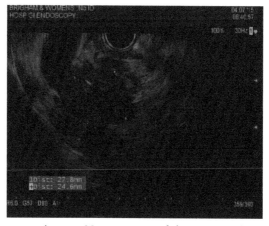

Fig. 17. EUS with pancreatic mass. Measurements of the mass are shown.

EUS often plays a pivotal role in the management of pancreatic cancer. Beyond identification of the pancreatic lesion, EUS can facilitate more sophisticated diagnostics as well.

Fine-needle aspiration EUS-guided FNA has been accepted as the optimal method for obtaining a tissue diagnosis (**Fig. 18**). EUS-FNA can identify pancreatic lesions that are too small to be characterized by CT or MRI and can sample pancreatic lesions that are inaccessible percutaneously because of adjacent vascular structures.[37]

A large meta-analysis in 2012 demonstrated that EUS-FNA for pancreatic cancer had sensitivity of 92% and specificity of 96%.[38] EUS-FNA can also sample regional lymph nodes (celiac, para-aortic, retroduodenopancreatic, or superior mesenteric), suspected metastases of the liver, and ascites.[39]

Referral for EUS-FNA typically occurs after discovery of a pancreatic mass concerning for malignancy, such that tissue diagnosis is needed before proceeding with surgery and/or chemotherapy. Complications from EUS-FNA are uncommon (see **Table 2**).

Staging

EUS is used for staging of pancreatic cancer and is especially useful in evaluating operative candidacy.[40] Within the TNM staging system, EUS provides tumor (T) staging (including vascular invasion) and nodal (N) staging (**Fig. 19**). Reported accuracy of EUS is 63% to 94% for T staging and 44% to 82% for N staging.[41,42]

Most clinicians follow a multimodal approach; a recent study showed that for resectability (ie, vascular invasion), correct assessment was performed in 86% of cases when both multidetector CT and EUS were used, an increase of greater than 20% compared with when either modality was used alone.[43]

Possible reasons for variability in EUS performance include reliance on skill of the endoscopist, endoscopist's knowledge of prior imaging, degree of anatomic distortion because of the cancer, and quality of EUS equipment.[41,42]

Novel techniques

Endoscopic retrograde cholangiopancreatography with intraductal ultrasonography In contrast to EUS, intraductal ultrasonography (IDUS) involves use of an endosonographic probe that can be advanced through the ERCP scope and into the bile or pancreatic duct to interrogate a stricture. When faced with a ductal stricture of unclear cause on ERCP and no clear pancreatic lesion on imaging, IDUS is

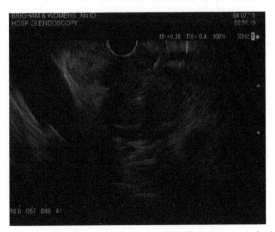

Fig. 18. EUS with FNA. FNA needle is shown accessing the pancreatic lesion.

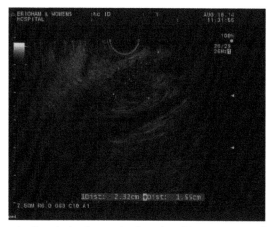

Fig. 19. EUS demonstrating lack of vascular invasion. Measurement of pancreatic mass is shown. Portal vein is noted as anechoic (black) structure; well-defined border separate from the mass indicates lack of invasion into the portal vein.

helpful in ruling out malignancy, in combination with brush cytology.[44] However, EUS would be necessary to specifically rule out a pancreatic lesion.

Endoscopic ultrasonography with trucut biopsy EUS-guided trucut biopsy (EUS-TCB) accomplishes tissue acquisition using a deployment method similar to EUS-FNA but with a cutting needle that is larger in caliber compared with a standard FNA needle. Larger tissue specimens are acquired, allowing analysis of histology and tissue architecture in addition to standard cytology.

Greater efficacy has not been definitively demonstrated for EUS-TCB compared with EUS-FNA, although safety is comparable.[45] Although EUS-TCB is not widely used, its performance characteristics and associated device development are areas of active research.[26]

Endoscopic ultrasonography with elastography EUS with elastography provides greater sophistication in characterizing pancreatic lesions in comparison to standard EUS, which cannot always differentiate between a neoplastic lesion and an area of inflammation. This technique provides potential histologic differentiation without more invasive tissue sampling.

A 2009 study demonstrated sensitivity and specificity for pancreatic cancer in 100% and 85.5%, respectively.[46] Although promising, EUS with elastography is not widely used at present.

Contrast-enhanced endoscopic ultrasonography Administration of intravenous US contrast agents can improve differentiation between benign and malignant lesions of the pancreas during EUS. The first feasibility study in 2001 with 23 patients showed sensitivity and specificity of 94% and 100%, respectively, for differentiation between pancreatic carcinoma and inflammatory changes.[47] This technique requires specialized expertise and has not gained widespread use as of yet.

Upper endoscopy with optical spectroscopy Spectroscopy during standard upper endoscopy has been developed to detect early mucosal changes heralding pancreatic cancer, without more invasive tissue sampling. According to field effect theory, by detecting microvascular changes in surrounding tissue, neoplastic lesions can be identified.

A pilot study including 14 patients with pancreatic cancer and 15 controls used fiber-optic spectroscopy during upper endoscopy to examine and assess the periampullary tissues. Spectroscopy was able to detect pancreatic cancer with a sensitivity of 92% and specificity of 86%.[48]

Treatment

The therapeutic role of endoscopy in the management of pancreatic cancer is traditionally supplemental, focusing on treatment of malignant complications. However, novel endoscopic techniques have also emerged that render treatment on the primary lesion itself.

Therapy for biliary obstruction

Endoscopic retrograde cholangiopancreatography with stenting Biliary strictures may be caused by the primary pancreatic malignancy, lymph nodes, and/or metastatic lesions, and decompression by ERCP with stenting is common.

The choice of stent material (plastic or metal), size, and coating (covered or uncovered) depends on the resectability of the pancreatic cancer, the patient's specific biliary anatomy, and the endoscopist's preference. Generally, compared with metal stents, plastic stents are usually easier to place but have higher occlusion rates and require more frequent exchange.

In planning for ERCP with stenting, tumor resectability must be considered, because resectable and unresectable pancreatic cancers represent 2 distinct populations (**Box 1**).

Endoscopic ultrasonography-assisted biliary drainage Pancreatic cancer may cause the biliary system to be inaccessible via traditional ERCP because of obstruction of the duodenal lumen, distortion of the ampulla, or both. A viable option in some cases is EUS-assisted biliary drainage, in which the bile duct is accessed via EUS-guided deployment with a transmural FNA needle from the stomach or duodenal bulb followed by biliary stent placement transmurally or across the major papilla (**Fig. 21**). Success rates have been shown to be 70% to 97% in large series, but use of this complex technique is currently limited to a few specialized centers.[51]

Therapy for other complications

Gastroduodenal obstruction: enteral stenting Endoscopic enteral stent placement is a viable nonsurgical alternative for gastroduodenal obstruction secondary to unresectable pancreatic cancer in patients with life expectancy less than 6 months (**Fig. 22**). Comparative data are limited, but outcomes in surgery versus stenting are similar, with shorter hospitalization/recovery time for stents. Enteral stents are not associated with improvement in survival.[25]

For patients with life expectancy greater than 6 months, surgical decompression (ie, gastrojejunostomy) is more effective because of risk of enteral stent occlusion.[52] In cases of multiple sites of bowel obstruction, stenting the proximal obstruction does not address more distal obstructions.

A comprehensive review of 32 case series (606 patients with pancreatic cancer and gastroduodenal obstruction) demonstrated successful advancement to soft mechanical diet in 87% of patients after enteral stent placement.[53] Rates of major complications are noted in **Table 2**.

Importantly, the major papilla usually cannot be accessed after gastroduodenal stenting. Thus, when gastroduodenal obstruction is present while biliary obstruction

---

Box 1
Biliary stenting in resectable versus unresectable pancreatic cancer

Resectable

- Benefit of preoperative ERCP with biliary stenting is controversial. On the one hand, placement of a preoperative plastic stent or distal metal stent does not interfere with surgery and doing so relieves jaundice, prevents cholestatic complications, and facilitates neoadjuvant chemotherapy (see **Fig. 20**). On the other hand, proceeding directly to surgery limits the number of invasive procedures and may decrease costs and complications.

- A seminal study of 202 patients demonstrated a much higher rate of serious complications—74% vs 39%—in patients undergoing preoperative biliary drainage followed by surgery compared with surgery alone; mortality rates did not differ. Of note, in the preoperative drainage group, ERCP-associated complications occurred at an unusually high rate (46%), and plastic stents were used exclusively.[49]

- A more recent study of 241 patients who underwent preoperative ERCP with placement of an uncovered metal stent demonstrated a significantly lower (18%) rate of complications associated with biliary drainage.[50]

- Many centers continue to endorse routine preoperative biliary drainage even when the diagnosis of pancreatic cancer is confirmed/presumed and surgery is planned. In such cases, short metal stents (placed most distally so as to not interfere with surgery) are usually the intervention of choice.

Unresectable

- In patients with no plan for surgery, goals are to provide biliary decompression to mitigate cholestatic symptoms, maximize quality of life, and facilitate palliative chemotherapy if indicated. These cases may be technically challenging, particularly if the lesion is large or if lymphadenopathy/metastases are present. Patients with advanced pancreatic cancer may also be quite frail, and the decision to pursue ERCP should be made with caution.

- Typically, biliary stenting for patients with unresectable disease uses a metal stent without plans for further ERCP. In a large meta-analysis of 24 studies containing 2436 patients comparing surgery, endoscopic plastic stent, and endoscopic metal stent for palliative relief of distal biliary obstruction, endoscopic metal stent was favored, with outcomes similar to those of using plastic stents but with improved patency rates.[40]

---

is suspected or impending, metal biliary stent placement should be done before gastroduodenal stent placement.[54]

Adjunctive therapy: endoscopic ultrasonography-guided fiducial placement
Fiducials are inert radiographic markers (small cylindrical or coil-shaped gold fragments) implanted to facilitate targeting of radiation therapy. Although traditionally placed percutaneously or surgically, EUS-guided fiducial placement in the pancreas has been shown to be feasible and safe, with complication rates comparable with those of EUS-FNA (see **Fig. 23**).[55]

Direct therapy: endoscopic ultrasonography-guided fine-needle injection
Moving beyond a diagnostic/supportive role, endoscopy's potential in direct therapy for pancreatic cancer has been demonstrated via EUS-guided fine-needle injection,

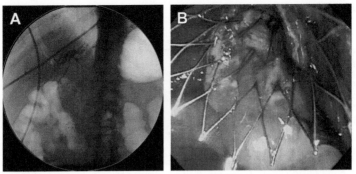

Fig. 20. ERCP with metal stent deployment for malignant stricture. Malignant stricture is seen in the distal common bile duct. One uncovered metal biliary stent is shown in position across the stricture, with fluoroscopic (*A*) and endoscopic (*B*) views.

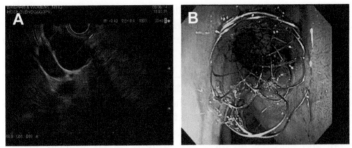

Fig. 21. EUS-guided choledochoduodenostomy with stent placement. Transduodenal puncture with FNA needle into the bile duct is seen on endosonographic view (*A*). Endoscopic view of successfully placed transmural covered metal biliary stent is shown (*B*).

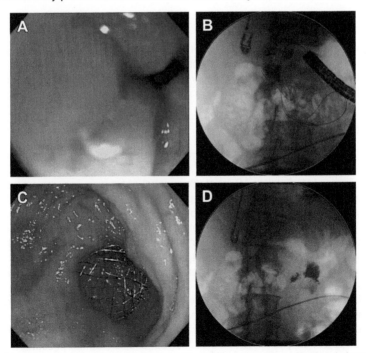

Fig. 22. Gastroduodenal obstruction treated with enteral stent. Gastroduodenal obstruction is shown with endoscopic view of narrowed lumen (*A*) and with fluoroscopic view of contrast pattern and guidewire across the stenosis (*B*). Enteral stent shown in good position, endoscopically protruding from the pylorus proximally (*C*) and traversing the stenosis fluoroscopically (*D*).

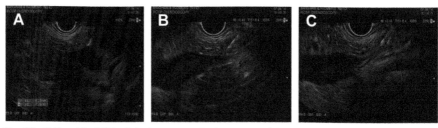

Fig. 23. EUS-guided fiducial placement. Endosonographic measurement of the pancreatic lesion is shown (*A*). FNA needle is deployed to the lesion, and fiducials are injected (*B*). Fiducials are in good position and are visible as hyperechoic (bright) objects in the lesion (*C*).

delivering a variety of therapeutic agents—allogenic mixed lymphocyte culture, modified viral vectors for drug delivery, immature dendritic cells, and DNA plasmids.[56–59] Unfortunately, significant tumor response and/or survival benefit has not yet been seen.

Endoscopy: Conclusion

The relationship between imaging and endoscopy in pancreatic cancer is a complementary one. Imaging may first detect the pancreatic lesion or its sequelae, and endoscopy can render both diagnosis and therapy as the next steps in management.

Newer endoscopic techniques such as cholangioscopy/pancreatoscopy, novel EUS imaging, and EUS-guided therapeutics have shown promise. As these techniques are further studied, their integration into the management of pancreatic cancer will become more defined.

SUMMARY

Noninvasive imaging and endoscopy offer a wealth of diagnostic and therapeutic tools for use throughout the management of pancreatic cancer. These tools provide complementary strengths when appropriately used as part of a multidisciplinary program of cancer care.

REFERENCES

1. Edge SB, Byrd DR, Compton CC, et al. AJCC cancer staging manual. 7th edition. New York: Springer; 2010.
2. Yu J, Turner MA, Fulcher AS, et al. Congenital anomalies and normal variants of the pancreaticobiliary tract and the pancreas in adults: part 2, Pancreatic duct and pancreas. AJR Am J Roentgenol 2006;187:1544–53.
3. Winston CB, Lee NA, Jarnagin WR, et al. CT angiography for delineation of celiac and superior mesenteric artery variants in patients undergoing hepatobiliary and pancreatic surgery. AJR Am J Roentgenol 2007;189:W13–9.
4. Baylin GJ, Weeks KD. Some Roentgen aspects of pancreatic necrosis. Radiology 1944;42:466–70.
5. Manfredi R, Costamagna G, Brizi MG, et al. Severe chronic pancreatitis versus suspected pancreatic disease: dynamic MR cholangiopancreatography after secretin stimulation. Radiology 2000;214:849–55.
6. Varadhachary GR, Tamm EP, Abbruzzese JL, et al. Borderline resectable pancreatic cancer: definitions, management, and role of preoperative therapy. Ann Surg Oncol 2006;13:1035–46.

7. Kamisawa T, Takuma K, Anjiki H, et al. Differentiation of autoimmune pancreatitis from pancreatic cancer by diffusion-weighted MRI. Am J Gastroenterol 2010; 105:1870–5.

8. Semelka RC, Kroeker MA, Shoenut JP, et al. Pancreatic disease: prospective comparison of CT, ERCP, and 1.5-T MR imaging with dynamic gadolinium enhancement and fat suppression. Radiology 1991;181:785–91.

9. Bilimoria KY, Bentrem DJ, Ko CY, et al. Validation of the 6th edition AJCC pancreatic cancer staging system: report from the National Cancer Database. Cancer 2007;110:738–44.

10. Callery MP, Chang KJ, Fishman EK, et al. Pretreatment assessment of resectable and borderline resectable pancreatic cancer: expert consensus statement. Ann Surg Oncol 2009;16:1727–33.

11. Tran Cao HS, Balachandran A, Wang H, et al. Radiographic tumor-vein interface as a predictor of intraoperative, pathologic, and oncologic outcomes in resectable and borderline resectable pancreatic cancer. J Gastrointest Surg 2014;18: 269–78 [discussion: 78].

12. Lu D, Reber HA, KraSny RM, et al. Local staging of pancreatic cancer: criteria for unresectability of major vessels as revealed by pancreatic-phase, thin-section helical CT. AJR Am J Roentgenol 1997;168:1439–43.

13. Katz MH, Marsh R, Herman JM, et al. Borderline resectable pancreatic cancer: need for standardization and methods for optimal clinical trial design. Ann Surg Oncol 2013;20:2787–95.

14. Tempero MA, Malafa MP, Behrman SW, et al. Pancreatic adenocarcinoma, version 2.2014: featured updates to the NCCN guidelines. J Natl Compr Canc Netw 2014;12:1083–93.

15. Cassinotto C, Mouries A, Lafourcade JP, et al. Locally advanced pancreatic adenocarcinoma: reassessment of response with CT after neoadjuvant chemotherapy and radiation therapy. Radiology 2014;273:108–16.

16. Katz MH, Fleming JB, Bhosale P, et al. Response of borderline resectable pancreatic cancer to neoadjuvant therapy is not reflected by radiographic indicators. Cancer 2012;118:5749–56.

17. Tempero MA, Malafa MP, Behrman SW, et al. Pancreatic adenocarcinoma, version 2.2014: featured updates to the NCCN guidelines. J Natl Compr Canc Netw 2014;12(8):1083–93.

18. Morgan DE. Dual-energy CT of the abdomen. Abdom Imaging 2014;39:108–34.

19. Patel BN, Thomas JV, Lockhart ME, et al. Single-source dual-energy spectral multidetector CT of pancreatic adenocarcinoma: optimization of energy level viewing significantly increases lesion contrast. Clin Radiol 2013;68:148–54.

20. Koay EJ, Truty MJ, Cristini V, et al. Transport properties of pancreatic cancer describe gemcitabine delivery and response. J Clin Invest 2014;124:1525–36.

21. Wang W, Shpaner A, Krishna SG, et al. Use of EUS-FNA in diagnosing pancreatic neoplasm without a definitive mass on CT. Gastrointest Endosc 2013;78:73–80.

22. Niederau C, Grendell JH. Diagnosis of pancreatic carcinoma. Imaging techniques and tumor markers. Pancreas 1992;7:66–86.

23. ASGE Standards of Practice Committee, Anderson MA, Fisher L, et al. Complications of ERCP. Gastrointest Endosc 2012;75:467–73.

24. Baron TH, Petersen BT, Mergener K, et al. Quality indicators for endoscopic retrograde cholangiopancreatography. Am J Gastroenterol 2006;101:892–7.

25. ASGE Technology Committee, Varadarajulu S, Banerjee S, et al. Enteral stents. Gastrointest Endosc 2011;74:455–64.

26. Iwashita T, Nakai Y, Samarasena JB, et al. High single-pass diagnostic yield of a new 25-gauge core biopsy needle for EUS-guided FNA biopsy in solid pancreatic lesions. Gastrointest Endosc 2013;77:909–15.

27. ASGE Standards of Practice Committee, Ben-Menachem T, Decker GA, et al. Adverse events of upper GI endoscopy. Gastrointest Endosc 2012;76:707–18.

28. ASGE Standards of Practice Committee, Early DS, Acosta RD, et al. Adverse events associated with EUS and EUS with FNA. Gastrointest Endosc 2013;77:839–43.

29. Alvarez-Sanchez MV, Jenssen C, Faiss S, et al. Interventional endoscopic ultrasonography: an overview of safety and complications. Surg Endosc 2014;28:712–34.

30. Fogel EL, Sherman S. How to improve the accuracy of diagnosis of malignant biliary strictures. Endoscopy 1999;31:758–60.

31. Glasbrenner B, Ardan M, Boeck W, et al. Prospective evaluation of brush cytology of biliary strictures during endoscopic retrograde cholangiopancreatography. Endoscopy 1999;31:712–7.

32. Parasher VK, Huibregtse K. Endoscopic retrograde wire-guided cytology of malignant biliary strictures using a novel scraping brush. Gastrointest Endosc 1998; 48:288–90.

33. Sugiyama M, Atomi Y, Wada N, et al. Endoscopic transpapillary bile duct biopsy without sphincterotomy for diagnosing biliary strictures: a prospective comparative study with bile and brush cytology. Am J Gastroenterol 1996;91:465–7.

34. Chen YK, Pleskow DK. SpyGlass single-operator peroral cholangiopancreatoscopy system for the diagnosis and therapy of bile-duct disorders: a clinical feasibility study (with video). Gastrointest Endosc 2007;65:832–41.

35. Kim HJ, Kim MH, Lee SK, et al. Tumor vessel: a valuable cholangioscopic clue of malignant biliary stricture. Gastrointest Endosc 2000;52:635–8.

36. Varadarajulu S, Eloubeidi MA. The role of endoscopic ultrasonography in the evaluation of pancreatico-biliary cancer. Surg Clin North Am 2010;90:251–63.

37. Harewood GC, Wiersema MJ. Endosonography-guided fine needle aspiration biopsy in the evaluation of pancreatic masses. Am J Gastroenterol 2002;97: 1386–91.

38. Chen J, Yang R, Lu Y, et al. Diagnostic accuracy of endoscopic ultrasound-guided fine-needle aspiration for solid pancreatic lesion: a systematic review. J Cancer Res Clin Oncol 2012;138:1433–41.

39. tenBerge J, Hoffman BJ, Hawes RH, et al. EUS-guided fine needle aspiration of the liver: indications, yield, and safety based on an international survey of 167 cases. Gastrointest Endosc 2002;55:859–62.

40. Moss AC, Morris E, Leyden J, et al. Malignant distal biliary obstruction: a systematic review and meta-analysis of endoscopic and surgical bypass results. Cancer Treat Rev 2007;33:213–21.

41. DeWitt J, Devereaux B, Chriswell M, et al. Comparison of endoscopic ultrasonography and multidetector computed tomography for detecting and staging pancreatic cancer. Ann Intern Med 2004;141:753–63.

42. Ahmad NA, Lewis JD, Siegelman ES, et al. Role of endoscopic ultrasound and magnetic resonance imaging in the preoperative staging of pancreatic adenocarcinoma. Am J Gastroenterol 2000;95:1926–31.

43. Arabul M, Karakus F, Alper E, et al. Comparison of multidetector CT and endoscopic ultrasonography in malignant pancreatic mass lesions. Hepatogastroenterology 2012;59:1599–603.

44. Levy MJ, Baron TH, Clayton AC, et al. Prospective evaluation of advanced molecular markers and imaging techniques in patients with indeterminate bile duct strictures. Am J Gastroenterol 2008;103:1263–73.

45. Varadarajulu S, Fraig M, Schmulewitz N, et al. Comparison of EUS-guided 19-gauge Trucut needle biopsy with EUS-guided fine-needle aspiration. Endoscopy 2004;36:397–401.
46. Iglesias-Garcia J, Larino-Noia J, Abdulkader I, et al. EUS elastography for the characterization of solid pancreatic masses. Gastrointest Endosc 2009;70: 1101–8.
47. Becker D, Strobel D, Bernatik T, et al. Echo-enhanced color- and power-Doppler EUS for the discrimination between focal pancreatitis and pancreatic carcinoma. Gastrointest Endosc 2001;53:784–9.
48. Patel M, Gomes A, Ruderman S, et al. Polarization gating spectroscopy of normal-appearing duodenal mucosa to detect pancreatic cancer. Gastrointest Endosc 2014;80(5):786–93.e1–2.
49. van der Gaag NA, Rauws EA, van Eijck CH, et al. Preoperative biliary drainage for cancer of the head of the pancreas. N Engl J Med 2010;362:129–37.
50. Siddiqui AA, Mehendiratta V, Loren D, et al. Self-expanding metal stents (SEMS) for preoperative biliary decompression in patients with resectable and borderline-resectable pancreatic cancer: outcomes in 241 patients. Dig Dis Sci 2013;58: 1744–50.
51. Dhir V, Artifon EL, Gupta K, et al. Multicenter study on endoscopic ultrasound-guided expandable biliary metal stent placement: choice of access route, direction of stent insertion, and drainage route. Dig Endosc 2014;26:430–5.
52. Jeurnink SM, Steyerberg EW, Hof G, et al. Gastrojejunostomy versus stent placement in patients with malignant gastric outlet obstruction: a comparison in 95 patients. J Surg Oncol 2007;96:389–96.
53. Dormann A, Meisner S, Verin N, et al. Self-expanding metal stents for gastroduodenal malignancies: systematic review of their clinical effectiveness. Endoscopy 2004;36:543–50.
54. Baron TH. Expandable metal stents for the treatment of cancerous obstruction of the gastrointestinal tract. N Engl J Med 2001;344:1681–7.
55. Sanders MK, Moser AJ, Khalid A, et al. EUS-guided fiducial placement for stereotactic body radiotherapy in locally advanced and recurrent pancreatic cancer. Gastrointest Endosc 2010;71:1178–84.
56. Chang KJ, Nguyen PT, Thompson JA, et al. Phase I clinical trial of allogeneic mixed lymphocyte culture (cytoimplant) delivered by endoscopic ultrasound-guided fine-needle injection in patients with advanced pancreatic carcinoma. Cancer 2000;88:1325–35.
57. Hecht JR, Bedford R, Abbruzzese JL, et al. A phase I/II trial of intratumoral endoscopic ultrasound injection of ONYX-015 with intravenous gemcitabine in unresectable pancreatic carcinoma. Clin Cancer Res 2003;9:555–61.
58. Irisawa A, Takagi T, Kanazawa M, et al. Endoscopic ultrasound-guided fine-needle injection of immature dendritic cells into advanced pancreatic cancer refractory to gemcitabine: a pilot study. Pancreas 2007;35:189–90.
59. Herman JM, Wild AT, Wang H, et al. Randomized phase III multi-institutional study of TNFerade biologic with fluorouracil and radiotherapy for locally advanced pancreatic cancer: final results. J Clin Oncol 2013;31:886–94.

Surgery for Pancreatic Cancer

Thomas E. Clancy, MD[a,b,c]

KEYWORDS

- Pancreatic cancer • Surgery • Pancreaticoduodenectomy • Whipple
- Distal pancreatectomy

KEY POINTS

- Surgical resection with negative margins offers the potential for cure for pancreatic cancer, although rates of local and systemic recurrence are high.
- Appropriate use of imaging and endoscopic techniques can determine resectability with high reliability.
- Surgery in high-volume centers can be performed with a perioperative mortality of 1% to 3% and 5-year survival approaching 20%, although surgical morbidity remains high.

INTRODUCTION

Pancreatic cancer is widely recognized as one of the most aggressive solid tumors and one of the most frequent causes of tumor-associated death in Western society. Surgical extirpation as part of a multimodality treatment course remains the only potentially curative therapy, although median survival is still only approximately 24 months in this select population.[1] Furthermore, only a minority of patients presenting with pancreatic cancer are candidates for surgical therapy due to the presence of either distant metastases or locally invasive disease.

Early skepticism for pancreatic surgery is seen in Moynihan's 1906 edition of "Abdominal Operations" in which he states that "the treatment of malignant disease of the pancreas by the surgeon can hardly be said to exist...the mechanical difficulties of the operation are well-nigh insuperable, and that if boldness and good fortune are the operator's gifts, the result to the patient hardly justifies the means."[2] Whipple's 1935 publication[3] describing surgical management of ampullary malignancy in 80 patients resulted in his name being commonly used to describe pancreaticoduodenectomy, although the anatomic and physiologic barriers to safe pancreatic surgery were

No disclosures.
[a] Division of Surgical Oncology, Brigham and Women's Hospital, 75 Francis Street, Boston, MA 02115, USA; [b] Pancreas and Biliary Tumor Center, Dana-Farber/Brigham and Women's Cancer Center, Boston, MA 02115-5450, USA; [c] Harvard Medical School, Boston, MA 02115, USA
E-mail address: tclancy@partners.org

Hematol Oncol Clin N Am 29 (2015) 701–716
http://dx.doi.org/10.1016/j.hoc.2015.04.001
0889-8588/15/$ – see front matter © 2015 Elsevier Inc. All rights reserved.

not realized until late in the twentieth century. Even in the mid 1960s, surgical morbidity of more than 60% and mortality of more than 25% persisted.[4]

Recent decades of progress in surgical and perioperative care have seen a decrease in perioperative morbidity to less than 35% and perioperative mortality to less than 2%.[5]

INDICATIONS/CONTRAINDICATIONS

Although surgical resection is the only potentially curative treatment for pancreatic cancer, benefit from surgical resection is limited to the subgroup of patients with localized disease in whom resection with negative surgical margins can be obtained. Patients with localized tumors are described as either "resectable," "unresectable," or "borderline resectable," largely based on involvement of local vasculature. With in-depth assessment of local and distant spread, at most 20% of patients are considered clearly candidates for up-front surgical resection.[6] See later in this article.

Thorough preoperative evaluation is essential before proceeding to surgical resection for pancreatic malignancy. Cross-sectional imaging and endoscopic techniques are used to assess involvement of nearby structures, and endoscopic retrograde cholangiopancreatography (ERCP) with biliary stenting may be required in the setting of preoperative biliary obstruction.

Imaging

Imaging studies must specifically address several pertinent points when considering patients candidates for surgical resection:

- Superior mesenteric vein/portal vein (SMV/PV) involvement
- Superior mesenteric artery involvement
- Celiac axis involvement
- Common/proper hepatic artery involvement
- Anatomic variants: origin of right and left hepatic artery, origin of common hepatic artery, presence of accessory hepatic arteries
- Regional and distant lymphadenopathy
- Local/regional invasion (inferior vena cava, left renal vein, left adrenal)
- Distant metastases (liver or lung)

Multiphase contrast-enhanced computed tomography (CT) timed to visualize both arterial and venous phases is generally the first preferred imaging method. The lack of local invasion or distant metastases can be predicted in most patients by using CT alone, particularly with multidetector helical CT scanners.[7] Contrast-enhanced MRI is often used interchangeably with multiphase CT scan for preoperative imaging.[8] MRI has the advantage of allowing magnetic resonance (MR) cholangiopancreatography, which offers superior visualization of the biliary or pancreatic duct. Published data do not convincingly demonstrate the superiority of either MR or CT as a cross-sectional imaging modality for detecting vascular involvement and local invasion.[9] Although PET-CT has the potential to detect occult metastases, it has a limited role in staging or pancreatic cancer. Sensitivity for disease is reported between 46% and 71%, with sensitivity between 63% and 100%.[10]

Endoscopic Evaluation

Endoscopic ultrasound (EUS) is useful for assessing small lesions and performing biopsy via fine-needle aspiration if pathology is required before surgical or medical therapy. EUS is useful in evaluation of resectability of pancreatic neoplasms, particularly involvement of the SMV/PV axis. EUS is particularly valuable with lesions smaller than 2 cm that may be particularly difficult to diagnose on cross-sectional imaging.[11] Although tissue biopsy may not be necessary in a patient in whom surgery is planned for a pancreatic mass, tissue biopsy is particularly important in cases of greater diagnostic uncertainty or if definitive or neoadjuvant chemotherapy is planned. Sensitivity of EUS is reported to be between 75% and 90%, with specificity of approximately 100% for pancreatic head tumors.[12] In a systematic review of more than 50 series of EUS for pancreatic neoplasms, the negative predictive value was only between 60% and 70%; thus, a negative biopsy must be interpreted within the appropriate clinical context and repeat biopsies may be needed if tissue diagnosis is essential to the treatment plan or clinical protocol.

ERCP is potentially useful for tumors of the pancreatic head. Cytology specimens via intraductal brushing can be of diagnostic use, although sensitivity is less than 50% for pancreatic cancer.[13] ERCP also provides the ability to relieve biliary obstruction. Routine biliary stent drainage is potentially useful in patients with biliary obstruction in those undergoing neoadjuvant chemotherapy or chemoradiotherapy. Otherwise, ERCP with biliary stenting is not used unless required for decompression of a severely obstructed biliary system.[14] Obstructive jaundice due to a periampullary mass can be associated with cholangitis impaired hepatic function, and altered coagulation due to decreased vitamin K absorption. Patients with bilirubin higher than 10 to 20 mg/dL or jaundice for more than 3 weeks are at particular risk for postoperative complications.[15] However, stent-related infections are associated with increased infectious complications after pancreatic surgery.[16] Randomized trials[17] and systematic reviews[18] have suggested no benefit to preoperative drainage. Preoperative biliary stenting is generally indicated for evidence cholangitis, complications of jaundice, coagulopathy, or anticipated delay to surgery, such as with the use of neoadjuvant chemotherapy. Otherwise, routine drainage has not been shown to be useful.[19]

Indications and Contraindications to Resection

More than 80% of patients with pancreatic cancer will present with unresectable disease,[20] and the vast majority of patients undergoing successful resection experience local or distant recurrence.[21] The primary factor determining management of newly diagnosed pancreatic cancers is therefore whether or not surgical resection can be obtained with a feasible chance at microscopically negative resection. In the past decade, several groups have attempted to define criteria of surgical resectability.[22–24] Criteria of resectability vary slightly among these proposed classifications.

Resectable disease is generally classified as the lack of vessel involvement of major vessels (SMV, PV, common hepatic artery, superior mesenteric artery, celiac trunk) (**Box 1**). Although the presence of an intact fat plane around vessels is often used to determine invasion, the lack of this radiographic finding is not universally consistent with invasion. Given the intimate association of the pancreatic parenchyma with the SMV and PV, tumors may frequently approach these vessels without invasion yet lack a radiographic fat plane. Descriptors such as "abutment" and "encasement" must often be interpreted cautiously as a result. In most classification systems, tumors are considered resectable with abutment of SMV or PV as long as there is no luminal narrowing or impingement (**Fig. 1**). Interpretation of localized lymphadenopathy is important when determining resectability. For instance, with spread to the hepatic artery lymph node, patient survival is similar to stage IV pancreatic cancer.[25]

The term "borderline resectable" was popularized by Maurer and colleagues[26] in 1999 and has evolved to include many tumors previously considered unresectable, such as those with more significant PV/SMV or superior mesenteric artery

> **Box 1**
> **Resectable pancreatic head tumor**
>
> - No locoregional vascular invasion
>   - Intact portal vein/superior mesenteric vein[a]
>   - No involvement of superior mesenteric artery
>   - No involvement of common hepatic artery or celiac trunk
> - No distant metastases
> - No metastatic lymphadenopathy outside boundaries of planned resection
> - Patient medically fit for major abdominal surgery
>
> [a] Differs in various classification systems. Tumor deemed resectable if it abuts vein but vein is patent,[22] if tumor abuts vein with no lumen narrowing or impingement,[24] or alternatively if there is no vessel contact.[23]

involvement. Resection of pancreatic tumors with venous reconstruction can provide survival benefits similar to resection without venous reconstruction,[27] although these benefits have not translated into similar confirmed benefit with arterial reconstruction. As noted, classification schemes of borderline-resectable tumors differ somewhat, particularly pertaining to degrees of SMV and celiac artery involvement.

Unresectable tumors are currently defined as those with more extensive vascular involvement (**Box 2**). All schemes consider encasement of the superior mesenteric or common hepatic artery to be unresectable disease (**Fig. 2**). Extrapancreatic disease is widely accepted as a strict contraindication to attempted curative surgical resection.

Diagnostic Laparoscopy

Diagnostic laparoscopy has the potential to identify small peritoneal disease that would not be identified by standard imaging techniques, and laparoscopy has therefore been

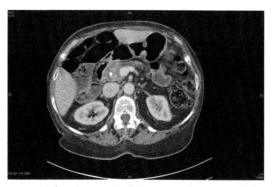

Fig. 1. Resectable pancreatic head tumor. Indistinct mass in pancreatic head is interpreted as abutting less than 180 degrees of SMV/PV junction. The tumor was thought to abut the vein, and no fat plane was seen between the tumor and the vein. Note the preserved architecture/shape of the PV. The tumor was removed with negative margins, without neoadjuvant chemotherapy.

Box 2
Contraindications to surgical therapy

- Locally unresectable tumor
  - Encasement of superior mesenteric or common hepatic artery
  - Invasion to inferior vena cava
- Distant metastases
- Metastatic lymphadenopathy beyond limits of resection
- Patient unfit for major abdominal surgery

used in the past before planned surgical resection so as to avoid unnecessary laparotomy in the patient with occult metastatic disease.[28] Occult metastatic disease has been described in up to 30% of patients on diagnostic laparoscopy, particularly in patients with locally invasive disease.[29,30] Although the incidence of occult metastatic disease may decrease with improved imaging, CT and MRI have lower sensitivity for small-volume disease. An alternative strategy of selective diagnostic laparoscopy has been advocated given the falling incidence of occult metastases, with laparoscopy used particularly for patients with a higher risk of metastases, such as in distal pancreatic neoplasms or locally invasive tumors.[31,32] Others have suggested a selective approach to diagnostic laparoscopy, with the use of laparoscopy for tumors larger than 3 cm; for all lesions in the neck, body, or tail of the pancreas[32]; or for patients with elevated preoperative levels of the tumor marker CA 19.9.[33]

TECHNIQUE/PROCEDURE

Surgery for pancreatic cancer primarily consists of 2 distinct operations, largely based on the anatomic location of the tumor to the right or left of the SMV/PV axis: pancreaticoduodenectomy for tumors of the pancreatic head, and left-sided or distal pancreatectomy for tumors of the pancreatic body or tail. Detailed descriptions of these surgical procedures are well-described in the literature and are beyond the scope of this review. The basic steps of each procedure are outlined.

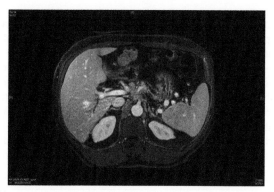

Fig. 2. Unresectable pancreatic head tumor. Clear involvement of the celiac axis renders this tumor unresectable.

Pancreaticoduodenectomy: Technical Considerations

Surgical exposure for a pancreaticoduodenectomy (Whipple procedure) is first obtained either through a vertical midline incision or bilateral subcostal incision. Several fundamental steps must be accomplished.

Exposure of anterior and posterior pancreatic head

An advantage of mobilizing the pancreatic head and duodenum early in the procedure is the ability to assess posterior invasion and more importantly to allow easier vascular control of the PV and SMV by direct compression. The peritoneum along the lateral duodenal border is divided from the porta hepatis to the third portion of the duodenum when the SMV is encountered, to allow sharp dissection underneath the pancreatic head and over the inferior vena cava.

Exposure of superior mesenteric vein

Traditional descriptions of pancreaticoduodenectomy have emphasized the importance of determining resectability of the tumor early in the operation by assessing involvement of the SMV and PV with tumor.[34] As SMV/PV involvement is not currently considered a strict contraindication to resection, other surgeons therefore delay any dissection underneath the pancreatic neck until later in the procedure, particularly when venous reconstruction is planned.[35]

Dissection of porta hepatis

Special attention must be given to arterial variants, such as accessory or replaced right hepatic arteries at this juncture. The PV is easily exposed after division of the gastroduodenal artery and division of the bile duct. The antrum of the stomach (or the postpyloric duodenum) is divided.

Inframesocolic dissection

The proximal jejunum is divided, dissected from the mesentery, and transferred beneath the mesenteric vessels to the right side of the abdomen.

Dissection of pancreatic head from mesenteric vessels

The pancreatic neck is sharply divided over the SMV-PV, and the specimen is dissected from the SMV and superior mesenteric artery. The specimen is oriented, and sent to pathology with or without frozen section analysis of the pancreatic neck margin.[36]

Reconstruction

Pancreaticojejunostomy is commonly performed with a duct-to-mucosa technique,[37] although others prefer a technique of invagination of the pancreatic neck into the jejunum.[38] A pancreatic duct stent is preferred by some to reduce pancreatic leak, although 2 meta-analyses have demonstrated that pancreatic duct stents do not change the rate of pancreatic fistula.[39,40] Anastomosis of the pancreatic stump to the posterior wall of the stomach is commonly used in some centers, with some studies demonstrating decreased risk of pancreatic fistula with pancreaticogastrostomy.[41] The hepaticojejunostomy is performed downstream from the pancreatic anastomosis in an end-to-side manner. Enteric continuity is established downstream from the hepaticojejunostomy, either within the lesser sac or in an antecolic manner.

Pancreaticoduodenectomy: Additional Considerations

Pylorus preservation

As classically described, pancreaticoduodenectomy entails removal of the pylorus and distal stomach. Pylorus-preserving pancreaticoduodenectomy (PPPD) was initially proposed as means of reducing the incidence of marginal ulceration at the gastroenterostomy.[42] Some have argued that PPPD may exacerbate the common postoperative complication of delayed gastric emptying.[43,44] However, retrospective studies have not confirmed this finding.[45]

PPPD has been compared with routine or standard Whipple in many studies, with outcome metrics including nutritional status, oncologic adequacy, morbidity, and surgical margins,[46–48] with most studies suggesting that PPPD does not impair oncologic margins or increase morbidity. Furthermore, several randomized studies comparing these procedures also have been reported,[49–52] demonstrating no difference in operative duration, mortality, length of stay, delayed gastric emptying, or oncologic outcome.

Vascular reconstruction

Although involvement of the SMV or PV with pancreatic tumors has previously been considered a contraindication to surgical resection, such involvement may be considered a function of anatomic proximity rather than necessarily of aggressive tumor biology.[53] Improved survival with PV resection versus palliative bypass has been demonstrated in a randomized study of patients with PV involvement with pancreatic adenocarcinoma.[54] Studies also have demonstrated increased frequency of postoperative complications after pancreaticoduodenectomy with vascular reconstruction.[55,56] Despite increased standardization in the diagnosis of borderline-resectable pancreatic malignancy,[22–24] variation remains even between high-volume pancreatic centers in terms of the degree of vascular involvement that constitutes a contraindication to surgery. Small defects in the SMV or PV may be closed primarily, otherwise reconstruction may be performed with an end-to-end anastomosis or vein grafts with internal jugular or left renal vein. Venous reconstruction is increasingly performed at high-volume centers for borderline-resectable tumors, although arterial reconstruction is shown to be associated with poor short-term and long-term outcomes, and is justified in only highly selected patients.[57]

Distal Pancreatectomy: Technical Considerations

Unlike tumors in the pancreatic head or neck, tumors in the body and tail of the pancreas do not require interruption and reconstruction of the bile duct or intestinal tract, nor is a pancreatic anastomosis required. The pancreas is removed left of the midline, up to or just to the right of the SMV/PV if necessary. Surgical mortality is considerably lower than with pancreaticoduodenectomy, although morbidity remains considerable with rates close to 50%; pancreatic leak or fistula from the pancreatic stump is one of the most commonly encountered complications.[58]

Splenectomy is often performed concurrently with distal pancreatectomy due to the close relationship between the pancreatic parenchyma and splenic artery and vein. Pancreatic resection performed while sparing these vessels could potentially lead to compromised surgical margins; thus, a vessel-sparing approach may be better suited to surgery for premalignant or benign disease. Distal pancreatectomy with spleen preservation is described with a technique to maintain spleen perfusion via the short gastric vessels off the greater curvature of the stomach.[59,60] Surgical splenectomy carries a small risk of postsplenectomy sepsis, and presplenectomy vaccination is recommended for pneumococcus, *Haemophilus influenzae*, and Neisseria meningitidis.

Open surgical exposure for distal pancreatectomy can be obtained either through a subcostal or midline incision. For either an open or minimally invasive approach, surgical steps are similar. The lesser sac is entered via the gastrocolic ligament between the stomach and the colon to expose the anterior pancreas. The splenic artery is isolated and divided on the anterior border of the pancreas, and the splenic vein is divided on the inferior surface of the pancreas. The pancreatic parenchyma may be divided either with surgical staplers, or sharply followed by mattress suture closure of the divided end. The remainder of the pancreatic parenchyma can then be dissected off the retroperitoneum with or without the spleen. Alternatively, the pancreatic tail and spleen can be mobilized from the retroperitoneum in a left-to-right manner before dividing the splenic vessels.

Fistula from the pancreatic duct is the most common complication after distal pancreatectomy.[61] Although single-institution studies have suggested decreased rates of pancreatic fistula by using various techniques such as staple line mesh reinforcement,[62] no method of pancreatic transection is universally demonstrated to be superior. Direct identification and suture control of the pancreatic duct may decrease the incidence of pancreatic leak,[63] although identification of the duct may be challenging, particularly after stapled transection.

Strasberg and colleagues[64] describe a modification of distal pancreatectomy referred to as "radical antegrade modular pancreaticosplenectomy" or RAMPS, with a goal of optimizing lymph node dissection and radial margins. The right-to-left dissection is primarily modified by ensuring a sufficiently deep posterior dissection behind anterior renal fascia and with or without removal of the adrenal gland and Gerota's fascia. Although these methods have not been compared in a randomized manner to standard techniques, single-institution studies report favorable 5-year survival compared with historical controls.[65]

COMPLICATIONS AND MANAGEMENT

Despite improvements in outcomes with pancreatic surgery over recent decades, morbidity remains more than 40% in most large series.[66] Improvements in surgery and postsurgical care have reduced perioperative mortality to less than 5% in high-volume centers, with many centers reporting perioperative mortality of less than 2%.[67]

Perioperative Mortality

Until relatively recently, pancreaticoduodenectomy was associated with postoperative mortality of more than 25%. With increase in experience and specialization, some centers began to report operative mortality rates of less than 5%.[68] The relationship between hospital and surgeon volume and outcomes has become well-established.[69–71] Birkmeyer and colleagues[72] demonstrated that pancreaticoduodenectomy shows among the strongest relationship between hospital volume and mortality for any procedure studied; mortality at hospitals defined as low-volume (performing <1 procedure per year) was 16.3%, contrasted to a rate of 3.8% for hospitals performing more than 16 Whipple procedures per year. Literature on the topic has been subject to methodologic criticism,[73] particularly due to the heterogeneity between studies. Definitions of what constitutes a high-volume hospital vary considerably between studies, from more than 6 pancreaticoduodenectomies per year[74] to more than 88 pancreaticoduodenectomies per year.[75] The precise nature of the relationship is also debated, with studies emphasizing the importance of individual surgeon experience[76] and complex systems of care within an institution.[77] Nevertheless, a strong correlation between surgeon and hospital volume and perioperative mortality is consistently demonstrated.[78] Specific high-volume centers have published postoperative mortality rates of 1% or less after pancreaticoduodenectomy.[79,80] Pancreaticoduodenectomy is associated with an approximately fourfold increased risk of postoperative mortality compared with distal pancreatectomy.[67]

Perioperative Morbidity

Pancreatic cancer surgery is associated with a significant rate of postoperative complications, yet measurement and reporting of complications is hampered by a lack of standardization in definitions and grading of severity.

Pancreatic fistula

Postoperative pancreatic fistula (POPF), or the leakage of pancreatic secretions from a pancreatic anastomosis or from the divided end of the pancreas, is one of the most frequent complications after pancreatic surgery. Variations in the precise definition of POPF has historically led to widely different rates of reported leak rates, from as low as 2% to more than 35%.[61,81] An internationally accepted definition was published in 2005,[82] defining a pancreatic fistula of any measurable fluid in a surgical drain on or after postoperative day 3 with amylase content greater than 3 times serum levels. Severity of the complication is also graded in this definition. Grade A fistulas are the most common; these are transient leaks requiring no significant change in management other than delayed removal of any surgical drains. Grade B fistulas may require hospitalization, treatment of infection, and somatostatin analogues. The more uncommon Grade C fistulas may require parenteral nutrition, percutaneous drainage, and extended hospitalization, and are associated with increased risk of mortality.

Delayed gastric emptying

Delayed gastric emptying in the absence of any mechanical obstruction can be seen after operations in the upper gastrointestinal tract, and is one of the most common postoperative complications after pancreatic surgery, seen in 19% to 57% of patients.[83,84] A standard definition is the inability to tolerate a regular oral diet after 1 postoperative week, and is also graded based on clinical impact.[84] In most cases, nutritional support is not required. More severe cases may require prokinetic agents or prolonged nasogastric drainage, usually with the need for nutritional support.

Postoperative hemorrhage

Significant bleeding in the postoperative period can be seen, with an incidence reported between 1% and 10%.[68,85] Early bleeding within 24 hours of surgery may require reoperation for hemostasis. Delayed bleeding more than 1 week after surgery may be related to pancreatic fistula with erosion into retroperitoneal vessels. This potentially lethal complication is best managed with early angiography with embolization or stenting when bleeding is recognized.[66] Bleeding from stress ulceration at the enteric anastomosis is diagnosed with endoscopic examination, and incidence can be reduced with the use of acid inhibitory medications.

OUTCOMES

Numerous large single-institution series have reported long-term outcomes after surgery for adenocarcinoma of the pancreas. Comparisons between studies over time is challenging due to differences in inclusion criteria and technique. Although modern imaging might theoretically lead to a more highly selected population undergoing surgery, contemporary series from high-volume centers may perform surgery on patients previously deemed inoperable for tumor characteristics, age, or medical comorbidity. Nevertheless, modern series repeatedly demonstrate 5-year survival in the range of approximately 20% in the select group of patients undergoing resection. A series from Massachusetts General Hospital reports actual 5- and 10-year survival after surgery for pancreatic cancer of 19% and 10%, respectively.[86] Surgeons from Johns Hopkins presented a series of 616 patients with pancreatic cancer over 15 years.[87] The overall survival was 63% at 1 year and 17% at 5 years, with a median survival of 17 months. Of note, survival for left-sided tumors at 1 and 5 years was 50% and 15%, respectively. A series of 1147 patients from Memorial Sloan-Kettering Cancer Center showed improved 1-year survival over 3 decades after pancreatic cancer surgery, but with similar overall median survival between 23.2 and 25.6 months. Five-year and 10-year actual survival rates were 18% and 11%, respectively.[88] Data from the Mayo Clinic also suggest 5-year and 10-year survival of 18% and 13% after pancreaticoduodenectomy.[89]

CONTROVERSIES/FUTURE CONSIDERATIONS
Minimally Invasive Surgery

The use of minimally invasive techniques, including laparoscopic and robotic techniques, to perform pancreatic surgery has been a topic of considerable debate. Minimally invasive surgery has the potential to decrease morbidity associated with incision-related complications, and thereby accelerate return to function with earlier administration of adjuvant therapy.

Minimally invasive procedures are particularly applicable to left-sided or distal pancreatectomy, as tumors less frequently involve local structures such as the SMV and no reconstruction or anastomoses are required. The use of laparoscopic pancreatectomy for distal tumors was examined in a meta-analysis demonstrating no difference in margin positivity between traditional open or laparoscopic procedures.[90] Other studies have confirmed the oncologic equivalence of laparoscopic and robotic distal pancreatectomy to open techniques,[91] although this had not been examined in a prospective controlled manner.

Application of minimally invasive techniques to pancreaticoduodenectomy has been more challenging. Series of minimally invasive pancreaticoduodenectomy are increasingly reported, including laparoscopic[92] and robotic[93] techniques for benign and malignant pancreatic head tumors. The benefits of minimally invasive pancreaticoduodenectomy have been questioned as the primary complications after Whipple procedure, specifically pancreatic fistula and delayed gastric emptying, are not related to the surgical approach.[94] Meta-analyses of published studies confirm the safety of minimally invasive pancreaticoduodenectomy with morbidity and mortality comparable to open techniques, although studies typically include highly selected patients with smaller tumors.[95]

Neoadjuvant Therapy for Resectable Tumors

Neoadjuvant therapy offers several theoretic benefits over a standard postoperative approach. Although increasingly used in patients with borderline-resectable tumors, neoadjuvant treatment has been proposed for all patients with pancreatic cancer. The presence of micrometastatic disease in most patients at the time of diagnosis is responsible for early recurrence. Neoadjuvant delivery allows more patients to receive chemotherapy in a timely manner, due to the delay for postoperative recovery and because up to 25% of patients do not receive postoperative therapy because of complications from surgery.[96] Numerous studies have evaluated the role of neoadjuvant chemotherapy or chemoradiotherapy in resectable tumors.[97] A comprehensive review of the topic exceeds the scope of this review, although despite the considerable theoretical benefits, little clear evidence supports the routine use of neo-adjuvant therapy in resectable pancreatic cancer. A systematic review and meta-analysis of 111 controlled trials showed no benefit to neoadjuvant therapy compared with adjuvant therapy in resectable pancreatic cancer.[98] Evaluation of studies is difficult because of differences in inclusion criteria, modalities, and regimens of neoadjuvant therapy. Properly addressing the issue of neoadjuvant therapy will require a randomized controlled trial using the most active combination chemotherapy regimens available.

SUMMARY

Surgical resection remains the only potentially curative therapy for pancreatic cancer, although only a minority of patients are candidates for resection. Recent decades have seen a dramatic decrease in perioperative mortality with refinement in surgical technique, improvement in patient selection and perioperative care, and concentration of pancreatic surgery to high-volume providers. Despite these improvements in mortality, pancreatic surgery remains associated with considerable morbidity. Minimally invasive and robotic surgical techniques have been applied with early success in pancreatic surgery, although it is unclear whether these techniques will be applicable in all patients with pancreatic cancer. Surgical resection with vascular reconstruction and after neoadjuvant therapy is increasingly considered in patients previously deemed unresectable because of local invasion. Despite surgical progress, pancreatic cancer has an extremely high rate of systemic recurrence, and further improvements in long-term outcomes for this disease will clearly depend on the availability of more effective systemic therapies.

REFERENCES

1. Neoptolemos JP, Stocken DD, Bassi C, et al. Adjuvant chemotherapy with fluoro-uracil plus folinic acid vs gemcitabine following pancreatic cancer resection: a randomized controlled trial. JAMA 2010;304(10):1073–81.
2. Clancy TE, Ashley SW. Pancreaticoduodenectomy (Whipple operation). Surg Oncol Clin N Am 2005;14(3):533–52, vii.
3. Whipple AO, Parsons WB, Mullins CR. Treatment of carcinoma of the ampulla of Vater. Ann Surg 1935;102(4):763–79.
4. Crile G Jr. The advantages of bypass operations over radical pancreatoduodenectomy in the treatment of pancreatic carcinoma. Surg Gynecol Obstet 1970; 130(6):1049–53.
5. Buchler MW, Wagner M, Schmied BM, et al. Changes in morbidity after pancreatic resection: toward the end of completion pancreatectomy. Arch Surg 2003; 138(12):1310–4 [discussion: 1315].
6. Konstantinidis IT, Warshaw AL, Allen JN, et al. Pancreatic ductal adenocarcinoma: is there a survival difference for R1 resections versus locally advanced unresectable tumors? What is a "true" R0 resection? Ann Surg 2013;257(4):731–6.
7. Smith SL, Rajan PS. Imaging of pancreatic adenocarcinoma with emphasis on multidetector CT. Clin Radiol 2004;59(1):26–38.
8. Clarke DL, Thomson SR, Madiba TE, et al. Preoperative imaging of pancreatic cancer: a management-oriented approach. J Am Coll Surg 2003;196(1):119–29.
9. Lee JK, Kim AY, Kim PN, et al. Prediction of vascular involvement and resectability by multidetector-row CT versus MR imaging with MR angiography in patients who underwent surgery for resection of pancreatic ductal adenocarcinoma. Eur J Radiol 2010;73(2):310–6.

10. Kauhanen SP, Komar G, Seppanen MP, et al. A prospective diagnostic accuracy study of 18F-fluorodeoxyglucose positron emission tomography/computed tomography, multidetector row computed tomography, and magnetic resonance imaging in primary diagnosis and staging of pancreatic cancer. Ann Surg 2009;250(6):957–63.

11. Wiersema MJ. Accuracy of endoscopic ultrasound in diagnosing and staging pancreatic carcinoma. Pancreatology 2001;1(6):625–32.

12. Helmstaedter L, Riemann JF. Pancreatic cancer–EUS and early diagnosis. Langenbecks Arch Surg 2008;393(6):923–7.

13. McGuire DE, Venu RP, Brown RD, et al. Brush cytology for pancreatic carcinoma: an analysis of factors influencing results. Gastrointest Endosc 1996;44(3):300–4.

14. Cohen S, Bacon BR, Berlin JA, et al. National Institutes of Health State-of-the-Science Conference Statement: ERCP for diagnosis and therapy, January 14–16, 2002. Gastrointest Endosc 2002;56(6):803–9.

15. Pitiakoudis M, Mimidis K, Tsaroucha AK, et al. Predictive value of risk factors in patients with obstructive jaundice. J Int Med Res 2004;32(6):633–8.

16. Mezhir JJ, Brennan MF, Baser RE, et al. A matched case-control study of preoperative biliary drainage in patients with pancreatic adenocarcinoma: routine drainage is not justified. J Gastrointest Surg 2009;13(12):2163–9.

17. Eshuis WJ, van der Gaag NA, Rauws EA, et al. Therapeutic delay and survival after surgery for cancer of the pancreatic head with or without preoperative biliary drainage. Ann Surg 2010;252(5):840–9.

18. Fang Y, Gurusamy KS, Wang Q, et al. Pre-operative biliary drainage for obstructive jaundice. Cochrane Database Syst Rev 2012;(9):CD005444.

19. Saleh MM, Norregaard P, Jorgensen HL, et al. Preoperative endoscopic stent placement before pancreaticoduodenectomy: a meta-analysis of the effect on morbidity and mortality. Gastrointest Endosc 2002;56(4):529–34.

20. Li D, Xie K, Wolff R, et al. Pancreatic cancer. Lancet 2004;363(9414):1049–57.

21. Yeo CJ, Abrams RA, Grochow LB, et al. Pancreaticoduodenectomy for pancreatic adenocarcinoma: postoperative adjuvant chemoradiation improves survival. A prospective, single-institution experience. Ann Surg 1997;225(5):621–33 [discussion: 633–6].

22. Varadhachary GR, Tamm EP, Abbruzzese JL, et al. Borderline resectable pancreatic cancer: definitions, management, and role of preoperative therapy. Ann Surg Oncol 2006;13(8):1035–46.

23. Callery MP, Chang KJ, Fishman EK, et al. Pretreatment assessment of resectable and borderline resectable pancreatic cancer: expert consensus statement. Ann Surg Oncol 2009;16(7):1727–33.

24. Tempero MA, Arnoletti JP, Behrman S, et al. Pancreatic adenocarcinoma. J Natl Compr Canc Netw 2010;8(9):972–1017.

25. LaFemina J, Chou JF, Gonen M, et al. Hepatic arterial nodal metastases in pancreatic cancer: is this the node of importance? J Gastrointest Surg 2013;17(6):1092–7.

26. Maurer CA, Zgraggen K, Buchler MW. Pancreatic carcinoma. Optimizing therapy by adjuvant and neoadjuvant therapy? Zentralbl Chir 1999;124(5):401–7.

27. Tseng JF, Raut CP, Lee JE, et al. Pancreaticoduodenectomy with vascular resection: margin status and survival duration. J Gastrointest Surg 2004;8(8):935–49 [discussion: 949–50].

28. Minnard EA, Conlon KC, Hoos A, et al. Laparoscopic ultrasound enhances standard laparoscopy in the staging of pancreatic cancer. Ann Surg 1998;228(2):182–7.

29. Jimenez RE, Warshaw AL, Rattner DW, et al. Impact of laparoscopic staging in the treatment of pancreatic cancer. Arch Surg 2000;135(4):409–14 [discussion: 414–5].
30. Liu RC, Traverso LW. Diagnostic laparoscopy improves staging of pancreatic cancer deemed locally unresectable by computed tomography. Surg Endosc 2005;19(5):638–42.
31. Hennig R, Tempia-Caliera AA, Hartel M, et al. Staging laparoscopy and its indications in pancreatic cancer patients. Dig Surg 2002;19(6):484–8.
32. Vollmer CM, Drebin JA, Middleton WD, et al. Utility of staging laparoscopy in subsets of peripancreatic and biliary malignancies. Ann Surg 2002;235(1):1–7.
33. Karachristos A, Scarmeas N, Hoffman JP. CA 19-9 levels predict results of staging laparoscopy in pancreatic cancer. J Gastrointest Surg 2005;9(9):1286–92.
34. Crist DW, Cameron JL. The current status of the Whipple operation for periampullary carcinoma. Adv Surg 1992;25:21–49.
35. Christians KK, Tsai S, Tolat PP, et al. Critical steps for pancreaticoduodenectomy in the setting of pancreatic adenocarcinoma. J Surg Oncol 2013;107(1):33–8.
36. Kooby DA, Lad NL, Squires MH 3rd, et al. Value of intraoperative neck margin analysis during Whipple for pancreatic adenocarcinoma: a multicenter analysis of 1399 patients. Ann Surg 2014;260(3):494–501 [discussion: 501–3].
37. Strasberg SM, McNevin MS. Results of a technique of pancreaticojejunostomy that optimizes blood supply to the pancreas. J Am Coll Surg 1998;187(6):591–6.
38. Zenilman ME. Use of pancreaticogastrostomy for pancreatic reconstruction after pancreaticoduodenectomy. J Clin Gastroenterol 2000;31(1):11–8.
39. Zhou Y, Zhou Q, Li Z, et al. Internal pancreatic duct stent does not decrease pancreatic fistula rate after pancreatic resection: a meta-analysis. Am J Surg 2013;205(6):718–25.
40. Xiong JJ, Altaf K, Mukherjee R, et al. Systematic review and meta-analysis of outcomes after intraoperative pancreatic duct stent placement during pancreaticoduodenectomy. Br J Surg 2012;99(8):1050–61.
41. Topal B, Fieuws S. Pancreaticogastrostomy after pancreaticoduodenectomy? Lancet Oncol 2013;14(9):e340–1.
42. Traverso LW, Longmire WP Jr. Preservation of the pylorus in pancreaticoduodenectomy. Surg Gynecol Obstet 1978;146(6):959–62.
43. Warshaw AL, Torchiana DL. Delayed gastric emptying after pylorus-preserving pancreaticoduodenectomy. Surg Gynecol Obstet 1985;160(1):1–4.
44. Hunt DR, McLean R. Pylorus-preserving pancreatectomy: functional results. Br J Surg 1989;76(2):173–6.
45. Yeo CJ, Barry MK, Sauter PK, et al. Erythromycin accelerates gastric emptying after pancreaticoduodenectomy. A prospective, randomized, placebo-controlled trial. Ann Surg 1993;218(3):229–37 [discussion: 237–8].
46. Patel AG, Toyama MT, Kusske AM, et al. Pylorus-preserving Whipple resection for pancreatic cancer. Is it any better? Arch Surg 1995;130(8):838–42 [discussion: 842–3].
47. Roder JD, Stein HJ, Huttl W, et al. Pylorus-preserving versus standard pancreatico-duodenectomy: an analysis of 110 pancreatic and periampullary carcinomas. Br J Surg 1992;79(2):152–5.
48. Grace PA, Pitt HA, Longmire WP. Pylorus preserving pancreatoduodenectomy: an overview. Br J Surg 1990;77(9):968–74.
49. Matsumoto I, Shinzeki M, Asari S, et al. A prospective randomized comparison between pylorus- and subtotal stomach-preserving pancreatoduodenectomy on postoperative delayed gastric emptying occurrence and long-term nutritional status. J Surg Oncol 2014;109(7):690–6.

50. Tran KT, Smeenk HG, van Eijck CH, et al. Pylorus preserving pancreaticoduode-nectomy versus standard Whipple procedure: a prospective, randomized, multi-center analysis of 170 patients with pancreatic and periampullary tumors. Ann Surg 2004;240(5):738–45.
51. Lin PW, Lin YJ. Prospective randomized comparison between pylorus-preserving and standard pancreaticoduodenectomy. Br J Surg 1999;86(5):603–7.
52. Lin PW, Shan YS, Lin YJ, et al. Pancreaticoduodenectomy for pancreatic head cancer: PPPD versus Whipple procedure. Hepatogastroenterology 2005;52(65):1601–4.
53. Fuhrman GM, Leach SD, Staley CA, et al. Rationale for en bloc vein resection in the treatment of pancreatic adenocarcinoma adherent to the superior mesenteric-portal vein confluence. Pancreatic Tumor Study Group. Ann Surg 1996;223(2):154–62.
54. Lygidakis NJ, Singh G, Bardaxoglou E, et al. Mono-bloc total spleno-pancreaticoduodenectomy for pancreatic head carcinoma with portal-mesenteric venous invasion. A prospective randomized study. Hepatogastroenterology 2004;51(56):427–33.
55. Castleberry AW, White RR, De La Fuente SG, et al. The impact of vascular resec-tion on early postoperative outcomes after pancreaticoduodenectomy: an anal-ysis of the American College of Surgeons National Surgical Quality Improvement Program database. Ann Surg Oncol 2012;19(13):4068–77.
56. Worni M, Castleberry AW, Clary BM, et al. Concomitant vascular reconstruction dur-ing pancreatectomy for malignant disease: a propensity score-adjusted, population-based trend analysis involving 10,206 patients. JAMA Surg 2013;148(4):331–8.
57. Mollberg N, Rahbari NN, Koch M, et al. Arterial resection during pancreatectomy for pancreatic cancer: a systematic review and meta-analysis. Ann Surg 2011;254(6):882–93.
58. Lillemoe KD, Kaushal S, Cameron JL, et al. Distal pancreatectomy: indications and outcomes in 235 patients. Ann Surg 1999;229(5):693–8 [discussion: 698–700].
59. Warshaw AL. Conservation of the spleen with distal pancreatectomy. Arch Surg 1988;123(5):550–3.
60. Ferrone CR, Konstantinidis IT, Sahani DV, et al. Twenty-three years of the War-shaw operation for distal pancreatectomy with preservation of the spleen. Ann Surg 2011;253(6):1136–9.
61. Irani JL, Ashley SW, Brooks DC, et al. Distal pancreatectomy is not associated with increased perioperative morbidity when performed as part of a multivisceral resection. J Gastrointest Surg 2008;12(12):2177–82.
62. Hamilton NA, Porembka MR, Johnston FM, et al. Mesh reinforcement of pancre-atic transection decreases incidence of pancreatic occlusion failure for left pancreatectomy: a single-blinded, randomized controlled trial. Ann Surg 2012;255(6):1037–42.
63. Bilimoria MM, Cormier JN, Mun Y, et al. Pancreatic leak after left pancreatec-tomy is reduced following main pancreatic duct ligation. Br J Surg 2003;90(2):190–6.
64. Strasberg SM, Drebin JA, Linehan D. Radical antegrade modular pancreatosple-nectomy. Surgery 2003;133(5):521–7.
65. Mitchem JB, Hamilton N, Gao F, et al. Long-term results of resection of adenocar-cinoma of the body and tail of the pancreas using radical antegrade modular pancreatosplenectomy procedure. J Am Coll Surg 2012;214(1):46–52.
66. Hartwig W, Werner J, Jager D, et al. Improvement of surgical results for pancreatic cancer. Lancet Oncol 2013;14(11):e476–85.

67. Mayo SC, Gilson MM, Herman JM, et al. Management of patients with pancreatic adenocarcinoma: national trends in patient selection, operative management, and use of adjuvant therapy. J Am Coll Surg 2012;214(1):33–45.
68. Mohammed S, Fisher WE. Quality metrics in pancreatic surgery. Surg Clin North Am 2013;93(3):693–709.
69. Lieberman MD, Kilburn H, Lindsey M, et al. Relation of perioperative deaths to hospital volume among patients undergoing pancreatic resection for malignancy. Ann Surg 1995;222(5):638–45.
70. Birkmeyer JD, Finlayson SR, Tosteson AN, et al. Effect of hospital volume on in-hospital mortality with pancreaticoduodenectomy. Surgery 1999;125(3):250–6.
71. Birkmeyer JD, Warshaw AL, Finlayson SR, et al. Relationship between hospital volume and late survival after pancreaticoduodenectomy. Surgery 1999;126(2):178–83.
72. Birkmeyer JD, Siewers AE, Finlayson EV, et al. Hospital volume and surgical mortality in the United States. N Engl J Med 2002;346(15):1128–37.
73. Wouters MW, Wijnhoven BP, Karim-Kos HE, et al. High-volume versus low-volume for esophageal resections for cancer: the essential role of case-mix adjustments based on clinical data. Ann Surg Oncol 2008;15(1):80–7.
74. Simunovic M, To T, Theriault M, et al. Relation between hospital surgical volume and outcome for pancreatic resection for neoplasm in a publicly funded health care system. CMAJ 1999;160(5):643–8.
75. Balzano G, Zerbi A, Capretti G, et al. Effect of hospital volume on outcome of pancreaticoduodenectomy in Italy. Br J Surg 2008;95(3):357–62.
76. Birkmeyer JD, Stukel TA, Siewers AE, et al. Surgeon volume and operative mortality in the United States. N Engl J Med 2003;349(22):2117–27.
77. Urbach DR, Baxter NN. Does it matter what a hospital is "high volume" for? Specificity of hospital volume-outcome associations for surgical procedures: analysis of administrative data. BMJ 2004;328(7442):737–40.
78. Gooiker GA, van Gijn W, Wouters MW, et al. Systematic review and meta-analysis of the volume-outcome relationship in pancreatic surgery. Br J Surg 2011;98(4):485–94.
79. Cameron JL, Riall TS, Coleman J, et al. One thousand consecutive pancreaticoduodenectomies. Ann Surg 2006;244(1):10–5.
80. Traverso LW, Shinchi H, Low DE. Useful benchmarks to evaluate outcomes after esophagectomy and pancreaticoduodenectomy. Am J Surg 2004;187(5):604–8.
81. Buchler MW, Friess H, Wagner M, et al. Pancreatic fistula after pancreatic head resection. Br J Surg 2000;87(7):883–9.
82. Bassi C, Dervenis C, Butturini G, et al. Postoperative pancreatic fistula: an international study group (ISGPF) definition. Surgery 2005;138(1):8–13.
83. Miedema BW, Sarr MG, van Heerden JA, et al. Complications following pancreaticoduodenectomy. Current management. Arch Surg 1992;127(8):945–9 [discussion: 949–50].
84. Wente MN, Bassi C, Dervenis C, et al. Delayed gastric emptying (DGE) after pancreatic surgery: a suggested definition by the International Study Group of Pancreatic Surgery (ISGPS). Surgery 2007;142(5):761–8.
85. Schafer M, Mullhaupt B, Clavien PA. Evidence-based pancreatic head resection for pancreatic cancer and chronic pancreatitis. Ann Surg 2002;236(2):137–48.
86. Ferrone CR, Pieretti-Vanmarcke R, Bloom JP, et al. Pancreatic ductal adenocarcinoma: long-term survival does not equal cure. Surgery 2012;152(3 Suppl 1):S43–9.

87. Sohn TA, Yeo CJ, Cameron JL, et al. Resected adenocarcinoma of the pancreas-616 patients: results, outcomes, and prognostic indicators. J Gastrointest Surg 2000;4(6):567–79.

88. Winter JM, Brennan MF, Tang LH, et al. Survival after resection of pancreatic adenocarcinoma: results from a single institution over three decades. Ann Surg Oncol 2012;19(1):169–75.

89. Schnelldorfer T, Ware AL, Sarr MG, et al. Long-term survival after pancreatoduodenectomy for pancreatic adenocarcinoma: is cure possible? Ann Surg 2008; 247(3):456–62.

90. Venkat R, Edil BH, Schulick RD, et al. Laparoscopic distal pancreatectomy is associated with significantly less overall morbidity compared to the open technique: a systematic review and meta-analysis. Ann Surg 2012;255(6):1048–59.

91. Magge D, Gooding W, Choudry H, et al. Comparative effectiveness of minimally invasive and open distal pancreatectomy for ductal adenocarcinoma. JAMA Surg 2013;148(6):525–31.

92. Kendrick ML, Cusati D. Total laparoscopic pancreaticoduodenectomy: feasibility and outcome in an early experience. Arch Surg 2010;145(1):19–23.

93. Zeh HJ, Zureikat AH, Secrest A, et al. Outcomes after robot-assisted pancreaticoduodenectomy for periampullary lesions. Ann Surg Oncol 2012;19(3):864–70.

94. Correa-Gallego C, Dinkelspiel HE, Sulimanoff I, et al. Minimally-invasive vs open pancreaticoduodenectomy: systematic review and meta-analysis. J Am Coll Surg 2014;218(1):129–39.

95. Cirocchi R, Partelli S, Trastulli S, et al. A systematic review on robotic pancreaticoduodenectomy. Surg Oncol 2013;22(4):238–46.

96. Spitz FR, Abbruzzese JL, Lee JE, et al. Preoperative and postoperative chemoradiation strategies in patients treated with pancreaticoduodenectomy for adenocarcinoma of the pancreas. J Clin Oncol 1997;15(3):928–37.

97. Belli C, Cereda S, Anand S, et al. Neoadjuvant therapy in resectable pancreatic cancer: a critical review. Cancer Treat Rev 2013;39(5):518–24.

98. Gillen S, Schuster T, Meyer Zum Buschenfelde C, et al. Preoperative/neoadjuvant therapy in pancreatic cancer: a systematic review and meta-analysis of response and resection percentages. PLoS Med 2010;7(4):e1000267.

Perioperative Therapy for Surgically Resectable Pancreatic Adenocarcinoma

Lingling Du, MD[a,b], Melissa DeFoe, MD[c],
Marianna B. Ruzinova, MD, PhD[d], Jeffrey R. Olsen, MD[e],
Andrea Wang-Gillam, MD, PhD[a,b],*

KEYWORDS

- Resectable pancreatic cancer • Adjuvant therapy • Neoadjuvant therapy
- Predictive biomarkers • hENT1

KEY POINTS

- Several landmark phase III studies have demonstrated a survival benefit with adjuvant systemic chemotherapy in patients with resected pancreatic cancer.
- The benefit of adjuvant chemoradiation in this population remains controversial.
- Understanding of the role of neoadjuvant treatment in resectable pancreatic cancer is largely limited by small early-phase studies.
- Predictive biomarkers, such as the human equilibrative nucleoside transporter 1 (hENT1), are emerging in the adjuvant setting.

Disclosure: The authors L. Du, M. DeFoe, M.B. Ruzinova have none. J.R. Olsen provided consultancy for DFine, Inc regarding the use of radiotherapy for palliation of bone metastases; he has grants/grants pending from RadioMed, Inc; he has received payment for lectures including service on Speakers' Bureaus for ViewRay, Inc and has received travel, accommodations, and meeting expenses reimbursements unrelated to activities listed by the RSNA Resident & Fellow Committee. A. Wang-Gillam served as consultant for Merrimack regarding the role of the MM-398 in pancreatic cancer.
This publication was supported by the Washington University Institute of Clinical and Translational Sciences grants UL1 TR000448 and KL2 TR000450 from the National Center for Advancing Translational Sciences. The content is solely the responsibility of the authors and does not necessarily represent official views of the National Institutes of Health.
[a] Division of Oncology, Department of Internal Medicine, Washington University School of Medicine, 660 South Euclid Avenue, St Louis, MO 63110, USA; [b] Division of Medical Oncology, Alvin J. Siteman Cancer Center, Washington University School of Medicine, 660 South Euclid Avenue, St Louis, MO 63110, USA; [c] Department of Internal Medicine, Washington University School of Medicine, 660 South Euclid Avenue, St Louis, MO 63110, USA; [d] Department of Pathology and Immunology, Washington University School of Medicine, 660 South Euclid Avenue, St Louis, MO 63110, USA; [e] Department of Radiation Oncology, Washington University School of Medicine, 660 South Euclid Avenue, St Louis, MO 63110, USA
* Corresponding author. Division of Oncology, Campus Box 8056, Washington University School of Medicine, 660 South Euclid Avenue, St Louis, MO 63110.
E-mail address: awang@dom.wustl.edu

INTRODUCTION

Pancreatic cancer is a highly lethal disease with a 5-year survival rate of less than 5%.[1] It is the fourth leading cause of cancer-related mortality in the United States[2] and is projected to rise to the second leading cause by 2030.[3] Surgical resection offers the only chance for cure in pancreatic cancer; unfortunately, only 10% to 20% of patients present with resectable disease at the time of diagnosis because of the lack of effective means of early detection and the presentation of only vague clinical symptoms. Even in patients who undergo curative surgical resections, the 5-year survival rate remains low at 10% to 20%.[4,5] Clinical studies have explored the role of perioperative therapy, including adjuvant and neoadjuvant treatment, and the survival benefits of adjuvant therapy have been well established over the past few years. The role of neoadjuvant therapy has been explored but remains largely undefined. Efforts to identify predictive and prognostic biomarkers have been intense with encouraging results. Moreover, promising novel therapies have been incorporated in the adjuvant and neoadjuvant settings that may potentially improve survival.

DEFINITION OF RESECTABLE PANCREATIC ADENOCARCINOMA

Traditionally, to better prognosticate patients with solid tumors, pathologic staging with the TNM (tumor, node, and metastases) classification system is commonly used. However, because most patients with pancreatic cancer are not eligible for resection, clinical staging is more practical than TNM staging, in particular for patients with localized disease, a group wherein the tumor's vascular involvement is the deciding factor for resection. An expert consensus group published its criteria on the resectability of pancreatic adenocarcinoma in 2009.[6] Using multidetector computed tomography with triple-phase study, patients without distant metastases or evidence of tumor extension to the superior mesenteric vein and portal vein, and with clear fat planes around the celiac axis, the hepatic artery, and superior mesenteric artery are categorized as resectable. These criteria have clearly distinguished resectable pancreatic cancer from borderline resectable and locally advanced disease, and they have been well recognized and incorporated into clinical trial design. The same criteria are adopted in the National Comprehensive Cancer Network guidelines.[7]

ADJUVANT THERAPY
Major Phase III Trials of Adjuvant Therapy

Pancreatic cancer has a high rate of early metastases. Even in patients with resectable pancreatic cancer who undergo surgical resection, up to 70% of recurrence occurs at distant sites.[8,9] The rationale of adjuvant treatment is to administer therapy systemically with the intent of eradicating occult metastases. The benefits of adjuvant therapy have been validated in several large phase III clinical trials (**Table 1**).

Gemcitabine was approved by the US Food and Drug Administration for its superior clinical benefit compared with 5-fluorouracil (5-FU) in advanced pancreatic cancer.[10] Since then, gemcitabine has become the cornerstone treatment for pancreatic cancer. The benefit of gemcitabine in the adjuvant setting was demonstrated in the CONKO-001 trial (Charité Onkologie 001).[11] This is the first phase III trial evaluating the role of adjuvant chemotherapy in patients with resectable pancreatic cancer, and it is a landmark study of this population.[11,12] In CONKO-001, 368 patients who underwent resection for pancreatic cancer in Germany and Austria were stratified by tumor stage, nodal status, and resection status. Patients were randomly assigned to receive either 6 cycles of gemcitabine 1000 mg/m^2 on days 1, 8, and 15 every 4 weeks or be

Table 1
Major phase III trials of adjuvant therapy in resectable pancreatic cancer

Trial	Year	Pts	Treatment	≥T3%	N+ %	R0%	Failure, % Local	Distant	Median Survival, mo	Survival Rate, %
CONKO-001[11,12]	2007, 2013	368	a. Gem b. Observation	86	72	83	38	53	22.8 vs 20.2 (P = .01)	20.7 vs 10.4 (5 y) 12.2 vs 7.7 (10 y)
ESPAC3[13]	2010	1088	a. Gem b. 5-FU/LCV	NA	72	65	NA	NA	23.6 vs 23.0 (P = .39)	49.1 vs 48.1 (2 y)
RTOG 9704[17]	2008	451	a. Gem→5-FU/RT→Gem b. 5-FU/LCV→5-FU/RT→5-FU/LCV	75	66	66	28	73	20.5 vs 17.1 (P = .08)	22 vs 18
JASPAC 01[16]	2013	378	a. Gem b. S-1	87	63	87	21	47	25.9 vs not matured (P<.0001)	53 vs 70 (2 y)

Abbreviations: CONKO-001, Charité Onkologie 001; ESPAC3, European Study Group for Pancreatic Cancer 3; Gem, gemcitabine; JASPAC 01, Japan Adjuvant Study Group of Pancreatic Cancer 01; LCV, leucovorin; N, regional lymph node metastasis; NA, not applicable; Pts, patients; RT, radiation therapy; RTOG 9704, Radiation Therapy Oncology Group 9704; R0, complete resection with no microscopic residual tumor; T, tumor.

observed without any treatment protocol. The primary endpoint was disease-free survival (DFS), and the secondary endpoints included overall survival (OS), toxicity, and quality of life. Results were first published in 2007.[11] Gemcitabine was well tolerated with rare adverse events. Grade 3 or 4 hematologic side effects were experienced in 3.8% of patients, and 3.1% had grade 3 or 4 nonhematologic adverse events. Of 186 patients in the gemcitabine group, 111 (62%) patients completed all 6 cycles of treatment. The gemcitabine group had a superior median DFS over observation alone (13.4 vs 6.9 months, $P<.001$). An updated result was later published in 2013, which not only confirmed the benefit in DFS, but more importantly, demonstrated a prolonged OS in the gemcitabine group (22.8 vs 20.2 months; $P = .01$).[12] The 5-year survival rate was 20.7% in the gemcitabine group compared with 10.4% in the observation group. The 10-year survival rate was 12.2% versus 7.7%, respectively. This is the first time an actual 10-year survival outcome was reported in patients with resectable pancreatic cancer. This study also established the pivotal role of adjuvant gemcitabine in treating this patient population.

Although gemcitabine was superior to 5-FU in advanced pancreatic cancer,[10] whether this survival advantage persisted in the adjuvant setting remained to be determined. The ESPAC-3 (European Study Group for Pancreatic Cancer 3) trial was initially designed to evaluate the survival benefit of adjuvant chemotherapy with either 5-FU and gemcitabine versus observation alone following resection for pancreatic cancer.[13] After the CONKO-001 trial demonstrated a survival benefit with gemcitabine in resectable pancreatic cancer,[14] the observation group in the ESPAC-3 study was removed. Therefore, this study directly compared the clinical efficacy of gemcitabine to 5-FU in the adjuvant setting.[13] In the ESPAC-3 study, 1088 patients who underwent resection for pancreatic cancer from 159 centers in Europe, Australia, Canada, and Japan were randomized to receive a 6-month course of adjuvant chemotherapy with 5-FU at 425 mg/m^2 plus leucovorin 20 mg/m^2 on days 1 to 5, or gemcitabine 1000 mg/m^2 on days 1, 8, and 15 every 28 days. The 5-FU was associated with more grade 3 or 4 gastrointestinal side effects (eg, stomatitis, diarrhea), whereas the gemcitabine arm had more grade 3 or 4 hematologic toxicities. Overall, gemcitabine was better tolerated with a severe adverse event rate of 7.5%, compared with 14.0% in the 5-FU group. It was speculated that the 5-FU schedule (bolus on days 1–5) was partially responsible for the higher rate of adverse events. There was no significant difference in DFS between the 2 groups. Median OS was 23.0 months for the 5-FU group and 23.6 months for the gemcitabine group, respectively, and this was not statistically significant. Therefore, this study demonstrated that adjuvant 5-FU is equally effective as gemcitabine in resectable pancreatic cancer. In a practical sense, patients with resectable pancreatic cancer who cannot tolerate gemcitabine may receive 5-FU as adjuvant therapy.

On the other side of the Pacific Ocean, Japanese researchers have been exploring the efficacy of S-1 in the treatment of pancreatic cancer. S-1 is an oral fluoropyrimidine that results in survival outcomes similar to gemcitabine in patients with advanced pancreatic cancer.[15] The JASPAC 01 (Japan Adjuvant Study Group of Pancreatic Cancer 01) trial was designed to assess the efficacy of S-1 compared with gemcitabine in the adjuvant setting.[16] In this study, 385 patients were assigned to receive either adjuvant gemcitabine (1000 mg/m^2, on days 1, 8, and 15, every 4 weeks for 6 courses) or S-1 (80, 100, or 120 mg/d depending on body surface area, days 1–28, every 6 weeks for 4 courses) after surgical resection for pancreatic cancer. The primary endpoint was OS. S-1 was well tolerated and associated with fewer hematologic adverse events. Median OS was 25.9 months in the gemcitabine group and not mature in the S-1 group when the results were presented at the American Society of Clinical

Oncology (ASCO) 2013 annual meeting. The 2-year survival rate was 53% for gemcitabine and 70% for S-1. S-1 demonstrated clear noninferiority when compared with gemcitabine (hazard ratio [HR] 0.56, P<.0001), and was even superior to gemcitabine (P<.0001). This study showed the promising role of S-1 as the new standard adjuvant treatment for resected pancreatic cancer in Japan, and longer follow-up is needed to confirm the survival benefit of S-1.

The RTOG 9704 (Radiation Therapy Oncology Group 9704) trial has incorporated radiation into adjuvant therapy. The study was designed to compare the effectiveness of gemcitabine and 5-FU as adjuvant chemotherapy in combination with radiation. Both groups had 5-FU–based chemoradiation as the backbone.[17] In this study, 451 patients with resected pancreatic cancer were treated with chemoradiation with 5-FU at 250 mg/m^2 per day concurrent with 50.4 Gy radiation after the surgery. In addition, they were assigned to receive either 5-FU at the same dose or gemcitabine (1000 mg/m^2 once weekly), which was given for 3 weeks before, and for 12 weeks after chemoradiation. The median OS was 20.5 months in the gemcitabine group, and 17.1 months in the 5-FU group; the 5-year survival was 22% and 18% for these 2 groups, respectively. The difference in survival was not statistically significant. Multivariate analysis revealed a trend toward better survival outcomes with gemcitabine over 5-FU (P = .08). Subgroup analysis showed a survival benefit in patients with tumors in the head of the pancreas (HR 0.80, 95% confidence interval 0.63–1.00; P = .05). Since the publication of this study, many institutions in the United States use this regimen of systemic gemcitabine plus 5-FU–based chemoradiation in the adjuvant treatment of resectable cancer in the head of the pancreas.

In summary, several large phase III studies have established the survival benefit of adjuvant chemotherapy in pancreatic cancer. Gemcitabine has been the most commonly used adjuvant agent, and 5-FU was found to have equal efficacy. S-1 was recently found to be noninferior, and even superior to gemcitabine in patients with resectable pancreatic cancer in Japan. Chemoradiation can be used as part of adjuvant therapy in patients with tumors in the head of the pancreas.

Controversy over Adjuvant Radiation Therapy

Although adjuvant chemotherapy was proven to improve survival in patients with resectable pancreatic cancer, the benefit of radiation therapy in the adjuvant setting remains debatable. In the 1980s, the Gastrointestinal Tumor Study Group first observed a survival benefit in 43 patients who received postoperative combined radiation therapy and 5-FU (n = 21) compared with observation alone (n = 22; OS 20 vs 11 months, P = .03).[18] This was followed by a European Organization for Research and Treatment of Cancer study, in which 218 patients with pancreatic head and periampullary cancers were randomized to receive adjuvant radiation therapy and 5-FU versus observation alone after resection.[19] The treatment group demonstrated a trend toward improved survival, but the data did not reach statistical significance (2-year survival rate of 34% vs 26%; P = .099).

The ESPAC-1 trial was a phase III study assessing the roles of adjuvant chemoradiation and chemotherapy, in which 541 patients were randomized by a 2-by-2 design to receive no treatment (observation arm), chemoradiation, chemotherapy, or combined chemoradiation and chemotherapy.[14,20] This study demonstrated an improved survival in patients who received chemotherapy compared with those who did not receive chemotherapy (5-year survival rate was 21% vs 8%, P = .009). In addition, adjuvant chemoradiation was found to be detrimental, with a 5-year survival rate of 10% in patients who received chemoradiation versus 20% in patients who did not (P = .05). However, this study was criticized for its study design and confounding factors.[21] For example, because of allowed modifications in the study, a significant number of patients in the "no chemotherapy" group and "chemotherapy only" group received chemoradiation, which confounds the interpretation of the results. Regardless, the incorporation of radiation therapy in the adjuvant setting after resection of pancreatic cancer has fallen out of favor among European researchers. However, in the United States, adjuvant radiation therapy is largely considered to be part of the ideal adjuvant therapy. The ongoing RTOG 0848 trial, which directly compares patients treated with chemotherapy alone versus chemotherapy plus chemoradiation may offer a definitive answer on the benefit of radiation therapy in resectable pancreatic cancer.

NEOADJUVANT THERAPY

As adjuvant chemotherapy has demonstrated improved survival, multiple studies also have explored the role of neoadjuvant therapy as an alternative to the standard adjuvant approach. Neoadjuvant therapy offers all patients the opportunity of receiving full courses of chemotherapy and/or radiation without the potential delay secondary to surgical complications or prolonged postoperative recovery. Additionally, it helps identify patients who are unlikely to benefit from surgery because of futility in the setting of early, subclinical metastatic spread. Furthermore, the neoadjuvant approach provides an opportunity to examine predictive biomarkers for novel agents in pancreatic cancer.

Most of the early pancreatic cancer neoadjuvant studies used 5-FU as a radiosensitizing agent. In a phase II trial published in 1992, 28 patients received preoperative chemoradiation with 5-FU, and 61% underwent resection.[22] No patients experienced a delay in surgery because of treatment toxicities. Evidence of tumor cell destruction was well appreciated on the resected specimens. Although the survival data were not reported, this study demonstrated the feasibility of preoperative chemoradiation. It was followed by several other studies incorporating a 5-FU–based regimen, and a wide range of OS results were observed.[23–27]

After gemcitabine demonstrated better survival over 5-FU in patients with advanced pancreatic cancer,[10] most clinical trials for patients with resectable pancreatic cancer switched to studying gemcitabine-based regimens. The efficacy of neoadjuvant gemcitabine 400 mg/m^2 with concurrent radiation in patients with resectable pancreatic cancer was evaluated and published in 2008.[28] Seventy-four percent of these patients underwent resection; the median OS was 34 months and 5-year survival rate was 36% for patients who underwent resection, and 22.7 months and 27%, respectively, for the overall cohort. A study of the same chemoradiation regimen with the addition of gemcitabine and cisplatin given before chemoradiation was published later in the same year, and it showed a resection rate of 66% among 90 patients with a median OS of 27.4 months for all patients and 31 months for those who underwent resection.[29] Direct comparison across the 2 studies was difficult given the slightly different patient population. However, the survival outcomes in both studies were quite encouraging, even compared with the CONKO-001 or ESPAC-3 studies.

Overall, most of the clinical studies of neoadjuvant therapy are phase II trials with small sample sizes. Several studies have demonstrated promising survival, but more consolidating evidence from large clinical studies using more effective treatment modalities is needed to validate the benefit of neoadjuvant therapy in resectable pancreatic cancer.

BIOMARKERS PREDICTIVE OF OUTCOME

With the growing understanding of the genomic profile of pancreatic cancer,[30] many studies have investigated molecular markers for their ability to predict treatment response and survival outcome. One of the most promising markers is the human equilibrative nucleoside transporter 1 (hENT1). hENT1 is a transmembrane glycoprotein that mediates the cellular uptake of cytotoxic nucleotides such as gemcitabine and capecitabine.[31,32] Early studies suggested that in patients treated with gemcitabine for pancreatic cancer, those with detectable hENT1 in their cancer cells had longer median survival compared with those with absent hENT1.[32–34] However, other studies failed to demonstrate the predictive or prognostic value of hENT1 in patients with pancreatic cancer.[35,36] The ESPAC study group recently published their results using the tumor samples of 380 patients from the ESPAC-3 trial.[37] The expression of hENT1 on these tumor samples was analyzed. In the gemcitabine arm, patients with low hENT1 expression had a significantly worse median OS compared with those with high hENT1 expression (17.1 vs 26.2 months, $P = .002$). In contrast, this predictive value of hENT1 expression was not observed in either the 5-FU or the observation group. These findings may help guide clinical decisions when considering adjuvant treatment regimens for patients with resectable pancreatic cancer (ie, patients who have low hENT1 expression in their resected tumors might be better treated with chemotherapeutic agents other than gemcitabine).

WHAT IS ON THE HORIZON

Recently, immunotherapy has emerged as a promising alternative treatment for pancreatic cancer. One approach is the "HyperAcute" immunotherapy using algenpantucel-L. Algenpantucel-L are allogeneic tumor cells modified to express the αGal xenoantigen, an antigen that is not normally present in humans. When these modified pancreatic tumor cells are introduced into patients with pancreatic cancer, they can trigger a profound immune reaction leading to hyperacute rejection of the tumor cells. In a phase II study presented at the 2013 ASCO annual meeting, 69 patients who underwent resection for pancreatic cancer received adjuvant gemcitabine and chemoradiation with 5-FU as per the RTOG 9704 protocol, with the addition of algenpantucel-L vaccination every 2 weeks for 6 months.[38] Patients were randomized into 2 groups: the low-dose arm (100 million cells) and the high-dose arm (300 million cells). This vaccine was well tolerated with the most frequent adverse events being mild skin reactions at injection sites. Patients who had ≥25% increase in the antimesothelin antibody (anti-MSLN Ab) demonstrated better survival over those without significant anti-MSLN Ab increase (median OS 42 vs 20 months). The 3-year DFS rate for the whole cohort was 26%, and the 3-year OS rate was 39%. These results are encouraging. Algenpantucel-L is currently being further evaluated in the IMPRESS trial, which is a phase III study comparing standard adjuvant gemcitabine and 5-FU–based chemoradiation with or without the algenpantucel-L immunotherapy in patients with surgically resected pancreatic cancer (National Library of Medicine [NLM] identifier: NCT01072981).

As discussed previously, the role of adjuvant chemoradiation in resectable pancreatic cancer remains controversial. The RTOG 0848 trial is designed to investigate whether the addition of adjuvant chemoradiation to chemotherapy improves survival (NLM Identifier: NCT01013649). This is a phase II/III study following a 2 × 2 randomization design. Patients who underwent resection for pancreatic cancer are first randomized to receive 6 cycles of chemotherapy with gemcitabine alone or gemcitabine plus erlotinib. The accrual to the gemcitabine plus erlotinib arm was closed in April 2014. Patients without progression at the end of 5 cycles of chemotherapy are further randomized to receive either 1 cycle of chemotherapy followed by capecitabine or 5-FU–based chemoradiation or 1 cycle of chemotherapy alone.

This study is estimated to complete data collection in August 2020, and hopefully will unveil the true role of adjuvant chemoradiation in resectable pancreatic cancer.

Recent advancements in the use of chemotherapeutic agents have shown an encouraging survival benefit in patients with advanced pancreatic cancer. In the metastatic setting, both gemcitabine plus nab-paclitaxel and FOLFIRINOX (leucovorin, 5-FU, irinotecan, oxaliplatin) have demonstrated better survival over gemcitabine alone.[39,40] Large clinical trials incorporating these 2 regimens in the adjuvant treatment after resection for pancreatic cancer are ongoing. The Nab-paclitaxel and Gemcitabine vs Gemcitabine Alone as Adjuvant Therapy for Patients With Resected Pancreatic Cancer (APACT) study is designed to evaluate the effect of gemcitabine plus nab-paclitaxel compared with gemcitabine alone as adjuvant chemotherapy in patients with resected pancreatic cancer (NLM identifier: NCT01964430). On the other hand, a randomized phase II/III study comparing FOLFIRINOX given in both the neoadjuvant and adjuvant settings versus adjuvant gemcitabine alone for patients with resectable pancreatic cancer is on the horizon (NLM identifier: NCT02172976).

Overall, recent advancements in chemotherapy and immunotherapy have provided researchers new modalities in treating resectable pancreatic cancer. Several phase III studies with the incorporation of newer regimens are ongoing and hopefully can improve the survival of patients with resectable pancreatic cancer.

SUMMARY

Resectable pancreatic adenocarcinoma represents 10% to 20% of all pancreatic adenocarcinomas. Although surgery offers the only opportunity for cure, treatment with surgery alone still provides poor survival outcomes. Adjuvant systemic chemotherapy has demonstrated improved survival over surgery alone. Whether the addition of chemoradiation in the adjuvant setting improves outcomes remains controversial. On the other hand, neoadjuvant therapy has shown survival improvements in several phase II studies, but more consolidating evidence is needed to demonstrate a true benefit. With the recent advancement in chemotherapeutic agent combinations and immunotherapy, large clinical studies with more effective treatment modalities should be explored in resectable pancreatic cancer.

REFERENCES

1. Sun H, Ma H, Hong G, et al. Survival improvement in patients with pancreatic cancer by decade: a period analysis of the SEER database, 1981-2010. Sci Rep 2014;4:6747.
2. Siegel R, Ma J, Zou Z, et al. Cancer statistics, 2014. CA Cancer J Clin 2014;64: 9–29.
3. Rahib L, Smith BD, Aizenberg R, et al. Projecting cancer incidence and deaths to 2030: the unexpected burden of thyroid, liver, and pancreas cancers in the United States. Cancer Res 2014;74:2913–21.
4. Trede M, Schwall G, Saeger HD. Survival after pancreatoduodenectomy. 118 consecutive resections without an operative mortality. Ann Surg 1990;211:447–58.
5. Nitecki SS, Sarr MG, Colby TV, et al. Long-term survival after resection for ductal adenocarcinoma of the pancreas. Is it really improving? Ann Surg 1995;221:59–66.
6. Callery MP, Chang KJ, Fishman EK, et al. Pretreatment assessment of resectable and borderline resectable pancreatic cancer: expert consensus statement. Ann Surg Oncol 2009;16:1727–33.
7. Tempero MA, Malafa MP, Behrman SW, et al. Pancreatic adenocarcinoma, version 2.2014. J Natl Compr Canc Netw 2014;12:1083–93.

8. Sperti C, Pasquali C, Piccoli A, et al. Recurrence after resection for ductal adeno-carcinoma of the pancreas. World J Surg 1997;21:195–200.

9. Raut CP, Tseng JF, Sun CC, et al. Impact of resection status on pattern of failure and survival after pancreaticoduodenectomy for pancreatic adenocarcinoma. Ann Surg 2007;246:52–60.

10. Burris HA 3rd, Moore MJ, Andersen J, et al. Improvements in survival and clinical benefit with gemcitabine as first-line therapy for patients with advanced pancreas cancer: a randomized trial. J Clin Oncol 1997;15:2403–13.

11. Oettle H, Post S, Neuhaus P, et al. Adjuvant chemotherapy with gemcitabine vs observation in patients undergoing curative-intent resection of pancreatic cancer: a randomized controlled trial. JAMA 2007;297:267–77.

12. Oettle H, Neuhaus P, Hochhaus A, et al. Adjuvant chemotherapy with gemcitabine and long-term outcomes among patients with resected pancreatic cancer: the CONKO-001 randomized trial. JAMA 2013;310:1473–81.

13. Neoptolemos JP, Stocken DD, Bassi C, et al. Adjuvant chemotherapy with fluoro-uracil plus folinic acid vs gemcitabine following pancreatic cancer resection: a randomized controlled trial. JAMA 2010;304:1073–81.

14. Neoptolemos JP, Dunn JA, Stocken DD, et al. Adjuvant chemoradiotherapy and chemotherapy in resectable pancreatic cancer: a randomised controlled trial. Lancet 2001;358:1576–85.

15. Ueno H, Ioka T, Ikeda M, et al. Randomized phase III study of gemcitabine plus S-1, S-1 alone, or gemcitabine alone in patients with locally advanced and metastatic pancreatic cancer in Japan and Taiwan: GEST study. J Clin Oncol 2013;31:1640–8.

16. Fukutomi A, Uesaka K, Boku N, et al. JASPAC 01: randomized phase III trial of adjuvant chemotherapy with gemcitabine versus S-1 for patients with resected pancreatic cancer. Jpn J Clin Oncol 2013;31(suppl 4;abstr 145).

17. Regine WF, Winter KA, Abrams R, et al. Fluorouracil-based chemoradiation with either gemcitabine or fluorouracil chemotherapy after resection of pancreatic adenocarcinoma: 5-year analysis of the U.S. Intergroup/RTOG 9704 phase III trial. Ann Surg Oncol 2011;18:1319–26.

18. Kalser MH, Ellenberg SS. Pancreatic cancer. Adjuvant combined radiation and chemotherapy following curative resection. Arch Surg 1985;120:899–903.

19. Klinkenbijl JH, Jeekel J, Sahmoud T, et al. Adjuvant radiotherapy and 5-fluoro-uracil after curative resection of cancer of the pancreas and periampullary region: phase III trial of the EORTC gastrointestinal tract cancer cooperative group. Ann Surg 1999;230:776–82 [discussion: 782–4].

20. Neoptolemos JP, Stocken DD, Friess H, et al. A randomized trial of chemoradio-therapy and chemotherapy after resection of pancreatic cancer. N Engl J Med 2004;350:1200–10.

21. Abrams RA, Lillemoe KD, Piantadosi S. Continuing controversy over adjuvant therapy of pancreatic cancer. Lancet 2001;358:1565–6.

22. Evans DB, Rich TA, Byrd DR, et al. Preoperative chemoradiation and pancreati-coduodenectomy for adenocarcinoma of the pancreas. Arch Surg 1992;127:1335–9.

23. Pisters PW, Abbruzzese JL, Janjan NA, et al. Rapid-fractionation preoperative chemoradiation, pancreaticoduodenectomy, and intraoperative radiation therapy for resectable pancreatic adenocarcinoma. J Clin Oncol 1998;16:3843–50.

24. Hoffman JP, Weese JL, Solin LJ, et al. A pilot study of preoperative chemoradia-tion for patients with localized adenocarcinoma of the pancreas. Am J Surg 1995;169:71–7 [discussion: 77–8].

25. Hoffman JP, Lipsitz S, Pisansky T, et al. Phase II trial of preoperative radiation therapy and chemotherapy for patients with localized, resectable adenocarcinoma of the pancreas: an Eastern Cooperative Oncology Group Study. J Clin Oncol 1998;16:317–23.

26. Le Scodan R, Mornex F, Partensky C, et al. Histopathological response to preoperative chemoradiation for resectable pancreatic adenocarcinoma: the French Phase II FFCD 9704-SFRO Trial. Am J Clin Oncol 2008;31:545–52.

27. Turrini O, Viret F, Moureau-Zabotto L, et al. Neoadjuvant 5 fluorouracil-cisplatin chemoradiation effect on survival in patients with resectable pancreatic head adenocarcinoma: a ten-year single institution experience. Oncology 2009;76:413–9.

28. Evans DB, Varadhachary GR, Crane CH, et al. Preoperative gemcitabine-based chemoradiation for patients with resectable adenocarcinoma of the pancreatic head. J Clin Oncol 2008;26:3496–502.

29. Varadhachary GR, Wolff RA, Crane CH, et al. Preoperative gemcitabine and cisplatin followed by gemcitabine-based chemoradiation for resectable adenocarcinoma of the pancreatic head. J Clin Oncol 2008;26:3487–95.

30. Biankin AV, Waddell N, Kassahn KS, et al. Pancreatic cancer genomes reveal aberrations in axon guidance pathway genes. Nature 2012;491:399–405.

31. Costello E, Greenhalf W, Neoptolemos JP. New biomarkers and targets in pancreatic cancer and their application to treatment. Nat Rev Gastroenterol Hepatol 2012;9:435–44.

32. Spratlin J, Sangha R, Glubrecht D, et al. The absence of human equilibrative nucleoside transporter 1 is associated with reduced survival in patients with gemcitabine-treated pancreas adenocarcinoma. Clin Cancer Res 2004;10:6956–61.

33. Marechal R, Bachet JB, Mackey JR, et al. Levels of gemcitabine transport and metabolism proteins predict survival times of patients treated with gemcitabine for pancreatic adenocarcinoma. Gastroenterology 2012;143:664–74.e1–6.

34. Farrell JJ, Elsaleh H, Garcia M, et al. Human equilibrative nucleoside transporter 1 levels predict response to gemcitabine in patients with pancreatic cancer. Gastroenterology 2009;136:187–95.

35. Fisher SB, Patel SH, Bagci P, et al. An analysis of human equilibrative nucleoside transporter-1, ribonucleoside reductase subunit M1, ribonucleoside reductase subunit M2, and excision repair cross-complementing gene-1 expression in patients with resected pancreas adenocarcinoma: implications for adjuvant treatment. Cancer 2013;119:445–53.

36. Kawada N, Uehara H, Katayama K, et al. Human equilibrative nucleoside transporter 1 level does not predict prognosis in pancreatic cancer patients treated with neoadjuvant chemoradiation including gemcitabine. J Hepatobiliary Pancreat Sci 2012;19:717–22.

37. Greenhalf W, Ghaneh P, Neoptolemos JP, et al. Pancreatic cancer hENT1 expression and survival from gemcitabine in patients from the ESPAC-3 trial. J Natl Cancer Inst 2014;106:djt347.

38. Rossi GR, Hardacre JM, Mulcahy MF, et al. Effect of algenpantucel-L immunotherapy for pancreatic cancer on anti-mesothelin antibody (Ab) titers and correlation with improved overall survival. J Clin Oncol 2013;31(suppl;abstr 3007).

39. Von Hoff DD, Ervin T, Arena FP, et al. Increased survival in pancreatic cancer with nab-paclitaxel plus gemcitabine. N Engl J Med 2013;369:1691–703.

40. Conroy T, Desseigne F, Ychou M, et al. FOLFIRINOX versus gemcitabine for metastatic pancreatic cancer. N Engl J Med 2011;364:1817–25.

Diagnosis and Management of Borderline Resectable Pancreatic Adenocarcinoma

Lilian Schwarz, MD, Matthew Harold G. Katz, MD*

KEYWORDS

- Borderline resectable • Pancreatic cancer • Pancreatoduodenectomy
- Neoadjuvant therapy • Chemotherapy • Chemoradiation

KEY POINTS

- Pancreatic cancers with borderline resectable anatomy are those at high risk for a microscopically positive (R1) resection when surgery is used as primary therapy.
- Local tumor anatomy is best assessed radiographically with high-quality computed tomography using a pancreatic protocol.
- Patients with clinical findings suggestive of metastatic disease or at high risk for pancreatic surgery also may be considered borderline resectable on the basis of nonanatomic parameters.
- Patients with borderline resectable pancreatic cancer should be treated with neoadjuvant therapy before planned surgical resection.
- Response to neoadjuvant therapy for pancreatic cancer is difficult to assess radiographically or serologically.
- Laparotomy with intent to resect the primary tumor should be performed for all patients with borderline resectable disease who have no evidence of disease progression and who have a performance status and comorbidity profile appropriate for major surgery after receipt of neoadjuvant therapy.

INTRODUCTION

A margin-negative resection of the primary tumor with a complete regional lymphadenectomy represents a necessary condition for cure of pancreatic ductal adenocarcinoma (PDAC).[1,2] The staging designation "borderline resectable" has been

---

Sources of support: none.
Department of Surgical Oncology, The University of Texas MD Anderson Cancer Center, 1400 Pressler St, 17th Floor, Houston, TX 77030, USA
* Corresponding author. Department of Surgical Oncology, The University of Texas MD Anderson Cancer Center, 1515 Holcombe Boulevard, Unit 1484, Houston, TX 77030.
E-mail address: mhgkatz@mdanderson.org

Hematol Oncol Clin N Am 29 (2015) 727–740
http://dx.doi.org/10.1016/j.hoc.2015.04.004
0889-8588/15/$ – see front matter © 2015 Elsevier Inc. All rights reserved.

hemonc.theclinics.com

historically used to characterize local tumor anatomy that confers high risk for a microscopically positive surgical resection and/or early treatment failure after an initial surgical approach. For this reason, borderline resectable disease has been considered an intermediate stage of disease on a spectrum of resectability delimited by "resectable" and "unresectable" PDAC.

Many definitions and criteria for this disease stage exist, however, and all have been used heterogeneously in the literature. Interpretation of existing data regarding diagnosis, treatment, and outcomes for patients with borderline resectable cancer is therefore difficult. Furthermore, no data from prospective trials have been generated to guide the evaluation, diagnosis, or management of patients with this stage of disease, so essentially all decision-making is directed by low-level data or consensus.[3–8]

Herein we describe current thinking regarding the classification, definition, diagnosis, and management of patients with borderline resectable PDAC and discuss ongoing controversies relevant to this disease stage.

DEFINITIONS
Anatomic Staging (Borderline Resectable Pancreatic Ductal Adenocarcinoma Type A)

It has long been recognized that the prognosis of patients who undergo surgical resection for PDAC is highly dependent on the histopathologic status of the surgical margins. Indeed, complete excision of the primary tumor to microscopically negative margins (R0 resection) is associated with the best postoperative outcome. In contrast, patients who undergo total gross excision but have histologically positive margins (R1 resection) have a shorter duration of overall survival in most series.[9–12] Moreover, patients with gross residual disease (R2) after surgery have a prognosis similar to that of patients who do not undergo resection and are treated with palliative intent.[1,2] For these reasons, the likelihood of attaining negative surgical margins is a critical consideration when determining whether or not a patient is a potential candidate for pancreatectomy.[13] A precise assessment of resectability represents the most critical component of the pretreatment workup (**Table 1**).[14]

As it was first described in the 1990s,[15–17] borderline resectability was an anatomic designation that was used to describe tumors that appeared to involve the superior mesenteric vein (SMV) and/or portal vein (PV), hepatic artery, superior mesenteric artery (SMA), or adjacent organs on cross-sectional imaging, because resection of cancers involving these peripancreatic structures was typically complicated by high rates of positive margins, postoperative complications, disease recurrence, and early

Table 1
Intergroup criteria for the clinical staging of localized PDAC

Vessel	Potentially Resectable	Borderline Resectable	Locally Advanced
SMV-PV	TVI <180	TVI ≥180 and/or reconstructible occlusion[a]	Unreconstructable occlusion
SMA	No TVI	TVI <180	TVI ≥180
CHA	No TVI	Reconstructible[a], short-segment TVI of any degree	Unreconstructable TVI
Celiac trunk	No TVI	TVI <180	TVI ≥180

Abbreviations: CHA, common hepatic artery; PDAC, pancreatic ductal adenocarcinoma; SMA, superior mesenteric artery; SMV-PV, superior mesenteric or portal vein; TVI; tumor-vessel interface.

[a] Normal vein or artery proximal and distal to the site of suggested tumor-vessel involvement suitable for vascular reconstruction.

death. Today, most definitions for this stage of disease continue to focus on the radiographic extent of involvement of the major mesenteric vascular structures by tumor.[8,15]

Two anatomic definitions of borderline resectable PDAC are most commonly used in the literature, and both are based on multidetector computed tomography (CT) images obtained before treatment: type A of the criteria put forward by investigators from the University of Texas MD Anderson Cancer Center (MDACC),[8] and criteria adopted at a consensus conference attended by members of the Americas Hepato-pancreatobiliary Association (AHPBA)/Society of Surgical Oncology (SSO)/Society for Surgery of the Alimentary Tract (SSAT)[5] (and subsequently modified by the National Comprehensive Cancer Network [NCCN][13]). Both of these sets of criteria designate tumors as resectable in the absence of evidence for significant mesenteric vein or arterial involvement, as borderline resectable in the presence of evidence for minor to moderate mesenteric venous or arterial involvement, and as unresectable in the presence of evidence for unreconstructable mesenteric venous occlusion or significant arterial involvement.

In 1997, Lu and colleagues,[15] reported that a radiographic interface between a primary pancreatic tumor and an adjacent vessel measuring at least 180° of the vessel's circumference was a specific indicator of necessitating resection of the vessel to remove the tumor. Recent studies using accurate imaging protocols have corroborated this observation. Furthermore, attempts at resection and reconstruction of the superior mesenteric artery or celiac trunk have been associated with high rates of perioperative morbidity and low rates of long-term survival, but surgical results with hepatic arterial resection have been more favorable.[18] Finally, tumors that narrow the SMV and/or PV unilaterally have been associated with a more favorable disease-specific survival than tumors that narrow the vein bilaterally or occlude it.[19,20] These data suggest that tumors that infiltrate the left side of the SMV-PV toward the SMA have a higher likelihood of a margin-positive resection and poor outcome following pancreatectomy whether or not concomitant venous resection is performed.

Based on these data, and in an attempt to standardize the language used to describe borderline resectable cancers, investigators from the Alliance for Clinical Trials in Oncology, the Southwest Oncology Group, the Eastern Cooperative Oncology Group, and the Radiation Therapy Oncology Group have proposed a comprehensive classification system that was used in the Alliance Trial A021101.[6] This classification system recognizes any one or more of the following as radiographic identifiers of borderline resectable PDAC:

- An interface between tumor and the SMV/PV measuring 180° or greater of the vessel wall circumference, and/or reconstructible venous occlusion;
- An interface between tumor and the SMA measuring less than 180° of the vessel wall circumference;
- A reconstructible, short-segment interface of any degree between tumor and the common hepatic artery; and/or
- An interface between tumor and the celiac trunk measuring less than 180° of the vessel wall circumference.

Anatomic, Biologic and Physiologic Criteria for Borderline Resectable Pancreatic Ductal Adenocarcinoma

In practice, the exclusive use of anatomic definitions of resectability have limited value with regard to estimating prognosis among patients with localized PDAC because each anatomically defined stage actually includes a clinically heterogeneous population within it. Indeed, more than 50% of patients with resectable cancers are unable to undergo surgery at all, and the survival duration of inoperable patients with resectable cancers is similar to that of patients with metastatic disease.[21–23] Moreover, although the rate of 5-year survival is approximately 30% among patients who complete multi-modality therapy including resection, recurrence within the first 2 years occurs in more than 50% of resected patients.[24] Thus, no existing anatomic staging systems can adequately identify patients most appropriate for surgery because those systems focus exclusively on *resectability* of the tumor as opposed to *operability* of the patient.

In an attempt to identify patients with primary tumor anatomy, cancer biology, or patient physiology that places them at the limits of compatibility with favorable results after potentially curative therapy including surgery, we have proposed 2 additional subsets of patients who often escape accurate classification into a specific stage of disease[25]: patients with suspicion for metastasis and patients with a suboptimal performance status or extensive medical comorbidities requiring prolonged evaluation or optimization. Inclusion of these latter 2 groups into the borderline resectable category allows for accurate staging of all patients who present with newly diagnosed pancreatic cancer. The MDACC criteria thus add to the anatomic (Type A) criteria described previously with 2 additional sets of criteria for Type B and Type C borderline resectable PDAC, as described in the following sections.

Borderline Resectable Pancreatic Ductal Adenocarcinoma (Type B)

Rapid recurrence of cancer after resection is frequently observed, whether or not patients receive adjuvant therapy.[26,27] This observation highlights both the prevalence and clinical significance of the preexisting micrometasases,[28] and/or undetected or incompletely treated disseminated cancer cells[26,27,29] that exist in most patients with radiographically localized PDAC. Indeed, one of the main concerns in treating patients with PDAC surgically is the risk of early recurrence following complete resection of the primary tumor.

Based on our initial definition and the recent literature, patients with borderline resectable type B PDAC have resectable or borderline resectable (Type A) tumor anatomy in association with clinical findings suspicious but not diagnostic for extrapancreatic disease. Such findings might include radiographically indeterminate liver lesions or distant lymph nodes,[30] a biopsy-proven involvement of regional lymph node,[31] or a serum carbohydrate antigen (CA) 19-9 level greater than 1000 units/mL (with a normal total bilirubin); any and all of these findings suggest a particularly high risk for early treatment failure when surgery is used as primary therapy.

Borderline Resectable Pancreatic Ductal Adenocarcinoma (Type C)

The risks and benefits of surgical resection must be critically evaluated in the context of a cancer that has a particularly poor prognosis regardless of the therapeutic approach initially chosen. Moreover, to the extent that postoperative complications are associated with a reduction in patients' likelihood of receiving adjuvant therapy and the duration of their survival, the performance of immediate pancreatectomy should be discouraged among patients at particularly high risk for surgery.

Using our definition, patients with borderline resectable PDAC are those with a marginal performance status or a severe preexisting comorbidity profile (including advanced age) that put them at high risk for a major surgical procedure. Although historically this has been a relatively subjective assessment, useful tools now exist with which a personalized assessment of risk based on age, comorbidities, and frailty can be calculated.[32,33] Patients with type C should be managed actively in a multidisciplinary group of expert physicians, including a dedicated pancreas program dietician, physical therapist, and members of the internal medicine faculty to appropriately risk stratify and optimize each patient for eventual surgery.

DIAGNOSIS AND STAGING
Computed Tomography and MRI

The characteristics used to define resectable, borderline resectable, and unresectable disease anatomically are based on the use of cross-sectional imaging and require the use of imaging techniques that optimize the visualization of tumor, its relationship to adjacent anatomic structures, and its possible spread to nodes outside the surgical field and/or distant sites, such as the liver, peritoneum, lung, and bone.[7,8]

The NCCN guidelines recommend pancreas-specific CT or MRI be performed for all patients with localized PDAC.[7] CT and MRI constitute the most commonly performed primary investigations used for the diagnosis and staging of pancreatic cancers, and they have equivalent accuracy with regard to the assessment of vascular involvement and resectability.[34,35] The studies generally can be used interchangeably[36]; the choice between CT or MRI should be determined by the availability of both the individual modality as well as the technical expertise in reading and reporting their results. MRI is more expensive and less available when compared with CT. Furthermore, the ability of most surgeons to interpret CT images is superior than their ability to interpret MRI. Thus, MRI is typically used as a secondary modality when CT cannot identify or characterize the pancreatic mass, when an indeterminate liver lesion exists, or in the presence of a CT contrast allergy.

Because the evaluation of resectability on cross-sectional imaging currently involves determining in cross section the degrees of circumferential involvement of regional arteries and veins by tumor and narrowing/occlusion of veins, CT angiography (preferably 16–detector row or greater) is the generally preferred staging modality. The most commonly used CT protocol is a biphasic examination, with preferably submillimeter sections (0.5–1 mm). The pancreatic phase is obtained approximately 40 to 50 seconds after the administration of intravenous contrast (preferably using high iodine concentration of at least 300 mg iodine/mL and at a relatively rapid rate of injection at 3–5 mL/s). In this phase, the pancreatic parenchyma enhances maximally, producing the highest contrast difference between the optimally enhanced pancreatic parenchyma and the usually hypodense pancreatic ductal adenocarcinoma. The peripancreatic arteries are usually well opacified in this phase allowing for their concomitant evaluation. The second acquisition is obtained in the portal venous phase, approximately 65 to 70 seconds after contrast administration. In this phase, the portomesenteric vessels are usually well opacified, allowing for better evaluation of the venous system. The hepatic parenchyma, a common site of metastasis, is also optimally enhanced in the portal venous phase allowing detection of metastatic deposits that are typically hypodense. The administration of positive oral contrast can affect the postprocessing of the CT examination and the generation of the volume-rendered images. A neutral or low Hounsfield units oral agent is preferred.[3]

Endoscopic Ultrasonography

Among the available imaging tools, endoscopic ultrasonography (EUS) has emerged as a useful modality in the diagnosis of pancreatic tumors because of its ability to facilitate the acquisition of tissue biopsies with fine-needle aspiration. But the role of EUS in staging is not clear. Indeed, in a systematic review of the literature, heterogeneous study designs, quality, and results have been reported and no definitive conclusions could be made.[37] Moreover, EUS is invasive and operator dependent. EUS thus serves as a complementary staging investigation to cross-sectional imaging with CT or MRI.[38]

Radiologic Reporting

Accurate anatomic staging of localized PDAC at the time of presentation may maximize the survival benefit for patients in whom complete resection can be achieved and minimize the morbidity from unnecessary laparotomy or major surgery in patients with high risk of residual disease after resection. The use of standardized descriptions of radiographic anatomy, as might be used in templated radiology reports, also can help to facilitate research and allow for comparison of stage-specific treatment results between different institutions.[3] Reporting of the imaging findings for patients with pancreatic cancer should include descriptions of the primary tumor's size and location, the extent of the circumferential interface (tumor-vessel interface) between the tumor and major vessels (in degrees), the presence or absence of vessel occlusion, variant vascular anatomy, an anatomic assessment of local tumor resectability (resectable, borderline resectable [**Fig. 1**A], or locally advanced [see **Fig. 1**B]), and extent and location of extrapancreatic disease.

MANAGEMENT

Borderline resectable PDAC is the most challenging stage of pancreatic cancer to manage. Multidisciplinary collaboration by pancreatic cancer specialists facilitates accurate staging, optimal management decisions, and timely initiation of therapy. The initial staging is crucial to determine to resectability status in terms of anatomic (Type A), or nonanatomic criteria (Types B and C). Ideally, all patients with localized pancreatic cancer should be managed in a comprehensive, coordinated care program. The general algorithm used at the MDACC is illustrated in **Fig. 2**.

Pancreatectomy performed at specialized, high-volume pancreatic cancer treatment centers by high-volume surgeons improves short-term and long-term outcomes.[39,40] Indeed, survival is maximized only with the completion of multimodality therapy that includes surgery.[7,41] Involvement of surgical oncologists, medical oncologists, and radiation oncologists is particularly critical on the diagnosis of a borderline resectable tumor because patients with these cancers are at high risk for positive surgical margins, early metastases, and poor overall survival in the absence of multimodality therapy.

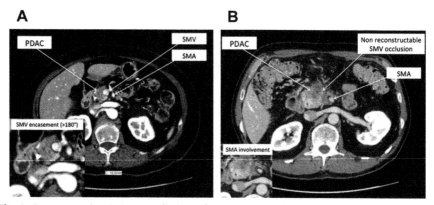

Fig. 1. Representative CT images distinguishing anatomically borderline from unresectable PDAC. (*A*) Borderline PDAC. (*B*) Locally advanced, unresectable PDAC.

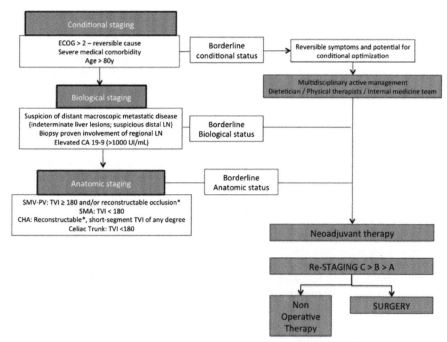

Fig. 2. General management algorithm used at the University of Texas MDACC. *, a segment of patent vessel exists both proximal and distal to the tumor sufficient for vascular control and vessel reconstruction. A, anatomic status; B, biological status; C, conditional status; CHA, common hepatic artery; LN, lymph node.

Rationale for Preoperative Therapy

The role of neoadjuvant treatment in patients with borderline resectable PDAC continues to be debated. A recently published European study based on a multi-institutional database reviewed a total of 492 patients, including 70 (14%) who underwent venous resection and 422 (86%) who did not undergo venous resection at pancreatectomy.[42] None of these patients received neoadjuvant therapy. No difference was found in survival following an R0 resection, nor was vein involvement shown to be a prognostic marker for survival. In consequence, the investigators questioned the indication for neoadjuvant treatment in the presence of major visceral venous involvement. The International Study Group of Pancreatic Surgery likewise does not support neoadjuvant therapy regimens in borderline resectable pancreatic cancer (BRPC) patients with isolated venous involvement if technical options of resections are possible.[4]

Nonetheless, despite a paucity of prospective data to support a standard treatment regimen for borderline resectable pancreatic cancer, neoadjuvant therapy is currently the preferred initial approach in the United States,[25,43-49] and was recommended by the expert consensus statement sponsored by the AHPBA, SSAT, and SSO.[41] The rationale for pursuing preoperative treatment for patients with borderline resectable PDAC is similar to that for patients with potentially resectable pancreatic cancer, but a greater emphasis is placed on maximizing the potential for R0 resection. Additional theoretic advantages to neoadjuvant treatment include early treatment of micrometastasis, giving most "adjuvant" therapy in the "neoadjuvant" setting when it is better tolerated,[50] and using this approach to gauge the aggressiveness of the cancer and thereby select patients for surgery who have the greatest likelihood of a favorable postoperative outcome.[45,51]

Therefore, although data are few with regard to the sequencing and duration of preoperative treatment modalities, most agree that a treatment schema that incorporates systemic chemotherapy and chemoradiation is the optimal strategy, and this notion has been embraced by several institutions and high-volume pancreatic cancer treatment centers (**Table 2**).[25,43–49]

Metrics of Response to Neoadjuvant Therapy

When neoadjuvant therapy is administered, patients should be staged before initiation and after completion of therapy (chemotherapy, chemoradiation, or both).[52,53] Changes in the patient's clinical or biologic status or the radiographic findings at the time of restaging may necessitate a reassessment of the treatment plan.

Although the resection rate has been used as a principal metric of comparison of the effects of different preoperative regimens for PDAC,[54,55] this metric is subjective and reflects biases not only in pretreatment and posttreatment staging, but also in preoperative and intraoperative decision-making processes. In a recent meta-analysis of neoadjuvant therapy, for example, 33% of patients with unresectable PDAC in the analysis were resected following neoadjuvant therapy. The investigators concluded that one-third of unresectable tumors can be converted to resectable tumors with neoadjuvant therapy. However, 53% of the studies included in the meta-analysis did not state the criteria used to stage disease and only 40% reported the criteria used to measure treatment response. The high resection rate reported likely reflected less "downstaging" by neoadjuvant therapy than an artifact of variability in staging and criteria used to indicate operative intervention.

Recently, objective radiographic response criteria have been tested as a reproducible metric to evaluate the outcome following neoadjuvant therapy in PDAC. At MDACC, only 12% of patients with borderline resectable cancers had a reduction in size sufficient to meet the definition of a Response Evaluation in Solid Tumors (RECIST) response following neoadjuvant therapy, and the tumor of only 1 patient was downstaged to meet a radiographic definition of potentially resectable.[56] Nonetheless, 66% of patients were able to undergo resection of their tumors with a 95% rate of microscopically negative margins. Cassinotto and colleagues[57] showed that neoadjuvant therapy significantly decreases the accuracy of CT scan in determining T-staging (39%) and resectability R0 (58%) of PDAC. In addition the investigators demonstrated that overestimation of tumor size and vascular invasion significantly reduces CT scan specificity after preoperative treatment.[57]

It is therefore critical to understand that RECIST criteria should not be used as a primary determinant of resectability after neoadjuvant therapy.

A recent retrospective study examined the trend in CA 19-9 levels of patients with borderline resectable pancreatic cancer who were undergoing neoadjuvant therapy and found that a decrease in CA 19-9 levels during neoadjuvant therapy had a positive predictive value of only 70% for successful resection but an 88% negative predictive value for predicting unresectability when CA 19-9 failed to decrease. Posttreatment CA 19-9 levels were a better predictor of metastases than pretreatment levels.[58] In addition, the study found that normalization of CA 19-9 during neoadjuvant therapy was associated with a longer overall survival in both resected and unresected patients.

Taken together, all these observations suggest that a laparotomy with intent to resect the primary tumor should be offered to all operable patients with borderline resectable disease in the absence of progressive metastasis after the administration of neoadjuvant therapy.

Table 2
Largest studies of borderline resectable PDAC (published between 2008 and 2014, with more than 40 cases)

First Author, Year (Ref)	Study Dates	N[a]	Type of Study	Definition	Neoadjuvant	Resected, n (%)	Negative Margins, %	Median OS, mo; All Borderline Resectable PDAC/Resected Only
Rose et al,[49] 2014	2008–2012	64	Retrospective, SC	AHPBA	Gem + Docetaxel-based CTX	31 (48)	87	24/81% alive after a median follow-up of 22 mo
Takahashi et al,[48] 2013	2002–2011	80	Prospective phase II	MDACC	Gem-based CRT	43 (54)	54	NA/25
Chuong et al,[47] 2013	2009–2011	57	Retrospective, SC	NCCN	Gem-based CRT	32 (56)	96	16/19
Katz et al,[25] 2008	1999–2006	84	Retrospective, SC	MDACC	Gem-based chemotherapy + CRT or CRT alone	32 (38)	97	21/40
Kang et al,[46] 2012	2000–2010	67	Retrospective, SC	NCCN	Gem-based CRT	32 (48)	87	NA/26
Stokes et al,[45] 2011	2005–2008	40	Retrospective, SC	MDACC	Cap-based CRT	16 (46)	75	12/23
Chun et al,[44] 2011	1990–2009	74	Retrospective, SC	Ishikawa	5-FU or Gem-based CRT	NA[b]	59	NA/23
Turrini et al,[43] 2009	1996–2006	49	Retrospective, SC	MDACC	5-FU-cisplatin–based CRT	18	100	NA/24

Abbreviations: 5-FU, 5-fluorouracil; AHPBA, Americas Hepatopancreatobiliary Association; Cap, capecitabine; CRT, chemoradiation; CTX, chemotherapy; Gem, Gemcitabine; MDACC, University of Texas MD Anderson Cancer Center; NA, not available; NCCN, National Comprehensive Cancer Network; OS, overall survival; PDAC, pancreatic ductal adenocarcinoma; SC, single center.

[a] Patients with borderline resectable PDAC who received neoadjuvant therapies.

[b] Only resected patients were included in the study.

SURGICAL ISSUES
Staging Laparoscopy

Staging laparoscopy is a rational study for this group of patients who are at high risk for occult metastatic disease to exclude such disease before the initiation of therapy otherwise perceived to be potentially curative.[59,60] Thus, staging laparoscopy may be considered in patients whose primary cancers are located in the pancreatic body or tail, are large or anatomically extensive, are associated with a high cancer antigen 19-9 level, are associated with equivocal CT findings of metastasis, and/or are associated with clinical findings suggesting advanced disease, such as marked weight loss or ascites.[60–63] In these scenarios, the use of staging laparoscopy is particularly encouraged[64,65] and should done either before the initiation of neoadjuvant chemotherapy or chemoradiation or before surgery.

Laparotomy After Neoadjuvant Therapy

Uniform criteria for proceeding to resection on completion of neoadjuvant therapy must be established. At our institution, attempted resection is offered to all patients with borderline resectable PDAC who have no evidence of cancer progression (either local or distant) on presurgical restaging studies, based on the fact that radiographic downstaging was rare after neoadjuvant therapy and that RECIST response was not effective for patients with borderline resectable pancreatic cancer.[56,57] Patients must have a physiologic status and comorbidity profile appropriate for major surgery.

Surgical Standards

Although the use of neoadjuvant therapy has been emphasized, the critical importance of a well-performed technical operation for patients with borderline resectable PDAC must not be dismissed. Given the frequent need for segmental resection and reconstruction of the SMV, PV, or hepatic artery to achieve negative resection margins among these patients, care must be provided by surgeons who are comfortable with techniques of vascular resection and reconstruction at pancreaticoduodenectomy. Moreover, particularly in this group in whom the primary cancer may abut the SMA, meticulous dissection along the periadventitial plane of the vessel at pancreaticoduodenectomy is absolutely essential to maximize the potential for a margin-negative resection.[66]

SUMMARY

Unfortunately, a uniformly accepted definition of borderline resectable PDAC still does not yet exist. Further well-designed studies are necessary to develop precise management algorithms for these difficult-to-treat patients. However, before that can be accomplished successfully, consensus must be achieved with regard to both definitions and standards of care.

REFERENCES

1. Sohn TA, Yeo CJ, Cameron JL, et al. Resected adenocarcinoma of the pancreas-616 patients: results, outcomes, and prognostic indicators. J Gastrointest Surg 2000;4:567–79.
2. Bilimoria KY, Talamonti MS, Sener SF, et al. Effect of hospital volume on margin status after pancreaticoduodenectomy for cancer. J Am Coll Surg 2008;207: 510–9.

3. Al-Hawary MM, Francis IR, Chari ST, et al. Pancreatic ductal adenocarcinoma radiology reporting template: consensus statement of the Society of Abdominal Radiology and the American Pancreatic Association. Gastroenterology 2014; 146:291–304.e1.

4. Bockhorn M, Uzunoglu FG, Adham M, et al. Borderline resectable pancreatic cancer: a consensus statement by the International Study Group of Pancreatic Surgery (ISGPS). Surgery 2014;155:977–88.

5. Callery MP, Chang KJ, Fishman EK, et al. Pretreatment assessment of resectable and borderline resectable pancreatic cancer: expert consensus statement. Ann Surg Oncol 2009;16:1727–33.

6. Katz MH, Marsh R, Herman JM, et al. Borderline resectable pancreatic cancer: need for standardization and methods for optimal clinical trial design. Ann Surg Oncol 2013;20:2787–95.

7. Tempero MA, Malafa MP, Behrman SW, et al. Pancreatic adenocarcinoma, version 2.2014: featured updates to the NCCN guidelines. J Natl Compr Canc Netw 2014;12:1083–93.

8. Varadhachary GR, Tamm EP, Abbruzzese JL, et al. Borderline resectable pancreatic cancer: definitions, management, and role of preoperative therapy. Ann Surg Oncol 2006;13:1035–46.

9. Chang DK, Johns AL, Merrett ND, et al. Margin clearance and outcome in resected pancreatic cancer. J Clin Oncol 2009;27:2855–62.

10. Merkow RP, Bilimoria KY, Bentrem DJ, et al. National assessment of margin status as a quality indicator after pancreatic cancer surgery. Ann Surg Oncol 2014;21: 1067–74.

11. Raut CP, Tseng JF, Sun CC, et al. Impact of resection status on pattern of failure and survival after pancreaticoduodenectomy for pancreatic adenocarcinoma. Ann Surg 2007;246:52–60.

12. Yeo CJ, Cameron JL, Sohn TA, et al. Six hundred fifty consecutive pancreaticoduodenectomies in the 1990s: pathology, complications, and outcomes. Ann Surg 1997;226:248–57 [discussion: 57–60].

13. Tempero MA, Arnoletti JP, Behrman S, et al. Pancreatic adenocarcinoma. J Natl Compr Canc Netw 2010;8:972–1017.

14. Halperin DM, Varadhachary GR. Resectable, borderline resectable, and locally advanced pancreatic cancer: what does it matter? Curr Oncol Rep 2014;16:366.

15. Lu DS, Reber HA, Krasny RM, et al. Local staging of pancreatic cancer: criteria for unresectability of major vessels as revealed by pancreatic-phase, thin-section helical CT. AJR Am J Roentgenol 1997;168:1439–43.

16. Maurer CA, Zgraggen K, Buchler MW. Pancreatic carcinoma. Optimizing therapy by adjuvant and neoadjuvant therapy? Zentralbl Chir 1999;124:401–7 [in German].

17. Mehta VK, Fisher G, Ford JA, et al. Preoperative chemoradiation for marginally resectable adenocarcinoma of the pancreas. J Gastrointest Surg 2001;5:27–35.

18. Mollberg N, Rahbari NN, Koch M, et al. Arterial resection during pancreatectomy for pancreatic cancer: a systematic review and meta-analysis. Ann Surg 2011; 254:882–93.

19. Tran Cao HS, Balachandran A, Wang H, et al. Radiographic tumor-vein interface as a predictor of intraoperative, pathologic, and oncologic outcomes in resectable and borderline resectable pancreatic cancer. J Gastrointest Surg 2014;18: 269–78 [discussion: 78].

20. Yamada S, Fujii T, Sugimoto H, et al. Aggressive surgery for borderline resectable pancreatic cancer: evaluation of National Comprehensive Cancer Network guidelines. Pancreas 2013;42:1004–10.

21. Baxter NN, Whitson BA, Tuttle TM. Trends in the treatment and outcome of pancreatic cancer in the United States. Ann Surg Oncol 2007;14:1320–6.
22. Bilimoria KY, Bentrem DJ, Ko CY, et al. National failure to operate on early stage pancreatic cancer. Ann Surg 2007;246:173–80.
23. Katz MH, Hwang R, Fleming JB, et al. Tumor-node-metastasis staging of pancreatic adenocarcinoma. CA Cancer J Clin 2008;58:111–25.
24. Katz MH, Wang H, Fleming JB, et al. Long-term survival after multidisciplinary management of resected pancreatic adenocarcinoma. Ann Surg Oncol 2009; 16:836–47.
25. Katz MH, Pisters PW, Evans DB, et al. Borderline resectable pancreatic cancer: the importance of this emerging stage of disease. J Am Coll Surg 2008;206: 833–46 [discussion: 46–8].
26. Fischer R, Breidert M, Keck T, et al. Early recurrence of pancreatic cancer after resection and during adjuvant chemotherapy. Saudi J Gastroenterol 2012;18:118–21.
27. Van den Broeck A, Sergeant G, Ectors N, et al. Patterns of recurrence after curative resection of pancreatic ductal adenocarcinoma. Eur J Surg Oncol 2009;35: 600–4.
28. Rhim AD, Mirek ET, Aiello NM, et al. EMT and dissemination precede pancreatic tumor formation. Cell 2012;148:349–61.
29. Takahashi S, Kinoshita T, Konishi M, et al. Borderline resectable pancreatic cancer: rationale for multidisciplinary treatment. J Hepatobiliary Pancreat Sci 2011; 18:567–74.
30. Schwarz L, Lupinacci RM, Svrcek M, et al. Para-aortic lymph node sampling in pancreatic head adenocarcinoma. Br J Surg 2014;101:530–8.
31. La Torre M, Nigri G, Lo Conte A, et al. Is a preoperative assessment of the early recurrence of pancreatic cancer possible after complete surgical resection? Gut Liver 2014;8:102–8.
32. Hill JS, Zhou Z, Simons JP, et al. A simple risk score to predict in-hospital mortality after pancreatic resection for cancer. Ann Surg Oncol 2010;17:1802–7.
33. Ragulin-Coyne E, Carroll JE, Smith JK, et al. Perioperative mortality after pancreatectomy: a risk score to aid decision-making. Surgery 2012;152:S120–7.
34. Karmazanovsky G, Fedorov V, Kubyshkin V, et al. Pancreatic head cancer: accuracy of CT in determination of resectability. Abdom Imaging 2005;30:488–500.
35. Tapper EB, Martin D, Adsay NV, et al. An MRI-driven practice: a new perspective on MRI for the evaluation of adenocarcinoma of the head of the pancreas. J Gastrointest Surg 2010;14:1292–7.
36. Bipat S, Phoa SS, van Delden OM, et al. Ultrasonography, computed tomography and magnetic resonance imaging for diagnosis and determining resectability of pancreatic adenocarcinoma: a meta-analysis. J Comput Assist Tomogr 2005; 29:438–45.
37. Dewitt J, Devereaux BM, Lehman GA, et al. Comparison of endoscopic ultrasound and computed tomography for the preoperative evaluation of pancreatic cancer: a systematic review. Clin Gastroenterol Hepatol 2006;4:717–25 [quiz: 664].
38. Goldberg J, Rosenblat J, Khatri G, et al. Complementary roles of CT and endoscopic ultrasound in evaluating a pancreatic mass. AJR Am J Roentgenol 2010;194:984–92.
39. Birkmeyer JD, Finlayson SR, Tosteson AN, et al. Effect of hospital volume on in-hospital mortality with pancreaticoduodenectomy. Surgery 1999;125:250–6.
40. Pawlik TM, Laheru D, Hruban RH, et al. Evaluating the impact of a single-day multidisciplinary clinic on the management of pancreatic cancer. Ann Surg Oncol 2008;15:2081–8.

41. Abrams RA, Lowy AM, O'Reilly EM, et al. Combined modality treatment of resectable and borderline resectable pancreas cancer: expert consensus statement. Ann Surg Oncol 2009;16:1751–6.

42. Kelly KJ, Winslow E, Kooby D, et al. Vein involvement during pancreaticoduodenectomy: is there a need for redefinition of "borderline resectable disease"? J Gastrointest Surg 2013;17:1209–17 [discussion: 17].

43. Turrini O, Viret F, Moureau-Zabotto L, et al. Neoadjuvant chemoradiation and pancreaticoduodenectomy for initially locally advanced head pancreatic adenocarcinoma. Eur J Surg Oncol 2009;35:1306–11.

44. Chun YS, Cooper HS, Cohen SJ, et al. Significance of pathologic response to preoperative therapy in pancreatic cancer. Ann Surg Oncol 2011;18:3601–7.

45. Stokes JB, Nolan NJ, Stelow EB, et al. Preoperative capecitabine and concurrent radiation for borderline resectable pancreatic cancer. Ann Surg Oncol 2011;18: 619–27.

46. Kang CM, Chung YE, Park JY, et al. Potential contribution of preoperative neoadjuvant concurrent chemoradiation therapy on margin-negative resection in borderline resectable pancreatic cancer. J Gastrointest Surg 2012;16:509–17.

47. Chuong MD, Springett GM, Freilich JM, et al. Stereotactic body radiation therapy for locally advanced and borderline resectable pancreatic cancer is effective and well tolerated. Int J Radiat Oncol Biol Phys 2013;86:516–22.

48. Takahashi H, Ohigashi H, Gotoh K, et al. Preoperative gemcitabine-based chemoradiation therapy for resectable and borderline resectable pancreatic cancer. Ann Surg 2013;258:1040–50.

49. Rose JB, Rocha FG, Alseidi A, et al. Extended neoadjuvant chemotherapy for borderline resectable pancreatic cancer demonstrates promising postoperative outcomes and survival. Ann Surg Oncol 2014;21:1530–7.

50. Tzeng CW, Tran Cao HS, Lee JE, et al. Treatment sequencing for resectable pancreatic cancer: influence of early metastases and surgical complications on multimodality therapy completion and survival. J Gastrointest Surg 2014;18: 16–24 [discussion: 5].

51. Tzeng CW, Fleming JB, Lee JE, et al. Defined clinical classifications are associated with outcome of patients with anatomically resectable pancreatic adenocarcinoma treated with neoadjuvant therapy. Ann Surg Oncol 2012;19:2045–53.

52. Evans DB, Varadhachary GR, Crane CH, et al. Preoperative gemcitabine-based chemoradiation for patients with resectable adenocarcinoma of the pancreatic head. J Clin Oncol 2008;26:3496–502.

53. Varadhachary GR, Wolff RA, Crane CH, et al. Preoperative gemcitabine and cisplatin followed by gemcitabine-based chemoradiation for resectable adenocarcinoma of the pancreatic head. J Clin Oncol 2008;26:3487–95.

54. Gillen S, Schuster T, Meyer Zum Buschenfelde C, et al. Preoperative/neoadjuvant therapy in pancreatic cancer: a systematic review and meta-analysis of response and resection percentages. PLoS Med 2010;7:e1000267.

55. Morganti AG, Massaccesi M, La Torre G, et al. A systematic review of resectability and survival after concurrent chemoradiation in primarily unresectable pancreatic cancer. Ann Surg Oncol 2010;17:194–205.

56. Katz MH, Fleming JB, Bhosale P, et al. Response of borderline resectable pancreatic cancer to neoadjuvant therapy is not reflected by radiographic indicators. Cancer 2012;118:5749–56.

57. Cassinotto C, Cortade J, Belleannee G, et al. An evaluation of the accuracy of CT when determining resectability of pancreatic head adenocarcinoma after neoadjuvant treatment. Eur J Radiol 2013;82:589–93.

58. Tzeng CW, Balachandran A, Ahmad M, et al. Serum carbohydrate antigen 19-9 represents a marker of response to neoadjuvant therapy in patients with borderline resectable pancreatic cancer. HPB (Oxford) 2014;16:430–8.
59. Contreras CM, Stanelle EJ, Mansour J, et al. Staging laparoscopy enhances the detection of occult metastases in patients with pancreatic adenocarcinoma. J Surg Oncol 2009;100:663–9.
60. Satoi S, Yanagimoto H, Toyokawa H, et al. Selective use of staging laparoscopy based on carbohydrate antigen 19-9 level and tumor size in patients with radiographically defined potentially or borderline resectable pancreatic cancer. Pancreas 2011;40:426–32.
61. Barabino M, Santambrogio R, Pisani Ceretti A, et al. Is there still a role for laparoscopy combined with laparoscopic ultrasonography in the staging of pancreatic cancer? Surg Endosc 2011;25:160–5.
62. Karachristos A, Scarmeas N, Hoffman JP. CA 19-9 levels predict results of staging laparoscopy in pancreatic cancer. J Gastrointest Surg 2005;9:1286–92.
63. Maithel SK, Maloney S, Winston C, et al. Preoperative CA 19-9 and the yield of staging laparoscopy in patients with radiographically resectable pancreatic adenocarcinoma. Ann Surg Oncol 2008;15:3512–20.
64. Ellsmere J, Mortele K, Sahani D, et al. Does multidetector-row CT eliminate the role of diagnostic laparoscopy in assessing the resectability of pancreatic head adenocarcinoma? Surg Endosc 2005;19:369–73.
65. Slaar A, Eshuis WJ, van der Gaag NA, et al. Predicting distant metastasis in patients with suspected pancreatic and periampullary tumors for selective use of staging laparoscopy. World J Surg 2011;35:2528–34.
66. Katz MH, Merchant NB, Brower S, et al. Standardization of surgical and pathologic variables is needed in multicenter trials of adjuvant therapy for pancreatic cancer: results from the ACOSOG Z5031 trial. Ann Surg Oncol 2011;18:337–44.

Treatment Approaches to Locally Advanced Pancreatic Adenocarcinoma

 CrossMark

Erqi L. Pollom, MD[a], Albert C. Koong, MD, PhD[a],
Andrew H. Ko, MD[b],*

KEYWORDS

- Pancreatic cancer • Locally advanced • Combined-modality therapy • Induction
- Stereotactic body radiation

KEY POINTS

- Locally advanced pancreatic cancer should be treated as a distinct entity separate from metastatic disease.
- The role, timing, and sequencing of radiation relative to systemic therapy for locally advanced pancreatic cancer remain uncertain, even more so with the development of more modern chemotherapy regimens that improves systemic disease control.
- Most clinical trials to date have evaluated initial chemoradiation followed by maintenance chemotherapy; this approach has produced mixed results in terms of whether it confers any survival benefit compared with chemotherapy alone.
- An emerging treatment paradigm for locally advanced pancreatic cancer involves induction chemotherapy, followed by consolidative chemoradiation in patients who do not progress. Dropout rates (ie, patients who do not go on to receive chemoradiation) with this strategy range from 13% to 39%.
- A large randomized phase III trial from Europe (LAP-07) did not indicate a survival benefit of sequential chemotherapy followed by chemoradiation, compared with chemotherapy alone. However, rates of locoregional control were higher for patients who received chemoradiation.
- Newer approaches for radiation, including reduction in target volumes and stereotactic body radiation, are increasingly used and warrant further exploration.

[a] Department of Radiation Oncology, Stanford Cancer Center, Stanford University, 875 Blake Wilbur Drive, MC5847, Stanford, CA 94305-5847, USA; [b] Division of Hematology/Oncology, University of California San Francisco, 1600 Divisadero Street, 4th Floor, Box 1705, San Francisco, CA 94115, USA
* Corresponding author.
E-mail address: andrewko@medicine.ucsf.edu

Hematol Oncol Clin N Am 29 (2015) 741–759
http://dx.doi.org/10.1016/j.hoc.2015.04.005
0889-8588/15/$ – see front matter © 2015 Elsevier Inc. All rights reserved.

INTRODUCTION

Most individuals diagnosed with pancreatic cancer are inoperable at the time of initial presentation, either because of metastatic dissemination of disease or based on the locoregional extent of their primary tumor.[1] Patients in this latter category, who do not have any radiographic evidence of distant metastases, are defined as having locally advanced disease. This article focuses on therapeutic considerations, including current controversies and areas of uncertainty that inform the current approach to patients with this stage of disease. Of note, borderline resectable pancreatic cancer, in which cytoreductive neoadjuvant therapy is used to maximize the chance of R0 resection, is being increasingly viewed as a distinct entity that warrants its own separate discussion from locally advanced disease[2] and is therefore covered elsewhere in the current issue of this journal.

DEFINITION OF LOCALLY ADVANCED PANCREATIC CANCER: ACCURATE DIAGNOSIS AND STAGING

Although nuanced differences exist among expert groups in defining locally advanced pancreatic cancer,[3,4] the primary basis on which resectability and unresectability is judged is the relationship of the primary pancreatic tumor to adjacent blood vessels. According to criteria outlined by the National Comprehensive Cancer Network (NCCN),[5] this includes (1) encasement of the superior mesenteric artery by greater than 180°; (2) encasement of the celiac axis by greater than 180° (for tumors of the body or tail) or any degree of celiac abutment (for tumors located at the pancreatic head); (3) superior mesenteric vein or portal vein occlusion without possibility of reconstruction; or (4) aortic invasion or encasement. Pancreatic protocol computed tomography (CT) using a multidetector scanner, which entails multiphasic imaging with thin cuts through the pancreas, is the primary diagnostic tool used to adjudicate this.[4,6] Although endoscopic ultrasound is also frequently used to gain additional information about the tumor and nodal staging of pancreatic cancers,[7,8] as well as to obtain a tissue diagnosis,[9] it should be considered an adjunct to high-quality CT scanning and not serve as the primary basis for staging and deciding on suitability for surgery.[5] Diagnostic laparoscopy can also be considered in the initial staging workup, because the presence of peritoneal metastases may influence treatment decisions, such as the role for, and relative importance of, locoregional therapy.

TREATMENT OF LOCALLY ADVANCED PANCREATIC CANCER

There remains much uncertainty regarding the optimal therapeutic approach for patients with locally advanced disease, including the respective roles, importance, and sequencing of chemotherapy and radiation, as well as many specifics regarding how best to deliver each of these modalities. Although such patients have often been grouped together with those with metastatic disease in chemotherapy clinical trials,[10–12] it is becoming increasingly clear that differences in biology and natural history warrant separate therapeutic approaches and studies for these patient subsets.[13]

Chemoradiation: Is There a Role?

One of the primary questions in locally advanced pancreatic cancer is the role that radiation plays and the importance of locoregional control. A postmortem study from Johns Hopkins indicated that up to 30% of patients with pancreatic cancer died of "locally destructive" rather than extensive metastatic disease, highlighting the potential importance of achieving locoregional control in this malignancy.[14]

There are conflicting data regarding the role of combined-modality therapy for locally advanced pancreatic cancer. In terms of concurrent administration of chemotherapy with radiation, an early study conducted by the Gastrointestinal Tumor Study Group (GITSG) demonstrated the superiority of chemotherapy (bolus 5-fluorouracil [5-FU]) administered together with radiation when compared with radiation alone in patients with locally advanced disease, with improved median survival, and with 1-year survival rates.[15] Although this informs the current practice standard of administering radiosensitizing doses of chemotherapy concurrently with radiation, it is worth noting that a much later published study conducted by the Eastern Cooperative Group (ECOG) failed to demonstrate any survival improvement when mitomycin C (MMC) and 5-FU were administered concurrently with radiation compared with radiation alone.[16]

The Question of Timing: Induction Chemoradiation

Most studies evaluating a treatment paradigm that includes chemoradiation for locally advanced disease have used it as part of initial therapy (**Table 1**). Several of these have used a randomized design to analyze whether sequential chemoradiation, followed by chemotherapy, is superior to chemotherapy alone (ie, what benefit is conferred by the addition of induction chemoradiation in this disease context). Notably, these trials have produced markedly discordant results: 2 trials demonstrated a survival advantage,[17,18] 1 trial showed no difference,[19] and 1 trial actually indicated a detrimental effect of using induction chemoradiation in this patient population.[20] These disparate findings may be potentially explained by several factors that could have affected clinical outcomes: different radiation doses and treatment plans, radiosensitizing agents, and stand-alone chemotherapy regimens. For example, in the one modern phase III study to demonstrate a shorter median survival with combined-modality therapy, conducted by the Federation Francophone de Cancerologie Digestive (FFCD) and the Societe Francophone de Radiotherapie Oncologique (SFRO),[20] induction chemoradiation consisted of 6000 cGy of radiation over 30 fractions with 2 concurrent cycles of cisplatin (20 $mg/m^2/d$ on days 1 through 5 during weeks 1 and 5) and continuous infusion 5-FU (300 $mg/m^2/d$, days 1 through 5 for 6 weeks). Not surprisingly, patients receiving this chemoradiation regimen incurred more frequent grade 3 to 4 toxicities when compared with those receiving chemotherapy alone, both during the corresponding induction periods and during the maintenance chemotherapy phase with gemcitabine, leading to early treatment interruption and shorter duration and lower cumulative dose of subsequent chemotherapy. Such factors may have contributed to the poorer outcomes, highlighting the importance of radiation treatment planning and selection of radiosensitizing agents, as is discussed later.

Delayed Chemoradiation Following Induction Chemotherapy

An emerging and promising treatment paradigm for locally advanced pancreatic cancer consists of delaying chemoradiation until after patients have completed a period of induction chemotherapy.[21] This strategy would address 2 important issues: (1) the need to optimally address systemic disease first, which is usually the most significant factor affecting longevity in most patients; and (2) limiting the use of radiation to that subgroup of patients whose tumors are well-controlled with this initial period of systemic therapy and do not develop metastatic disease. This approach would spare a subset of individuals the potential toxicities associated with radiation.

Support for this strategy came from the Groupe Cooperateur Multidisciplinaire en Oncologie (GERCOR), which performed a retrospective analysis on 181 patients with locally advanced pancreatic cancer who had participated in several separate

Table 1
Clinical trials evaluating induction chemoradiation in locally advanced pancreatic cancer

| Study | N | Induction Chemoradiation | | Maintenance Chemotherapy After RT? | Median Survival | | (For Randomized Trials): | | |
		Radiation (Dose/Schedule)	Concurrent Chemotherapy			n	Comparator Arm (RT Alone or Chemo Alone)	Median Survival	Statistically Significant?
Randomized trials vs radiation alone									
GITSG 9273[15]	169	4000 or 6000 cGy (split course)	Bolus 5-FU	Bolus 5-FU	40 wk	25	RT	23 wk	Yes, in favor of chemoRT (P<.01)
ECOG 8282[16]	55	5940 cGy	MMC/5-FU	No	8.4 mo	49	RT	7.1 mo	No
Randomized trials vs chemotherapy alone									
ECOG (1985)[19]	47	4000 cGy	Bolus 5-FU	Bolus 5-FU	8.3 mo	44	Bolus 5-FU	8.2 mo	No
GITSG 9283[17]	54	5400 cGy	Bolus 5-FU	Streptozocin, MMC, 5-FU	42 wk		Streptozocin, MMC, 5-FU	32 wk	Yes, in favor of induction chemoRT (P<.02)
FFCD/SFRO[20]	59	6000 cGy	Cisplatin/5-FU	Gemcitabine	8.6 mo	60	Gemcitabine	13.0 mo	Yes, in favor of chemo alone (P = .03)
ECOG 4201[18]	34	5040 cGy	Gemcitabine	Gemcitabine	11.1 mo	37	Gemcitabine	9.2 mo	Yes, in favor of induction chemoRT (P = .034)
Nonrandomized trials									
RTOG 9812[42]	122	5040 cGy	Paclitaxel	No	11.3 mo	N/A			
RTOG PA 0020[84]	154	5040 cGy	Paclitaxel/gemcitabine	R115777 (farnesyl transferase inhibitor)	11.7 mo				
RTOG PA-0411[85]	94	5040 cGy	Capecitabine/bevacizumab	Capecitabine/bevacizumab	11.9 mo				
CALGB 80003[86]	81	5040 cGy	Gemcitabine/infusional 5-FU	Gemcitabine	12.2 mo				

phase II or phase III trials and received initial chemotherapy with a gemcitabine-based combination regimen for 3 months or more.[22] For those patients who showed good disease control (70.7%, n = 128), the treating investigator was then permitted to decide whether to continue with the same chemotherapy or proceed onto consolidative chemoradiation. Seventy-two (56%) patients received consolidative radiation (5500 cGy with concurrent infusional 5-FU), whereas the remaining 56 (44%) patients continued with chemotherapy alone. Patients receiving chemoradiation had longer rates of overall survival (OS) and progression-free survival (PFS) (median OS 15.0 vs 11.7 months, $P = .0009$; median PFS 10.8 vs 7.4 months, $P = .005$).

Krishnan and colleagues[23] similarly performed a retrospective analysis of 323 patients with locally advanced pancreatic cancer treated at M.D. Anderson Cancer Center, 76 of whom received gemcitabine-based induction chemotherapy (for a median duration of 2.5 months) before chemoradiation.[23] These patients, when compared with those who had received chemoradiation as part of their initial treatment, were found to have significantly longer OS and PFS rates (median OS, 11.9 vs 8.5 months, $P<.001$; median PFS, 6.4 vs 4.2 months, $P<.001$, respectively).

Although intriguing, the retrospective nature of both these analyses prevents any definitive conclusions about the benefit of delayed chemoradiation compared with either no chemoradiation or induction chemoradiation. Data are now available from several prospectively designed phase II studies,[24–28] and most recently, a large randomized phase III study,[29] that have analyzed this sequential approach of induction chemotherapy followed by chemoradiation (**Table 2**). These studies have highlighted several important findings: (1) approximately 13% to 39% of patients receiving induction chemotherapy will not be candidates for subsequent chemoradiation, most commonly due to disease progression; and (2) patients who successfully undergo sequential chemotherapy followed by chemoradiation typically have survival outcomes greater than 1 year.

More recently, this strategy of delayed chemoradiation was attempted to be addressed more definitively via a phase III European study conducted by GERCOR (LAP-07).[29] In this trial, patients with locally advanced pancreatic cancer were initially randomized to receive gemcitabine with or without the epidermal growth factor receptor inhibitor erlotinib for 4 months. Patients who did not progress during this initial treatment were then included in the second randomization step, which involved either continuation of systemic therapy for 2 more months (patients receiving erlotinib could be maintained on this agent indefinitely) versus chemoradiation (54 Gy in 30 fractions, with concurrent capecitabine at 800 mg/m^2 twice a day). Results of this 442-patient study were initially presented by Hammel and colleagues[29] at the 2013 annual American Society of Clinical Oncology meeting. Of 442 patients enrolled to this study, 269 reached the second randomization step, representing a 39% dropout rate following induction chemotherapy (primarily due to progressive disease). Updated efficacy results in 2014[30] indicated that patients assigned to receive chemoradiation experienced no improvement in survival compared with those continuing with chemotherapy alone (median OS, 15.2 vs 16.5 months, respectively; log-rank $P = .829$), although there was a trend toward improved PFS in the chemoradiation-treated patients (median PFS 9.9 vs 8.4 months, log-rank $P = .055$). Not surprisingly, patterns of disease progression differed between the 2 arms: patients receiving chemoradiation did have a lower rate of subsequent local progression as well as a longer treatment-free interval before having to resume therapy at a later time. As the systemic therapy used in LAP-07 (gemcitabine ± erlotinib) is no longer commonly given, it is unclear whether the results of this trial will still be applicable, and whether newer and more effective modern chemotherapy regimens administered in the induction setting

Table 2
Select clinical trials evaluating induction chemotherapy followed by chemoradiation in locally advanced pancreatic cancer

Author	N	Induction Chemotherapy Regimen (Duration)	Patients NOT Receiving ChemoRT (%)[a]	Chemoradiation Regimen	Additional Chemo After ChemoRT Complete?	Median Survival (mo)
Ko et al,[24] 2007	25	Gemcitabine, cisplatin (6 mo)	32	50.4 Gy + capecitabine	No	13.5
Moureau-Zabotto et al,[25] 2008	59	Gemcitabine, oxaliplatin (2 mo)	15	55 Gy + 5-FU + oxaliplatin	No	12.2
Crane et al,[26] 2011	69	Gemcitabine, oxaliplatin, cetuximab (2 mo)	13	50.4 Gy + capecitabine + cetuximab	Cetuximab × 1 mo	19.2
Ch'ang et al,[87] 2011	50	Gemcitabine, 5-FU, oxaliplatin (3 mo)	40	50.4 Gy + gemcitabine	Gemcitabine, 5-FU, oxaliplatin until progression	
Kim et al,[27] 2012	37	Gemcitabine, cisplatin (9 wk)	19	55.8 Gy + capecitabine	Gemcitabine × 3 cycles	16.8
Mukherjee (SCALOP) et al,[28] 2013	114	Gemcitabine, capecitabine (12 wk)	35	50.4 Gy + (gemcitabine or capecitabine)	No	14.5
Hammel (LAP-07) et al,[29] 2013	442 (133)[b]	Gemcitabine ± erlotinib (4 mo)	39	54 Gy + capecitabine	Erlotinib (for patients on gemcitabine/erlotinib arm)	15.3

[a] Due to disease progression, toxicity, or doctor/patient choice.
[b] 442 represents all patients enrolled in study; 133 includes only patients demonstrating nonprogressive disease after induction chemotherapy who were randomized to receive chemoradiation. Survival result reflects only this limited subset.

will attenuate or magnify any potential benefits associated with radiation in this patient population.

SYSTEMIC THERAPY IN LOCALLY ADVANCED PANCREATIC CANCER
Selection of Chemotherapy Administered Independently of Radiation

Two regimens have emerged as front-line standards of care for the treatment of metastatic pancreatic cancer: FOLFIRINOX (a biweekly regimen consisting of 5-FU administered over 48 hours plus leucovorin, irinotecan, and oxaliplatin); and the combination of gemcitabine and nab-paclitaxel. Both of these regimens demonstrated significantly prolonged survival times compared with gemcitabine monotherapy in randomized phase III trials[31,32] (FOLFIRINOX vs gemcitabine, median OS 11.1 vs 6.8 months; hazard ratio [HR] 0.57, $P<.001$; gemcitabine/nab-paclitaxel vs gemcitabine, median OS 8.5 vs 6.7 months; HR 0.72, $P<.001$), as well as improvements in other clinically relevant endpoints including PFS and objective response rate. However, it is important to recognize that both of these trials enrolled patients exclusively with metastatic disease, and hence, use of either of these regimens in the locally advanced setting requires some extrapolation as the experience to date in this context has been limited to small single-institution series.[33–35] Of note, NCCN guidelines do not make a distinction in choice of chemotherapy between patients with metastatic versus locally advanced disease.[5] In a recently opened national cooperative group trial (RTOG 1201), all patients will receive induction chemotherapy with the combination of gemcitabine and nab-paclitaxel, followed by a randomization to 1 of 3 arms: continued chemotherapy, standard-fractionation radiation, or higher-dose intensity-modulated radiation (ClinicalTrials.gov NCT01921751).

Selection of Radiosensitizing Agents

Historically, most studies for locally advanced pancreatic cancer have delivered fluoropyrimidine- or gemcitabine-based therapies concurrent with radiation. Older trials used bolus 5-FU, but administration of fluoropyrimidine therapy continuously throughout the course of radiation (either as infusional 5-FU or as the oral prodrug capecitabine), rather than in bolus fashion, may provide superior radiosensitization[36–38] and represents the currently accepted standard of care. Although gemcitabine is a more potent radiosensitizer, rates of severe toxicity may be higher with gemcitabine-based chemoradiation, as suggested from a retrospective analysis by Crane and colleagues[39] of patients with locally advanced disease treated at M.D. Anderson. However, other data have shown that full doses of gemcitabine, if delivered with limited volume and highly conformal radiotherapy, can be well-tolerated and efficacious.[40] A comparison of fluoropyrimidine-based versus gemcitabine-based chemoradiation was performed in the context of a randomized phase II study (the SCALOP trial),[28] in which 74 patients with locally advanced disease were randomized, after a 12-week course of induction chemotherapy with gemcitabine/capecitabine, to receive radiation (5040 cGy over 28 fractions) with either concurrent capecitabine (830 mg/m^2 twice a day Monday through Friday) or gemcitabine (300 mg/m^2 weekly). Median OS was significantly superior in the former group (15.2 vs 13.4 months; adjusted HR 0.39, $P = .012$), suggesting that a capecitabine-based regimen may be the preferred choice in the context of consolidative chemoradiation.

Other radiosensitizing agents that have been explored for locally advanced pancreatic cancer include new oral fluoropyrimidine derivatives (S-1[41]), taxanes,[42] epidermal growth factor receptor inhibitors (erlotinib,[43] cetuximab[26,44]), anti-angiogenic therapy (bevacizumab[45]), and protease inhibitors (nelfinavir[46]); however, at present, these should only be administered in the context of a clinical trial. One interesting recent study intending to enhance the effects of radiation involved localized injection of TNFerade, a replication-deficient adenoviral vector expressing the transgene tumor necrosis factor-α, regulated by the radiation-inducible promoter Egr-1. However, final results of a 187-patient randomized phase III trial[47] demonstrated that the addition of TNFerade to 5-FU-based chemoradiation did not prolong survival compared with standard of care therapy (median OS 10.0 vs 10.0 months; HR 0.90, $P = .26$).

ADVANCES IN PANCREATIC RADIATION TECHNIQUES

With continued progress in systemic therapy and improved control of distant disease, radiation therapy and achieving local control may become even more important in the management of locally advanced pancreas cancer. Delivery of effective radiation doses to the pancreas, however, is limited by the radiosensitivity of normal tissues in the abdomen, including liver, kidneys, spinal cord, and bowel. Technological advances, including image guidance, respiratory-motion management, and better treatment planning and delivery systems, have enabled 3-dimensional conformal radiotherapy (3D-CRT) and safer delivery of radiation. Intensity-modulated radiation treatment (IMRT), a 3D-CRT technique, has been shown to decrease dose to organs at risk and to be well-tolerated in patients with pancreatic cancer in multiple series.[48–52] However, these newer techniques add more complexity to the treatment planning and delivery process and require advanced procedures for their implementation.

Treatment Volumes

The earlier landmark trials of chemoradiation in locally advanced pancreatic cancer[15,17] treated large volumes covering the pancreatic tumor and draining lymph nodes with a 2-field technique, with concurrent chemotherapy. Because of the toxicities associated with combined radiotherapy and chemotherapy, the treatment course consisted of 2 weeks of radiotherapy, followed by a 2-week recovery period, followed by 2 more weeks of radiotherapy. Despite this suboptimal method of delivering radiotherapy, these studies demonstrated a significant benefit in favor of radiotherapy.

More recent data suggest that reduction in these treatment volumes improves the tolerability of radiotherapy. Multiple series using limited volumes including only gross disease, without elective nodal coverage, show improved toxicity rates and no compromise in local progression rates.[40,53–56] Avoiding prophylactic nodal irradiation may allow intensification of therapy without exceeding normal tissue constraints. Murphy and colleagues[40] were able to deliver radiation with concurrent full-dose gemcitabine by treating gross tumor volume (GTV) plus 1-cm margin only and found that only 5% of these patients experienced peripancreatic lymph node failures. These data are compelling, indicating that prophylactic nodal irradiation may be omitted in certain clinical scenarios.

With more focal radiation fields, target volumes as well as organs at risk must be accurately delineated. High-quality biphasic (early arterial and portal venous phase) CT and fluorodeoxyglucose (FDG)-PET imaging are both useful in helping to identify pancreatic tumors and to distinguish tumor from adjacent organs and vessels. In addition to intravenous contrast, dilute oral contrast can be used to define the pancreatic head better against the duodenum.

Respiratory-Motion Management

More conformal treating planning requires consideration of target motion. Pancreatic tumors, as with any upper abdominal organ, are subject to respiratory motion. The magnitude of motion for pancreatic tumors has been shown to be more significant in the cranio-caudal direction and can be as much as 2 to 3 cm from inspiration to expiration.[57] Four-dimensional (4D) CT should be obtained at simulation to characterize this tumor motion during the respiratory cycle and subsequently construct an internal tumor volume (ITV). If the tumor motion is significantly great, construction of a large ITV can result in much larger treatment fields and potentially increased toxicity. Given this, multiple strategies can be used to reduce the expansion of treatment volume without compromising tumor coverage. Respiratory gating may be used to limit treatment to only specific phases of the respiratory cycle whereby tumor motion is minimal[58,59] or during a phase when the overlap between planning treatment volume (PTV) and organ at risk is minimal.[60] Mechanical techniques, such as abdominal compression to limit diaphragmatic excursion and active breathing control breath-holding technique, can also be used to minimize respiratory and tumor motion.[61,62]

STEREOTACTIC BODY RADIOTHERAPY

Despite modern radiation techniques, outcomes are still poor with conventionally fractionated radiation, with local control rates of only 40% to 55% and median survival of 5 to 24 months.[24,40,53–56,63–65] Local progression of pancreatic cancers can result in considerable morbidity, including gastric outlet obstruction and pain.[66] Although more conformal delivery of radiation has enabled dose-escalation, most series have used 50.4 or 54 Gy at 1.8 to 2 Gy per fraction with concurrent radiosensitizing chemotherapy, because higher doses have been associated with increased morbidity and mortality.[20,53] Efforts to increase radiation dose to the pancreatic tumor without risking normal tissue injury have generally required relatively invasive techniques, such as interstitial implantation of radioactive sources or intraoperative radiotherapy.[67,68]

Stereotactic radiosurgery has long been used to treat small lesions in the brain,[69] but only more recently has this treatment concept been able to be safely applied to extracranial targets. Stereotactic body radiotherapy (SBRT), also referred to as stereotactic ablative therapy, allows accurate and conformal delivery of much higher biologically effective doses and provides an opportunity to improve on local outcomes. The rapid dose fall-off at the target periphery allows significant reduction in the volume of normal tissue irradiated, thus allowing ablative radiation doses to be delivered while minimizing potential toxicity.

Technical Considerations of Stereotactic Body Radiotherapy

Given the high doses used near critical organs, accurate target localization as previously discussed is critically important in SBRT. The GTV and ITV are delineated using the biphasic CT, respiratory-correlated 4D-CT scan, and the FDG-PET/CT scan. An expansion of 2 to 3 mm is typically added for a PTV to account for uncertainties in planning and treatment delivery. Again, respiratory gating and mechanical techniques are important strategies to reduce this final treatment volume. Dose is prescribed to the periphery of the PTV, and the treatment may be delivered using coplanar fields or conformal arcs. Flattening filter–free mode, where the flattening filter is removed, can be used to increase dose rate and allow high doses to be delivered quickly, reducing time of treatment and the risk of intrafraction patient movement.[70] **Fig. 1** shows a representative pancreas SBRT plan.

As tumors are not well-visualized with on-board imaging, metallic markers are generally placed as surrogates for tumor position during treatment delivery. These markers allow for fluoroscopic verification as well as real-time tracking of tumor motion with respiration during treatment delivery. In addition, respiratory tracking, which

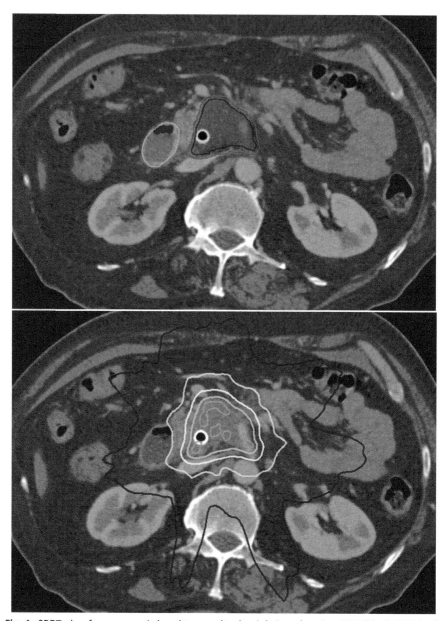

Fig. 1. SBRT plan for pancreatic head tumor: (*top*) axial view showing GTV (*blue*), PTV (*red*), and duodenum (*pale green*); and (*bottom*) isodose distribution with 40 Gy in 5 fractions prescribed to the periphery of the PTV (*orange* = 45 Gy; *green* = 40 Gy; *yellow* = 30 Gy; *cyan* = 20 Gy; *dark blue* = 10 Gy).

synchronizes radiation delivery with target motion, can be used based on the position of implanted markers[71] and to correct for daily setup error.[72,73] Implantation of these markers into the tumor or tumor periphery can be performed via endoscopic ultrasound or percutaneously with low complication rates.[74,75]

Table 3
Reported series of stereotactic body radiotherapy for locally advanced or unresectable pancreas cancer

Study	n	Dose per Fraction (Gy) × Number of Fractions	Chemotherapy	Grade 3 or Higher Toxicity	Local Control (at 1 y) (%)	Median Survival (mo)
Koong et al,[76] 2004	15	15–25 Gy × 1	None	0%	100	11
Koong et al,[79] 2005	16	25 Gy × 1 (boost to 45 Gy IMRT)	5-FU concurrent with IMRT	12.5%	94	8.3
Hoyer et al,[88] 2005	22 (3 had SBRT after resection for recurrent disease)	15 Gy × 3	None	79% ≥ Grade 2	57	5.4
Schellenberg et al,[78] 2011	20	25 Gy × 1	Induction and post-SBRT gemcitabine	5%	94	11.8
Schellenberg et al,[77] 2008	16	25 Gy × 1	Induction and post-SBRT gemcitabine	18.8%	100	11.4
Didolkar et al,[89] 2010	85 (14 had SBRT after resection for recurrent disease)	5–10 Gy × 3	Post-SBRT gemcitabine	22.3%	92	18.6
Rwigema et al,[90] 2011	71 (23 had SBRT after resection for recurrent disease)	20–24 Gy × 1 or 10 Gy × 3	90% received chemotherapy (various regimens)	4.2%	48.5	10.3
Mahadevan et al,[91] 2010	36	8–12 Gy × 3	Post-SBRT gemcitabine	8%	78	14.3
Mahadevan et al,[92] 2011	39	8–12 Gy × 3	Induction gemcitabine	9%	85	20

(continued on next page)

Table 3
(continued)

Study	n	Dose per Fraction (Gy) × Number of Fractions	Chemotherapy	Grade 3 or Higher Toxicity	Local Control (at 1 y) (%)	Median Survival (mo)
Seo et al,[93] 2009	30	2 Gy × 20 followed by 14, 15, 16, or 17 Gy × 1 SBRT	15 patients received concurrent chemo (various regimens) with EBRT	3%	70.2	14
Polistina et al,[94] 2010	23	10 Gy × 3	Induction gemcitabine	0%	50	10.6
Goyal et al,[95] 2012	19 (2 had SBRT after resection for recurrent disease)	20–25 Gy × 1 8–10 Gy × 3	68% received 5-FU or gemcitabine-based chemo	16%	81	14.4
Lominska et al,[96] 2012	28	All patients had EBRT before SBRT using 4–8 Gy × 3–5	5-FU or gemcitabine before SBRT	7%	86	5.9
Gurka et al,[97] 2013	10	5 Gy × 5	Concurrent gemcitabine	0%	40	12.2
Chuong et al,[98] 2013	73 (57 were borderline resectable)	5–10 Gy × 5	65.8% received induction chemo, 83.6% received adjuvant chemo, various regimens	5%	81	16.4 (borderline resectable), 15 (locally advanced)
Pollom et al,[82] 2014	76	25 Gy × 1	85.5% received neoadjuvant/adjuvant chemo, various regimens	12.3%	9.5	13.6
	91	5–9 Gy × 3–5	89.0% received neoadjuvant/adjuvant chemo, various regimens	5.6%	11.7	14.0

Efficacy and Toxicity

Koong and colleagues[76] published the first prospective clinical report on SBRT in the treatment of pancreatic cancer in 2004, showing 100% local control with up to 25 Gy in a single fraction. This report was followed by several phase II studies of SBRT integrated with gemcitabine chemotherapy, also reporting excellent local control rates.[77,78] Other groups have since reported their experiences using pancreatic SBRT with various fractionation schemes, also showing excellent local control compared with conventionally fractionated radiotherapy, with outcomes listed in **Table 3**.

Toxicity associated with SBRT is a concern given the close proximity of tumor, and thus high dose, to organs at risk, including the stomach and duodenum. A significant number of late gastrointestinal (GI) toxicities, such as upper GI bleed and ulcerations, after SBRT were initially reported.[77–80] Better understanding of duodenal tolerance has allowed SBRT to become safer with increased follow-up and study.[81,82] In addition, recent single- and multi-institutional studies show that GI toxicity is significantly less using a multifraction radiation schedule compared with single-fraction radiation schedule.[82,83]

Compared with conventionally fractionated radiotherapy, SBRT has been shown to be a more effective local control modality. In addition, because SBRT is well-tolerated and can be given in a shortened course, it minimizes interruptions in systemic treatment. As systemic therapies become more effective in this disease, these gains in local control may have a more meaningful impact on survival. The role of SBRT for treatment of locally advanced pancreatic cancer is currently being evaluated in the setting of more aggressive systemic therapy (FOLFIRINOX) in a multi-institutional phase III trial (ClinicalTrials.gov NCT01926197).

SUMMARY/DISCUSSION

The optimal treatment paradigm for locally advanced pancreatic cancer remains controversial. Unresolved questions include the importance and timing of radiation in this disease context. Multiple studies evaluating initial chemoradiation have produced equivocal results, possibly because of the selection and intensity of the prescribed chemoradiation regimen. Meanwhile, the theoretic advantage of deferring chemoradiation until after a period of induction chemotherapy, to select for the subgroup of patients likely to benefit from such treatment, has been an increasingly popular strategy; however, the largest trial to date evaluating this approach (LAP-07) failed to demonstrate a survival benefit compared with chemotherapy alone. More effective chemotherapy regimens such as FOLFIRINOX and gemcitabine/nab-paclitaxel that are commonly used for metastatic disease need to be tested further in the locally advanced setting. Moreover, newer radiation techniques, in particular SBRT, that offer theoretic and practical advantages over conventionally fractionated radiation also warrant further study in prospective, randomized trial design. Finally, secondary considerations relating to novel radiosensitizing agents, the optimal duration of systemic therapy, and the role of "maintenance" therapy should be explored.

REFERENCES

1. Siegel R, Ma J, Zou Z, et al. Cancer statistics, 2014. CA Cancer J Clin 2014;64: 9–29.
2. Katz MH, Marsh R, Herman JM, et al. Borderline resectable pancreatic cancer: need for standardization and methods for optimal clinical trial design. Ann Surg Oncol 2013;20:2787–95.

3. Varadhachary GR, Tamm EP, Abbruzzese JL, et al. Borderline resectable pancreatic cancer: definitions, management, and role of preoperative therapy. Ann Surg Oncol 2006;13:1035–46.

4. Callery MP, Chang KJ, Fishman EK, et al. Pretreatment assessment of resectable and borderline resectable pancreatic cancer: expert consensus statement. Ann Surg Oncol 2009;16:1727–33.

5. Wong ET, Huberman M, Lu XQ, et al. Bevacizumab reverses cerebral radiation necrosis. J Clin Oncol 2008;26:5649–50.

6. McNulty NJ, Francis IR, Platt JF, et al. Multi–detector row helical CT of the pancreas: effect of contrast-enhanced multiphasic imaging on enhancement of the pancreas, peripancreatic vasculature, and pancreatic adenocarcinoma. Radiology 2001;220:97–102.

7. Nawaz H, Fan CY, Kloke J, et al. Performance characteristics of endoscopic ultrasound in the staging of pancreatic cancer: a meta-analysis. JOP 2013;14:484–97.

8. Luz LP, Al-Haddad MA, Sey MS, et al. Applications of endoscopic ultrasound in pancreatic cancer. World J Gastroenterol 2014;20:7808–18.

9. Wang W, Shpaner A, Krishna SG, et al. Use of EUS-FNA in diagnosing pancreatic neoplasm without a definitive mass on CT. Gastrointest Endosc 2013;78:73–80.

10. Berlin JD, Catalano P, Thomas JP, et al. Phase III study of gemcitabine in combination with fluorouracil versus gemcitabine alone in patients with advanced pancreatic carcinoma: Eastern Cooperative Oncology Group Trial E2297. J Clin Oncol 2002;20:3270–5.

11. Louvet C, Labianca R, Hammel P, et al. Gemcitabine in combination with oxaliplatin compared with gemcitabine alone in locally advanced or metastatic pancreatic cancer: results of a GERCOR and GISCAD phase III trial. J Clin Oncol 2005;23:3509–16.

12. Moore MJ, Goldstein D, Hamm J, et al. Erlotinib plus gemcitabine compared with gemcitabine alone in patients with advanced pancreatic cancer: a phase III trial of the National Cancer Institute of Canada Clinical Trials Group. J Clin Oncol 2007;25:1960–6.

13. Philip PA, Mooney M, Jaffe D, et al. Consensus report of the national cancer institute clinical trials planning meeting on pancreas cancer treatment. J Clin Oncol 2009;27:5660–9.

14. Iacobuzio-Donahue CA, Fu B, Yachida S, et al. DPC4 gene status of the primary carcinoma correlates with patterns of failure in patients with pancreatic cancer. J Clin Oncol 2009;27:1806–13.

15. Moertel CG, Frytak S, Hahn RG, et al. Therapy of locally unresectable pancreatic carcinoma: a randomized comparison of high dose (6000 rads) radiation alone, moderate dose radiation (4000 rads + 5-fluorouracil), and high dose radiation + 5-fluorouracil: The Gastrointestinal Tumor Study Group. Cancer 1981;48:1705–10.

16. Cohen SJ, Dobelbower R Jr, Lipsitz S, et al. A randomized phase III study of radiotherapy alone or with 5-fluorouracil and mitomycin-C in patients with locally advanced adenocarcinoma of the pancreas: Eastern Cooperative Oncology Group study E8282. Int J Radiat Oncol Biol Phys 2005;62:1345–50.

17. Treatment of locally unresectable carcinoma of the pancreas: comparison of combined-modality therapy (chemotherapy plus radiotherapy) to chemotherapy alone. Gastrointestinal Tumor Study Group. J Natl Cancer Inst 1988;80:751–5.

18. Loehrer PJ Sr, Feng Y, Cardenes H, et al. Gemcitabine alone versus gemcitabine plus radiotherapy in patients with locally advanced pancreatic cancer: an Eastern Cooperative Oncology Group trial. J Clin Oncol 2011;29:4105–12.

19. Klaassen DJ, MacIntyre JM, Catton GE, et al. Treatment of locally unresectable cancer of the stomach and pancreas: a randomized comparison of 5-fluorouracil alone with radiation plus concurrent and maintenance 5-fluorouracil–an Eastern Cooperative Oncology Group study. J Clin Oncol 1985;3:373–8.

20. Chauffert B, Mornex F, Bonnetain F, et al. Phase III trial comparing intensive induction chemoradiotherapy (60 Gy, infusional 5-FU and intermittent cisplatin) followed by maintenance gemcitabine with gemcitabine alone for locally advanced unresectable pancreatic cancer. Definitive results of the 2000-01 FFCD/SFRO study. Ann Oncol 2008;19:1592–9.

21. Huguet F, Girard N, Guerche CS, et al. Chemoradiotherapy in the management of locally advanced pancreatic carcinoma: a qualitative systematic review. J Clin Oncol 2009;27:2269–77.

22. Huguet F, Andre T, Hammel P, et al. Impact of chemoradiotherapy after disease control with chemotherapy in locally advanced pancreatic adenocarcinoma in GERCOR phase II and III studies. J Clin Oncol 2007;25:326–31.

23. Krishnan S, Rana V, Janjan NA, et al. Induction chemotherapy selects patients with locally advanced, unresectable pancreatic cancer for optimal benefit from consolidative chemoradiation therapy. Cancer 2007;110:47–55.

24. Ko AH, Quivey JM, Venook AP, et al. A phase II study of fixed-dose rate gemcitabine plus low-dose cisplatin followed by consolidative chemoradiation for locally advanced pancreatic cancer. Int J Radiat Oncol Biol Phys 2007;68:809–16.

25. Moureau-Zabotto L, Phelip JM, Afchain P, et al. Concomitant administration of weekly oxaliplatin, fluorouracil continuous infusion, and radiotherapy after 2 months of gemcitabine and oxaliplatin induction in patients with locally advanced pancreatic cancer: a Groupe Coordinateur Multidisciplinaire en Oncologie phase II study. J Clin Oncol 2008;26:1080–5.

26. Crane CH, Varadhachary GR, Yordy JS, et al. Phase II trial of cetuximab, gemcitabine, and oxaliplatin followed by chemoradiation with cetuximab for locally advanced (T4) pancreatic adenocarcinoma: correlation of Smad4(Dpc4) immunostaining with pattern of disease progression. J Clin Oncol 2011;29:3037–43.

27. Kim JS, Lim JH, Kim JH, et al. Phase II clinical trial of induction chemotherapy with fixed dose rate gemcitabine and cisplatin followed by concurrent chemoradiotherapy with capecitabine for locally advanced pancreatic cancer. Cancer Chemother Pharmacol 2012;70:381–9.

28. Mukherjee S, Hurt CN, Bridgewater J, et al. Gemcitabine-based or capecitabine-based chemoradiotherapy for locally advanced pancreatic cancer (SCALOP): a multicentre, randomised, phase 2 trial. Lancet Oncol 2013;14:317–26.

29. Hammel P, Huguet F, Van Laethem J, et al. Comparison of chemoradiotherapy (CRT) and chemotherapy (CT) in patients with a locally advanced pancreatic cancer (LAPC) controlled after 4 months of gemcitabine with or without erlotinib: final results of the international phase III LAP 07 study. J Clin Oncol 2013; 31(Suppl) [abstract: LBA4003].

30. Huguet F, Hammel P, Vernerey D, et al. Impact of chemoradiotherapy (CRT) on local control and time without treatment in patients with locally advanced pancreatic cancer (LAPC) included in the international phase III LAP 07 study. J Clin Oncol 2014;32(Suppl) [abstract: 4001].

31. Conroy T, Desseigne F, Ychou M, et al. FOLFIRINOX versus gemcitabine for metastatic pancreatic cancer. N Engl J Med 2011;364:1817–25.

32. Von Hoff DD, Ervin T, Arena FP, et al. Increased survival in pancreatic cancer with nab-paclitaxel plus gemcitabine. N Engl J Med 2013;369:1691–703.

33. Faris JE, Blaszkowsky LS, McDermott S, et al. FOLFIRINOX in locally advanced pancreatic cancer: the Massachusetts General Hospital Cancer Center experience. Oncologist 2013;18:543–8.

34. Boone BA, Steve J, Krasinskas AM, et al. Outcomes with FOLFIRINOX for borderline resectable and locally unresectable pancreatic cancer. J Surg Oncol 2013; 108:236–41.

35. Gunturu KS, Yao X, Cong X, et al. FOLFIRINOX for locally advanced and metastatic pancreatic cancer: single institution retrospective review of efficacy and toxicity. Med Oncol 2013;30:361.

36. O'Connell MJ, Martenson JA, Wieand HS, et al. Improving adjuvant therapy for rectal cancer by combining protracted-infusion fluorouracil with radiation therapy after curative surgery. N Engl J Med 1994;331:502–7.

37. Rich TA, Lokich JJ, Chaffey JT. A pilot study of protracted venous infusion of 5-fluorouracil and concomitant radiation therapy. J Clin Oncol 1985;3:402–6.

38. Sawada N, Ishikawa T, Sekiguchi F, et al. X-ray irradiation induces thymidine phosphorylase and enhances the efficacy of capecitabine (Xeloda) in human cancer xenografts. Clin Cancer Res 1999;5:2948–53.

39. Crane CH, Abbruzzese JL, Evans DB, et al. Is the therapeutic index better with gemcitabine-based chemoradiation than with 5-fluorouracil-based chemoradiation in locally advanced pancreatic cancer? Int J Radiat Oncol Biol Phys 2002; 52:1293–302.

40. Murphy JD, Adusumilli S, Griffith KA, et al. Full-dose gemcitabine and concurrent radiotherapy for unresectable pancreatic cancer. Int J Radiat Oncol Biol Phys 2007;68:801–8.

41. Sudo K, Yamaguchi T, Ishihara T, et al. Phase II study of oral S-1 and concurrent radiotherapy in patients with unresectable locally advanced pancreatic cancer. Int J Radiat Oncol Biol Phys 2011;80:119–25.

42. Rich T, Harris J, Abrams R, et al. Phase II study of external irradiation and weekly paclitaxel for nonmetastatic, unresectable pancreatic cancer: RTOG-98-12. Am J Clin Oncol 2004;27:51–6.

43. Jiang Y, Mackley HB, Kimchi ET, et al. Phase I dose escalation study of capecitabine and erlotinib concurrent with radiation in locally advanced pancreatic cancer. Cancer Chemother Pharmacol 2014;74:205–10.

44. Chakravarthy AB, Tsai CJ, O'Brien N, et al. A phase I study of cetuximab in combination with gemcitabine and radiation for locally advanced pancreatic cancer. Gastrointest Cancer Res 2012;5:112–8.

45. Small W Jr, Mulcahy MF, Rademaker A, et al. Phase II trial of full-dose gemcitabine and bevacizumab in combination with attenuated three-dimensional conformal radiotherapy in patients with localized pancreatic cancer. Int J Radiat Oncol Biol Phys 2011;80:476–82.

46. Brunner TB, Geiger M, Grabenbauer GG, et al. Phase I trial of the human immunodeficiency virus protease inhibitor nelfinavir and chemoradiation for locally advanced pancreatic cancer. J Clin Oncol 2008;26:2699–706.

47. Herman JM, Wild AT, Wang H, et al. Randomized phase III multi-institutional study of TNFerade biologic with fluorouracil and radiotherapy for locally advanced pancreatic cancer: final results. J Clin Oncol 2013;31:886–94.

48. Milano MT, Chmura SJ, Garofalo MC, et al. Intensity-modulated radiotherapy in treatment of pancreatic and bile duct malignancies: toxicity and clinical outcome. Int J Radiat Oncol Biol Phys 2004;59:445–53.

49. van der Geld YG, van Triest B, Verbakel WF, et al. Evaluation of four-dimensional computed tomography-based intensity-modulated and respiratory-gated

radiotherapy techniques for pancreatic carcinoma. Int J Radiat Oncol Biol Phys 2008;72:1215–20.

50. Ben-Josef E, Shields AF, Vaishampayan U, et al. Intensity-modulated radiotherapy (IMRT) and concurrent capecitabine for pancreatic cancer. Int J Radiat Oncol Biol Phys 2004;59:454–9.

51. Yovino S, Poppe M, Jabbour S, et al. Intensity-modulated radiation therapy significantly improves acute gastrointestinal toxicity in pancreatic and ampullary cancers. Int J Radiat Oncol Biol Phys 2011;79:158–62.

52. Abelson JA, Murphy JD, Minn AY, et al. Intensity-modulated radiotherapy for pancreatic adenocarcinoma. Int J Radiat Oncol Biol Phys 2012;82:e595–601.

53. McGinn CJ, Zalupski MM, Shureiqi I, et al. Phase I trial of radiation dose escalation with concurrent weekly full-dose gemcitabine in patients with advanced pancreatic cancer. J Clin Oncol 2001;19:4202–8.

54. Muler JH, McGinn CJ, Normolle D, et al. Phase I trial using a time-to-event continual reassessment strategy for dose escalation of cisplatin combined with gemcitabine and radiation therapy in pancreatic cancer. J Clin Oncol 2004;22: 238–43.

55. Goldstein D, Van Hazel G, Walpole E, et al. Gemcitabine with a specific conformal 3D 5FU radiochemotherapy technique is safe and effective in the definitive management of locally advanced pancreatic cancer. Br J Cancer 2007;97:464–71.

56. Jackson AS, Jain P, Watkins GR, et al. Efficacy and tolerability of limited field radiotherapy with concurrent capecitabine in locally advanced pancreatic cancer. Clin Oncol 2010;22:570–7.

57. Bussels B, Goethals L, Feron M, et al. Respiration-induced movement of the upper abdominal organs: a pitfall for the three-dimensional conformal radiation treatment of pancreatic cancer. Radiother Oncol 2003;68:69–74.

58. Minohara S, Kanai T, Endo M, et al. Respiratory gated irradiation system for heavy-ion radiotherapy. Int J Radiat Oncol Biol Phys 2000;47:1097–103.

59. Ohara K, Okumura T, Akisada M, et al. Irradiation synchronized with respiration gate. Int J Radiat Oncol Biol Phys 1989;17:853–7.

60. Taniguchi CM, Murphy JD, Eclov N, et al. Dosimetric analysis of organs at risk during expiratory gating in stereotactic body radiation therapy for pancreatic cancer. Int J Radiat Oncol Biol Phys 2013;85:1090–5.

61. Wang X, Zhong R, Bai S, et al. Lung tumor reproducibility with active breath control (ABC) in image-guided radiotherapy based on cone-beam computed tomography with two registration methods. Radiother Oncol 2011;99:148–54.

62. Wong JW, Sharpe MB, Jaffray DA, et al. The use of active breathing control (ABC) to reduce margin for breathing motion. Int J Radiat Oncol Biol Phys 1999;44: 911–9.

63. Small W Jr, Berlin J, Freedman GM, et al. Full-dose gemcitabine with concurrent radiation therapy in patients with nonmetastatic pancreatic cancer: a multicenter phase II trial. J Clin Oncol 2008;26:942–7.

64. Shinchi H, Takao S, Noma H, et al. Length and quality of survival after external-beam radiotherapy with concurrent continuous 5-fluorouracil infusion for locally unresectable pancreatic cancer. Int J Radiat Oncol Biol Phys 2002;53:146–50.

65. Haddock MG, Swaminathan R, Foster NR, et al. Gemcitabine, cisplatin, and radiotherapy for patients with locally advanced pancreatic adenocarcinoma: results of the North Central Cancer Treatment Group Phase II Study N9942. J Clin Oncol 2007;25:2567–72.

66. Willett CG, Czito BG, Bendell JC, et al. Locally advanced pancreatic cancer. J Clin Oncol 2005;23:4538–44.

67. Crane CH, Beddar AS, Evans DB. The role of intraoperative radiotherapy in pancreatic cancer. Surg Oncol Clin N Am 2003;12:965–77.
68. Willett CG, Del Castillo CF, Shih HA, et al. Long-term results of intraoperative electron beam irradiation (IOERT) for patients with unresectable pancreatic cancer. Ann Surg 2005;241:295–9.
69. Leksell L. The stereotaxic method and radiosurgery of the brain. Acta Chir Scand 1951;102:316–9.
70. Scorsetti M, Alongi F, Castiglioni S, et al. Feasibility and early clinical assessment of flattening filter free (FFF) based stereotactic body radiotherapy (SBRT) treatments. Radiat Oncol 2011;6:113.
71. Schweikard A, Shiomi H, Adler J. Respiration tracking in radiosurgery. Med Phys 2004;31:2738–41.
72. Jayachandran P, Minn AY, Van Dam J, et al. Interfractional uncertainty in the treatment of pancreatic cancer with radiation. Int J Radiat Oncol Biol Phys 2010;76: 603–7.
73. Minn AY, Schellenberg D, Maxim P, et al. Pancreatic tumor motion on a single planning 4D-CT does not correlate with intrafraction tumor motion during treatment. Am J Clin Oncol 2009;32:364–8.
74. Kothary N, Heit JJ, Louie JD, et al. Safety and efficacy of percutaneous fiducial marker implantation for image-guided radiation therapy. J Vasc Interv Radiol 2009;20:235–9.
75. Park WG, Yan BM, Schellenberg D, et al. EUS-guided gold fiducial insertion for image-guided radiation therapy of pancreatic cancer: 50 successful cases without fluoroscopy. Gastrointest Endosc 2010;71:513–8.
76. Koong AC, Le QT, Ho A, et al. Phase I study of stereotactic radiosurgery in patients with locally advanced pancreatic cancer. Int J Radiat Oncol Biol Phys 2004;58:1017–21.
77. Schellenberg D, Goodman KA, Lee F, et al. Gemcitabine chemotherapy and single-fraction stereotactic body radiotherapy for locally advanced pancreatic cancer. Int J Radiat Oncol Biol Phys 2008;72:678–86.
78. Schellenberg D, Kim J, Christman-Skieller C, et al. Single-fraction stereotactic body radiation therapy and sequential gemcitabine for the treatment of locally advanced pancreatic cancer. Int J Radiat Oncol Biol Phys 2011;81:181–8.
79. Koong AC, Christofferson E, Le QT, et al. Phase II study to assess the efficacy of conventionally fractionated radiotherapy followed by a stereotactic radiosurgery boost in patients with locally advanced pancreatic cancer. Int J Radiat Oncol Biol Phys 2005;63:320–3.
80. Chang DT, Schellenberg D, Shen J, et al. Stereotactic radiotherapy for unresectable adenocarcinoma of the pancreas. Cancer 2009;115:665–72.
81. Murphy JD, Christman-Skieller C, Kim J, et al. A dosimetric model of duodenal toxicity after stereotactic body radiotherapy for pancreatic cancer. Int J Radiat Oncol Biol Phys 2010;78:1420–6.
82. Pollom EL, Alagappan M, von Eyben R, et al. Single- versus multifraction stereotactic body radiation therapy for pancreatic adenocarcinoma: outcomes and toxicity. Int J Radiat Oncol Biol Phys 2014;90:918–25.
83. Herman JM, Chang DT, Goodman KA, et al. Phase II multi-institutional trial evaluating gemcitabine and stereotactic body radiation therapy for locally advanced unresectable pancreatic adenocarcinoma. Cancer 2015;121(7):1128–37.
84. Rich TA, Winter K, Safran H, et al. Weekly paclitaxel, gemcitabine, and external irradiation followed by randomized farnesyl transferase inhibitor R115777 for locally advanced pancreatic cancer. Onco Targets Ther 2012;5:161–70.

85. Crane CH, Winter K, Regine WF, et al. Phase II study of bevacizumab with concurrent capecitabine and radiation followed by maintenance gemcitabine and bevacizumab for locally advanced pancreatic cancer: Radiation Therapy Oncology Group RTOG 0411. J Clin Oncol 2009;27:4096–102.
86. Mamon HJ, Niedzwiecki D, Hollis D, et al. A phase 2 trial of gemcitabine, 5-fluorouracil, and radiation therapy in locally advanced nonmetastatic pancreatic adenocarcinoma: cancer and Leukemia Group B (CALGB) 80003. Cancer 2011;117:2620–8.
87. Ch'ang HJ, Lin YL, Wang HP, et al. Induction chemotherapy with gemcitabine, oxaliplatin, and 5-fluorouracil/leucovorin followed by concomitant chemoradiotherapy in patients with locally advanced pancreatic cancer: a Taiwan cooperative oncology group phase II study. Int J Radiat Oncol Biol Phys 2011;81:e749–57.
88. Hoyer M, Roed H, Sengelov L, et al. Phase-II study on stereotactic radiotherapy of locally advanced pancreatic carcinoma. Radiother Oncol 2005;76:48–53.
89. Didolkar MS, Coleman CW, Brenner MJ, et al. Image-guided stereotactic radiosurgery for locally advanced pancreatic adenocarcinoma results of first 85 patients. J Gastrointest Surg 2010;14:1547–59.
90. Rwigema JC, Parikh SD, Heron DE, et al. Stereotactic body radiotherapy in the treatment of advanced adenocarcinoma of the pancreas. Am J Clin Oncol 2011;34:63–9.
91. Mahadevan A, Jain S, Goldstein M, et al. Stereotactic body radiotherapy and gemcitabine for locally advanced pancreatic cancer. Int J Radiat Oncol Biol Phys 2010;78:735–42.
92. Mahadevan A, Miksad R, Goldstein M, et al. Induction gemcitabine and stereotactic body radiotherapy for locally advanced nonmetastatic pancreas cancer. Int J Radiat Oncol Biol Phys 2011;81:e615–22.
93. Seo Y, Kim MS, Yoo S, et al. Stereotactic body radiation therapy boost in locally advanced pancreatic cancer. Int J Radiat Oncol Biol Phys 2009;75:1456–61.
94. Polistina F, Costantin G, Casamassima F, et al. Unresectable locally advanced pancreatic cancer: a multimodal treatment using neoadjuvant chemoradiotherapy (gemcitabine plus stereotactic radiosurgery) and subsequent surgical exploration. Ann Surg Oncol 2010;17:2092–101.
95. Goyal K, Einstein D, Ibarra RA, et al. Stereotactic body radiation therapy for nonresectable tumors of the pancreas. J Surg Res 2012;174:319–25.
96. Lominska CE, Unger K, Nasr NM, et al. Stereotactic body radiation therapy for reirradiation of localized adenocarcinoma of the pancreas. Radiat Oncol 2012; 7:74.
97. Gurka MK, Collins SP, Slack R, et al. Stereotactic body radiation therapy with concurrent full-dose gemcitabine for locally advanced pancreatic cancer: a pilot trial demonstrating safety. Radiat Oncol 2013;8:44.
98. Chuong MD, Springett GM, Freilich JM, et al. Stereotactic body radiation therapy for locally advanced and borderline resectable pancreatic cancer is effective and well tolerated. Int J Radiat Oncol Biol Phys 2013;86:516–22.

Therapeutic Approaches for Metastatic Pancreatic Adenocarcinoma

Douglas A. Rubinson, MD, PhD[a,b], Brian M. Wolpin, MD, MPH[b,c],*

KEYWORDS

- Pancreatic cancer • Metastatic disease • Gemcitabine • FOLFIRINOX
- Nab-paclitaxel • Targeted therapy

KEY POINTS

- Over 50% of patients with pancreatic cancer present with metastatic disease, when treatment is palliative and consists primarily of systemic chemotherapy.
- Recent studies have identified 2 combination chemotherapy programs that impart improved survival times compared with gemcitabine monotherapy for patients with adequate functional status: FOLFIRINOX (folinic acid, 5-fluorouracil, irinotecan, oxaliplatin) and gemcitabine plus nab-paclitaxel.
- New treatment approaches that leverage a growing understanding of pancreatic cancer biology are under development, including those that modify tumor-associated stroma, inhibit signaling from mutant *KRAS*, augment host immune response to the cancer, and exploit defects in tumor DNA repair mechanisms.

INTRODUCTION

Among 46,420 estimated new cases of pancreatic cancer in the United States in 2014, the majority of patients are diagnosed with metastatic disease at presentation.[1] Among the patients able to undergo a potentially curative resection, most experience disease relapse, necessitating palliative therapy. Thus, the 5-year survival rate among all patients diagnosed with pancreatic ductal adenocarcinoma (PDAC) remains estimated at 6.7%, with pancreatic cancer projected to become the second leading cause of cancer death in the United States by 2020.[2]

Since the US Food and Drug Administration (FDA) approval of gemcitabine monotherapy in 1996,[3] multiple randomized trials have failed to demonstrate improved

These authors have nothing to disclose.
[a] Department of Medical Oncology, Dana-Farber Cancer Institute, 450 Brookline Avenue, Boston, MA 02215, USA; [b] Harvard Medical School, 25 Shattuck St, Boston, MA 02115, USA; [c] Pancreas and Biliary Tumor Center, Department of Medical Oncology, Dana-Farber Cancer Institute, 450 Brookline Avenue, Boston, MA 02215, USA
* Corresponding author.
E-mail address: bwolpin@partners.org

survival for combination chemotherapy programs in advanced PDAC. However, in the past several years, clinical trials of FOLFIRINOX[4] and gemcitabine plus nab-paclitaxel[5] have demonstrated improved outcomes compared with gemcitabine alone in patients with metastatic PDAC. Targeted therapies and immunotherapy building upon these new chemotherapy backbones hold great promise for future improvements in patient outcomes.

PATIENT EVALUATION AND PROGNOSTIC MARKERS

Suspicion for metastatic PDAC typically results from symptomatic complaints and the radiologic appearance of a pancreatic mass associated with a characteristic pattern of metastatic spread. Presenting symptoms relate either to the local effects of the primary pancreatic mass, such as with biliary obstruction, epigastric pain, and weight loss, or from symptoms due to metastatic deposits, which most commonly occur in the liver, peritoneum, and lungs. Initial evaluation consists of computed tomographic scan encompassing the chest, abdomen, and pelvis and biopsy of the primary tumor or a metastatic site to confirm invasive adenocarcinoma. Histologic evaluation is important because less-common malignancies can resemble metastatic PDAC but require distinct management. These malignancies include less-common pancreatic malignancies such as pancreatic neuroendocrine tumors and nonpancreatic malignancies such as high-grade lymphomas or metastatic implants to the pancreas.

Immunohistochemistry (IHC) of a metastatic biopsy can be helpful in confirming the diagnosis when the primary pancreatic mass is difficult to visualize on imaging studies. PDAC typically demonstrates reactivity against cytokeratin (CK) 7, CK19, and carcinoembryonic antigen (CEA) and often lacks reactivity to CK20.[6] IHC analysis for loss of Smad4 expression, which occurs in approximately 50% of PDAC tumors, as well as mutation analysis of the *KRAS* oncogene, which is mutated at codons 12 or 61 in 80% to 95% of tumors, can also be useful in defining a pancreatic origin when the primary site is radiologically indistinct.

The serum markers carbohydrate antigen 19-9 (CA19-9) and CEA should be assessed at diagnosis, and if their levels are elevated, they can be followed serially during therapy as a disease surrogate. CA19-9 is a sialylated Lewis blood group antigen that requires fucosyltransferase 3 (FUT3) activity for its production. Almost 10% of the population bears a germline polymorphism in *FUT3*, making them Lewis-antigen negative and incapable of producing CA19-9.[7] For individuals capable of CA19-9 production, low serum CA19-9 levels at diagnosis and declines in CA19-9 levels with initiation of chemotherapy are associated with improved outcomes.[8,9] Additional clinical, circulating, and histologic factors are associated with poorer prognosis in patients undergoing chemotherapy for metastatic PDAC, including older age, poor performance status, high serum C-reactive protein (CRP) levels, high metastatic burden, presence of peritoneal carcinomatosis, and high-grade histology.[10,11]

Molecular alterations have also been associated with prognosis in PDAC. Pancreatic cancers are typified by genetic alterations in *KRAS*, *TP53*, *CDKN2A*, and *SMAD4*, with approximately 40% of tumors possessing alterations in all 4 genes.[12] Initial studies have demonstrated a poorer prognosis for patients with tumors possessing a greater number of these alterations.[12] Furthermore, a comprehensive sequencing analysis of resected pancreatic cancers identified a survival disadvantage to the presence of somatic alterations in axon guidance genes.[13]

GEMCITABINE

Gemcitabine is a nucleoside analog whose metabolic product, difluorodeoxycytidine triphosphate competes with deoxycytidine for incorporation into DNA, inhibiting DNA synthesis.[14] US FDA approval of gemcitabine in 1996 for patients with advanced PDAC followed the report of a trial involving 126 patients randomized to weekly gemcitabine (1000 mg/m² weekly × 7 followed by a week of rest, and then weekly for 3 of every 4 weeks) or weekly bolus of 5-fluorouracil at 600 mg/m².[3] The primary outcome of the trial was clinical benefit as assessed by a composite of pain measurement, Karnofsky performance status (KPS), and weight loss. Clinical benefit was seen in 23.8% of patients receiving gemcitabine compared with 4.8% of those receiving 5-fluorouracil ($P = .0022$). Median overall survival (OS) was superior in the gemcitabine group at 5.65 months compared with 4.41 months in the 5-fluorouracil group ($P = .0025$).[3] Furthermore, the 12-month survival rate was 18% for patients receiving gemcitabine versus 2% for those receiving 5-fluorouracil. This trial established single-agent gemcitabine as the standard of care for first-line treatment of patients with advanced PDAC.

Strategies to Improve Gemcitabine Effectiveness

In an attempt to improve upon the efficacy of weekly gemcitabine at 1000 mg/m² administered over 30 minutes, prolonged gemcitabine infusions were evaluated. A phase 1 pharmacokinetic study demonstrated saturation of the rate-limiting deoxycytidine-kinase-driven enzymatic conversion of gemcitabine to its active metabolite with an optimal dose rate of 10 mg/m²/min.[15] Thus, it was hypothesized that prolonged infusion of gemcitabine could maximize production of the active nucleotide analog and improve efficacy for a given dose of gemcitabine. A fixed dose rate (FDR) gemcitabine strategy of 10 mg/m²/min over 150 minutes was assessed in phase 2 trials and suggested improved response rates compared with standard infusion rates.[16] Nevertheless, a randomized phase 3 clinical trial demonstrated no statistically significant improvement in survival for FDR gemcitabine compared with standard gemcitabine infusion in patients with advanced PDAC.[17]

One mechanism that may explain de novo resistance of PDAC to gemcitabine is low tumor expression of human equilibrative nucleoside transporter 1 (hENT1), a transporter protein that facilitates gemcitabine entry into cells. CO-101 is a lipid-drug conjugate of gemcitabine that allows hENT1-independent entry of gemcitabine into tumor cells. A large phase 2 trial dichotomized patients with metastatic PDAC into hENT1-high and hENT1-low subgroups based on tumor staining for hENT1 by IHC, with the hypothesis that patients with low hENT1 expression may derive benefit from CO-101. Unfortunately, no difference was observed in survival between patients who received gemcitabine and those who received CO-101 in the hENT1-low subgroup or the overall study population.[18]

Gemcitabine Treatment Doublets

Gemcitabine-based chemotherapy doublets have been extensively explored in patients with advanced PDAC, with the goal of improving upon the modest efficacy of gemcitabine monotherapy (**Table 1**). The combination of gemcitabine with 5-fluorouracil[19] or its orally available prodrug capecitabine[20,21] failed to demonstrate statistically significant improvements in OS in several individual trials. However, a meta-analysis of 3 randomized trials evaluating gemcitabine plus capecitabine versus gemcitabine monotherapy in patients with advanced PDAC demonstrated statistical significance with a hazard ratio (HR) of 0.86 (95% confidence interval [CI],

Table 1
Selected phase 3 clinical trials of gemcitabine-based cytotoxic chemotherapy in advanced pancreatic adenocarcinoma

Study	No. of Patients	Treatment Arms	Progression-Free Survival			Overall Survival		
			Median (mo)	HR (95% CI)	Log-Rank P Value	Median (mo)	HR (95% CI)	Log-Rank P Value
Berlin et al,[19] 2002	327	Gemcitabine	2.2			5.4		
		Gemcitabine + 5-fluorouracil	3.4	NA	.02	6.7	NA	.09
Rocha Lima et al,[26] 2004	360	Gemcitabine	3.0			6.6		
		Gemcitabine + irinotecan	3.5	NA	.35	6.3	NA	.79
Louvet et al,[25] 2005	313	Gemcitabine	3.7			7.1		
		Gemcitabine + oxaliplatin	5.8	1.29 (1.01–1.69)	.04	9.0	1.20 (0.95–1.54)	.13
Oettle et al,[28] 2005	565	Gemcitabine	3.3			6.3		
		Gemcitabine + pemetrexed	3.9	NA	.11	6.2	0.98 (0.82–1.18)	.85
Abou-Alfa et al,[27] 2006	349	Gemcitabine	3.8			6.2		
		Gemcitabine + exatecan	3.7	NA	.22	6.7	NA	.52
Heinemann et al,[24] 2006	195	Gemcitabine	3.1			6.0		
		Gemcitabine + cisplatin	5.3	0.75 (NA)	.05	7.5	0.80 (NA)	.15
Herrmann et al,[21] 2007	319	Gemcitabine	3.9			7.2		
		Gemcitabine + capecitabine	4.3	NA	.10	8.4	0.87 (0.67–1.10)	.23
Cunningham et al,[20] 2009	533	Gemcitabine	3.8			6.2		
		Gemcitabine + capecitabine	5.3	0.78 (0.66–0.93)	.004	7.1	0.86 (0.72–1.02)	.08
Poplin et al,[17] 2009	832	Gemcitabine	2.6			4.9		
		Gemcitabine FDR	3.5	NA	.04[a]	6.2	0.83 (0.69–1.00)	.04[a]
		Gemcitabine + oxaliplatin	2.7	NA	.10	5.7	0.88 (0.73–1.05)	.22
Colucci et al,[23] 2010	400	Gemcitabine	3.9			8.3		
		Gemcitabine + cisplatin	3.8	0.97 (0.80–1.19)	.80	7.2	1.10 (0.89–1.35)	.38
Ueno et al,[22] 2013	554	Gemcitabine	4.1			8.8		
		Gemcitabine + S-1	5.7	0.66 (0.54–0.81)	<.001	10.1	0.88 (0.71–1.08)	.15
Von Hoff et al,[5] 2013	861	Gemcitabine	3.7			6.7		
		Gemcitabine + nab-paclitaxel	5.5	0.69 (0.58–0.82)	<.001	8.5	0.72 (0.62–0.83)	<.001

Abbreviations: CI, confidence interval; HR, hazard ratio; NA, not available.
[a] P values did not meet the study-defined thresholds for statistical significance.

0.75–0.98).[20] Nevertheless, the improvement in median OS with the combination was less than 1 month (6.2 vs 7.1 months) and patients receiving gemcitabine plus capecitabine experienced increased neutropenia and hand-foot syndrome. The oral fluoropyrimidine analog S-1 has been studied primarily in Asia in patients with gastrointestinal malignancies. In patients with advanced PDAC, a phase 3 trial conducted in Japan and Taiwan compared gemcitabine monotherapy to either S-1 monotherapy or gemcitabine plus S-1. Monotherapy with S-1 was noninferior to gemcitabine, but the trial failed to demonstrate a significant improvement in OS with the gemcitabine plus S-1 combination compared with gemcitabine alone.[22]

Clinical trials assessing gemcitabine combined with other cytotoxic agents have been similarly disappointing (see **Table 1**). Phase 3 studies assessing combination therapy of gemcitabine with platinum compounds including cisplatin[23,24] and oxaliplatin[17,25] failed to recapitulate the suggested synergy observed in preclinical and phase 2 studies. In addition, phase 3 studies adding irinotecan,[26] exatecan,[27] or pemetrexed[28] to gemcitabine were unable to demonstrate improved survival with combination treatment programs compared with gemcitabine alone.

In addition to cytotoxic doublets, phase 3 trials have also assessed several molecularly targeted agents in combination with gemcitabine (**Table 2**). The dense tumor stroma and poor vascularity of PDAC suggested that inhibition of tumor-derived angiogenesis could normalize the vascular microenvironment of pancreatic tumors and permit improved chemotherapy delivery.[29] Several trials assessed the addition to gemcitabine of antiangiogenic agents, including bevacizumab, ziv-aflibercept, and axitinib.[30–33] Bevacizumab is a monoclonal antibody to vascular endothelial growth factor (VEGF)-A, while ziv-aflibercept binds to VEGF-A, VEGF-B, and placental growth factor and axitinib binds to VEGF receptors, inhibiting receptor signaling. No statistically significant survival benefit was seen for these agents in randomized phase 3 trials of gemcitabine plus placebo versus gemcitabine plus the antiangiogenic agent.[30–33] A randomized phase 3 trial also failed to demonstrate benefit of adding sorafenib, an agent thought to inhibit downstream signaling from *KRAS* and with antiangiogenic activity, to gemcitabine.[34] Agents targeting other molecular pathways have also been combined with gemcitabine in large randomized phase 3 trials with negative results, including ganitumab[35] and cetuximab[36] monoclonal antibodies to the insulinlike growth factor 1 receptor and epidermal growth factor receptor (EGFR), respectively.

Gemcitabine and Erlotinib

The observation of EGFR overexpression in PDAC and data suggesting that EGFR overexpression is associated with poorer outcomes[37] led to the evaluation of erlotinib, a small-molecule EGFR inhibitor, in patients with pancreatic cancer. A phase 3 trial (PA.3) randomized 569 patients to receive gemcitabine monotherapy or gemcitabine plus erlotinib and demonstrated an improvement in median OS for the combination arm from 5.91 months to 6.24 months (HR, 0.82; 95% CI, 0.69–0.99; $P = .038$).[38] This improvement in survival was accompanied by increased rates of diarrhea of any grade (56% vs 41%) and rash of any grade (72% vs 29%) in the gemcitabine plus erlotinib arm. Given the modest survival benefit and increased toxicity of gemcitabine plus erlotinib, uptake of this regimen by the oncology community was not widespread.

Experience with EGFR inhibition in other malignancies has suggested that the development of acneiform rash is predictive of improved patient survival.[39] The phase 2 RACHEL (Dose-Escalation to Rash for Erlotinib Plus Gemcitabine for Metastatic Pancreatic Cancer) study attempted to dose-escalate erlotinib from 100 mg daily by 50 mg every 2 weeks to a maximum of 250 mg daily in combination with gemcitabine

Table 2
Selected phase 3 clinical trials of targeted agents in advanced pancreatic adenocarcinoma

Study	No. of Patients	Treatment Arms	Progression-Free Survival			Overall Survival		
			Median (mo)	HR (95% CI)	Log-Rank P Value	Median (mo)	HR (95% CI)	Log-Rank P Value
Bramhall et al,[57] 2002	239	Gemcitabine Gemcitabine + marimastat	3.2 3.0	0.95 (0.73–1.23)	.68	5.4 5.4	0.99 (0.76–1.30)	.95
Van Cutsem et al,[58] 2004	688	Gemcitabine Gemcitabine + tipifarnib	3.6 3.7	1.03 (0.87–1.22)	.72	6.0 6.3	1.03 (0.86–1.23)	.75
Moore et al,[38] 2007	569	Gemcitabine Gemcitabine + erlotinib	3.6 3.8	0.77 (0.64–0.92)	.004	5.9 6.2	0.82 (0.69–0.99)	.04
Van Cutsem et al,[31] 2009	301	Gemcitabine + erlotinib Gem + erlotinib + bevacizumab	3.6 4.6	0.73 (0.61–0.86)	.0002	6.0 7.1	0.89 (0.74–1.07)	.21
Kindler et al,[30] 2010	602	Gemcitabine Gemcitabine + bevacizumab	2.9 3.8	NA	.08	5.9 5.8	1.04 (0.88–1.24)	.95
Phillip et al,[36] 2010	745	Gemcitabine Gemcitabine + cetuximab	3.0 3.4	1.07 (0.93–1.24)	.18	5.9 6.3	1.06 (0.91–1.23)	.23
Kindler et al,[33] 2011	632	Gemcitabine Gemcitabine + axitinib	4.4 4.4	1.01 (0.78–1.30)	.52	8.3 8.5	1.01 (0.79–1.31)	.54
Goncalves et al,[34] 2012	104	Gemcitabine Gemcitabine + sorafenib	5.7 3.8	1.04 (0.70–1.55)	.90	9.2 8.0	1.27 (0.84–1.93)	.23
Rougier et al,[32] 2013	546	Gemcitabine Gemcitabine + ziv-aflibercept	3.7 3.7	1.02 (0.83–1.25)	.86	7.8 6.5	1.17 (0.92–1.47)	.20

Abbreviation: NA, not available.

or until development of a rash of grade 2 or more. Nevertheless, this erlotinib dose-escalation strategy failed to improve outcomes in patients with metastatic PDAC compared with standard erlotinib administration.[40] Most pancreatic cancers (80%–95%) possess activating mutations in the KRAS oncogene.[13] Clinical benefit from EGFR inhibition in colorectal and lung cancer is limited to tumors lacking an activating KRAS mutation.[41,42] To assess whether KRAS mutations conferred resistance to erlotinib therapy in pancreatic cancer, posthoc analyses were performed of the PA.3 trial and a second trial involving erlotinib, known as AIO-PK0104 (Arbeitsgemeinschaft Internistische Onkologie - PK0104).[38,43] The latter trial compared gemcitabine followed by capecitabine at disease progression with capecitabine followed by gemcitabine at disease progression, with erlotinib administered in the first-line regimen in both arms. Unfortunately, these subgroup analyses had modest power and failed to show statistically significant interactions between somatic KRAS mutations and patient survival while receiving erlotinib.[44,45]

FOLINIC ACID, 5-FLUOROURACIL, IRINOTECAN, OXALIPLATIN

The report of the PRODIGE-4/ACCORD-11 (Partenarait de Recherche en Oncologie Digestive-4 / Actions Concertées dans les Cancers Colo-Rectaux et Digestifs-11) phase 3 trial comparing FOLFIRINOX with gemcitabine altered the therapeutic landscape for patients with metastatic PDAC.[4] Patients were eligible if they were aged 18 to 75 years and had previously untreated metastatic PDAC, Eastern Cooperative Oncology Group (ECOG) performance status of 0 or 1, and adequate liver function (bilirubin levels $\leq$1.5 times the upper limit of normal). Patients were randomized to receive gemcitabine or FOLFIRINOX, which was given every 2 weeks and consisted of oxaliplatin 85 mg/m^2, irinotecan 180 mg/m^2, leucovorin 400 mg/m^2, and 5-fluorouracil 400 mg/m^2 bolus followed by an intravenous infusion of 2400 mg/m^2 over 46 hours.

The OS significantly improved with FOLFIRINOX (HR, 0.57; 95% CI, 0.45–0.73; $P<.001$), with median OS of 11.1 months for patients receiving FOLFIRINOX compared with 6.8 months for patients receiving gemcitabine (**Table 3**). Improvements were also noted in 1-year survival rate (48.4% vs 20.6%), median progression-free survival (PFS) (6.4 months vs 3.3 months), and response rate (31.6% vs 9.4%). However, FOLFIRINOX was associated with increased rates of several toxicities, including grade 3 or 4 sensory neuropathy, diarrhea, neutropenia, febrile neutropenia, and thrombocytopenia (**Table 4**). The PRODIGE trial also included regular assessments of quality of life using the European Organization for the Research and Treatment of Cancer quality of life core questionnaire (QLQ-C30). Despite increased toxicities from chemotherapy, patients reported a significant improvement in global health status and a delay in time until deterioration of health status with FOLFIRINOX,[46] likely reflecting the ability of FOLFIRINOX to ameliorate cancer-related symptoms and delay disease progression. Attempts to modify FOLFIRINOX to improve tolerability have assessed elimination of the bolus dose of 5-fluorouracil, modification of irinotecan or oxaliplatin doses, and standard inclusion of growth factor support.[47,48] Nevertheless, the efficacy of these modified programs has not been definitively demonstrated in comparison with the FOLFIRINOX program tested in the PRODIGE trial.

GEMCITABINE PLUS NAB-PACLITAXEL

The pancreatic tumor stroma and microenvironment have been proposed as barriers to therapy, and pancreatic cancer-associated fibroblasts generate an environment rich in the secreted protein SPARC, an albumin-binding protein.[49] To target the tumor stroma, an albumin-bound formulation of paclitaxel (nab-paclitaxel) was designed and

Table 3
Patient characteristics and outcomes in the PRODIGE and MPACT trials

| Outcome or Characteristic | PRODIGE Trial | | MPACT Trial | |
	FOLFIRINOX (N = 171)	Gemcitabine (N = 171)	Gemcitabine (N = 430)	Gemcitabine + Nab-paclitaxel (N = 431)
Overall survival				
HR (95% CI)	0.57 (0.45–0.73)		0.72 (0.62–0.83)	
Log-rank P value	<.001		<.001	
Median, mo	11.1	6.8	6.7	8.5
12 mo, %	48.4	20.6	22	35
Progression-free survival				
HR (95% CI)	0.47 (0.37–0.59)		0.69 (0.58–0.82)	
Log-rank P value	<.001		<.001	
Median, mo	6.4	3.3	3.7	5.5
Response rate, %	31.6	9.4	7	23
Median age, y (range)	61 (25–76)	61 (34–75)	63 (32–88)	62 (27–86)
Male gender, %	62.0	61.4	60	57
ECOG PS or KPS, %				
0 or 100	37.4	38.6	16	16
1 or 80/90	61.9	61.4	76	77
2 or 60/70	0.6	0	8	7
Primary head tumor, %	39.2	36.8	42	44
Biliary stent, %	15.8	12.9	16	19
Serum CA19-9, %				
Normal	14.6	13.9	15	16
Elevated, <59 times the ULN	43.9	39.4	32	32
Elevated, ≥59 times the ULN	41.5	46.7	52	52
Unknown	4.1	3.5	0	0
Metastatic organ involvement, %				
Liver	87.6	87.7	84	85
Lung	19.4	28.7	43	35
Peritoneum	19.4	18.7	2	4

Abbreviations: PS, performance status; ULN, upper limit of normal.

evaluated in patients with advanced PDAC. In a single-arm phase 2 study of patients with metastatic PDAC, gemcitabine plus nab-paclitaxel demonstrated a 12.2-month median OS with a response rate of 42%. Although this was a nonrandomized study and subject to bias because of patient selection, the results prompted an 861-patient phase 3 trial of gemcitabine monotherapy versus gemcitabine plus nab-paclitaxel.[5] The MPACT trial demonstrated a statistically significant improvement in survival for gemcitabine plus nab-paclitaxel compared with gemcitabine monotherapy with median OS of 8.5 months versus 6.7 months (HR, 0.72; 95% CI, 0.62–0.83; P<.001) (see **Table 3**). Improvements were also seen for the combination regimen in PFS (HR, 0.69; 95% CI, 0.58–0.82; P<.001) and response rate (23% vs 7%; P<.001). Grade 3 or 4 toxicities that had higher rates in the gemcitabine plus nab-paclitaxel arm compared with the gemcitabine monotherapy arm included peripheral neuropathy (17% vs 1%), neutropenia (38% vs 27%), diarrhea (6% vs 1%), and fatigue (17% vs

Table 4
Selected grade 3 or greater adverse events in the PRODIGE and MPACT trials

Adverse Event	PRODIGE Trial		MPACT Trial	
	FOLFIRINOX	Gemcitabine	Gemcitabine	Gemcitabine + Nab-paclitaxel
Neutropenia (%)	45.7	21.0	27	38
Febrile neutropenia (%)	5.4	1.2	1	3
Thrombocytopenia (%)	9.1	3.6	9	13
Peripheral neuropathy (%)	9.0	0.0	1	17
Diarrhea (%)	12.7	1.8	1	6
Fatigue (%)	23.6	17.8	7	17

7%) (see **Table 4**). Quality of life data were not systematically collected from patients enrolled to the MPACT (Metastatic Pancreatic Adenocarcinoma Clinical Trial) trial.

Growing molecular evidence suggests that the mechanism of activity for nab-paclitaxel when administered with gemcitabine may be independent of SPARC expression in the tumor microenvironment. The deletion of SPARC in genetically engineered mouse models of PDAC did not alter intratumoral concentrations of paclitaxel or tumor response during treatment of mice with nab-paclitaxel.[50] Alternative hypotheses for nab-paclitaxel activity are under investigation and will be important for future drug development efforts.

FOLINIC ACID, 5-FLUOROURACIL, IRINOTECAN, OXALIPLATIN VERSUS GEMCITABINE PLUS NAB-PACLITAXEL

The emergence of 2 active combination chemotherapy programs for the treatment of pancreatic cancer is an exciting development, but it also leads to questions as to how best to use these regimens for individual patients. In the absence of a formal randomized trial of FOLFIRINOX versus gemcitabine plus nab-paclitaxel, the comparison of results across the PRODIGE and MPACT trials is understandable. However, cross-trial comparisons have significant limitations and can lead to incorrect conclusions. The PRODIGE trial was limited to patients 75 years old or younger and with ECOG performance status of 0 or 1. In contrast, in the MPACT trial 10% of patients were older than 75 years and 7.6% had a KPS of 60 or 70, roughly equivalent to an ECOG performance status of 2. However, fewer patients in the MPACT study had peritoneal metastases compared with the PRODIGE study (3% vs 19%), a factor associated with shorter survival. In addition, the PRODIGE trial was conducted at 48 centers in France, whereas MPACT was a global trial conducted at 151 centers in 11 countries, suggesting the potential for further unmeasured differences across the 2 patient populations.

Despite identified and potentially unrecognized differences in trial and patient characteristics, a comparison of the gemcitabine control arms between the 2 trials suggests that the enrolled populations were similar in terms of patient outcomes (see **Table 3**). Median OS in the gemcitabine arm was 6.8 months (95% CI, 5.5–7.6) in the PRODIGE trial and 6.7 months (95% CI, 6.0–7.2) in the MPACT trial, and similar response rates and median PFS times were also seen. Although these data do not eliminate concerns regarding cross-trial comparison, they at least suggest that the base populations in these trials were overall similar in their outcomes. As no clinical trial to directly compare FOLFIRINOX and gemcitabine plus nab-paclitaxel is currently underway in patients with metastatic PDAC, the field for the foreseeable future is limited to the available data from the PRODIGE and MPACT trials, which grossly suggest that FOLFIRINOX may have some increase in efficacy compared with gemcitabine plus nab-paclitaxel, but at the cost of some increase in toxicity. Thus, appropriate patient selection and local expertise will remain paramount in choosing first-line chemotherapy programs in patients with metastatic PDAC.

Aside from choosing which combination chemotherapy program to use in the first-line setting, a consideration that has yet to be examined formally is the ability to sequentially use FOLFIRINOX and gemcitabine plus nab-paclitaxel. Small studies have suggested the feasibility of this approach,[51,52] but definitive data remain to be generated for both efficacy and tolerability with sequential administration of these treatment regimens.

SECOND-LINE THERAPY

Although second-line treatment with FOLFIRINOX or gemcitabine plus nab-paclitaxel has not yet undergone rigorous evaluation in clinical trials, several randomized studies have evaluated 5-fluorouracil-based regimens in this setting. The CONKO-003 (Charité Onkologie 003) trial assessed the addition of oxaliplatin to folinic acid and 5-fluorouracil in 168 patients with gemcitabine-refractory, advanced PDAC.[53] The addition of oxaliplatin was associated with an improvement in median OS from 3.3 to 5.9 months (HR, 0.66; 95% CI, 0.48–0.91; $P = .01$), with similar toxicities aside from an increase in neurotoxicity with the use of oxaliplatin. The PANCREOX (Randomized phase 3 study of 5FU/LV with or without oxaliplatin for second-line advanced pancreatic cancer in patients who have received gemcitabine-based chemotherapy) trial compared mFOLFOX6 (folinic acid, 5-fluorouracil, and oxaliplatin) with folinic acid and infusional 5-fluorouracil in 108 patients with advanced PDAC after disease progression on gemcitabine.[54] No improvements were seen in PFS or OS in the mFOLFOX6 arm, with significantly more patients withdrawing because of adverse events in the mFOLFOX6 arm (20.4% vs 1.9%). Although these study results seem contradictory, they suggest that selection of a robust patient population will be necessary to realize improved patient survival with second-line combination chemotherapy.

A three-arm phase 3 study of MM-398, a nanoliposomal encapsulation of irinotecan was recently reported in 417 patients with metastatic PDAC previously treated with gemcitabine.[55] Patients were randomly assigned to receive MM-398 with 5-fluorouracil and folinic acid, MM-398 alone, or 5-fluorouracil and folinic acid alone. The addition of MM-398 to 5-fluorouracil and folinic acid demonstrated improved median OS from 4.2 months in the 5-fluorouracil and folinic acid arm to 6.1 months in the combination arm containing MM-398 (HR, 0.67; 95% CI, 0.49–0.92; $P = .012$). Nevertheless, it remains unclear whether the nanoliposomal encapsulation of irinotecan provided benefit beyond what would have been seen with standard delivery of irinotecan. Also of interest in the second-line setting are results from the recently reported phase 2 RECAP (Randomized Phase 2 Study of Ruxolitinib Efficacy and Safety in Combination with Capecitabine for Subjects with Recurrent or Treatment Refractory Metastatic Pancreatic Cancer) trial, which randomized 127 patients to capecitabine alone or capecitabine plus ruxolitinib, an oral inhibitor of Janus kinase 1 (JAK1)/JAK2.[56] Results favored the combination arm for PFS and OS, particularly in a subgroup with high systemic inflammation defined by elevated serum CRP levels. A phase 3 study of ruxolitinib in second-line therapy is now underway for patients with advanced PDAC refractory to first-line therapy.

NEW APPROACHES

Further assessments of cytotoxic combination chemotherapy may offer modest incremental improvements in survival but are unlikely to yield large improvements in patient outcomes. The next era of therapies are working to exploit our knowledge of pancreatic cancer biology derived from ongoing genomic, proteomic, and epigenomic studies, in addition to studies of genetically engineered mouse models. Broadly, these ongoing efforts fall into one of the following categories: (1) modification of tumor-induced stroma, (2) inhibition of signaling from mutant *KRAS*, (3) induction or augmentation of the host immune response to the cancer, (4) exploitation of defects in tumor DNA repair mechanisms, and (5) modulation of key signaling pathways, such as JAK/signal transducer and activator of transcription, Notch, and transforming growth factor β. These ongoing studies hold great hope for leveraging the increasing understanding of pancreatic cancer biology to improve quality of life and survival for patients with metastatic PDAC.

SUMMARY

The recent studies examining FOLFIRINOX and gemcitabine plus nab-paclitaxel reflect nearly 2 decades of work to improve upon the efficacy of gemcitabine monotherapy and provide exciting new treatment options for patients with metastatic PDAC. Furthermore, recent trials have defined treatment options for patients after progression of their cancer on first-line therapy. Thus, patients and medical oncologists now have several treatment regimens to choose from (**Tables 5** and **6**), with new hope for better patient quality of life and longer survival. Nevertheless, despite the important gains achieved by these new treatment programs, most patients with

Table 5
Systemic treatment options for patients with metastatic pancreatic adenocarcinoma

	Favored Options	**Less-Active Options**
First-Line Treatment		
ECOG PS = 0 or 1	FOLFIRINOX Gemcitabine plus nab-paclitaxel Clinical trial	Gemcitabine plus capecitabine Gemcitabine plus erlotinib
ECOG PS ≥2	Gemcitabine Best supportive care Clinical trial	5-fluorouracil and folinic acid Capecitabine
Second-Line Treatment		
ECOG PS = 0 or 1	FOLFOX Gemcitabine FOLFIRINOX Gemcitabine plus nab-paclitaxel Clinical trial	5-fluorouracil and folinic acid Capecitabine
ECOG PS ≥2	Gemcitabine Best supportive care Clinical trial	5-fluorouracil and folinic acid Capecitabine
Third-Line Treatment		
ECOG PS = 0 or 1	Best supportive care Clinical trial	—

Abbreviation: PS, performance status.

Table 6
Systemic treatment programs for patients with metastatic pancreatic adenocarcinoma

Treatment Program	Doses and Schedule	Cycle Length
Gemcitabine[3]	Gemcitabine 1000 mg/m² IV, days 1, 8, 15, 22, 29, 36, and 43; 1 wk rest (cycle 1); followed by days 1, 8, and 15 every 28 d (cycles ≥2) or Gemcitabine 1000 mg/m² IV, days 1, 8, and 15	28-d cycle
Gemcitabine plus capecitabine[20]	Gemcitabine 1000 mg/m² IV, days 1, 8, and 15 Capecitabine 830 mg/m² po bid, days 1–21	28-d cycle
Gemcitabine plus erlotinib[38]	Gemcitabine 1000 mg/m² IV, days 1, 8, and 15 Erlotinib 100 mg po qd, days 1–28	28-d cycle
Gemcitabine plus nab-paclitaxel[5]	Gemcitabine 1000 mg/m² IV, days 1, 8, and 15 Nab-paclitaxel 125 mg/m² IV, days 1, 8, and 15	28-d cycle
FOLFIRINOX[4]	Oxaliplatin 85 mg/m² IV, day 1 Irinotecan 180 mg/m² IV, day 1 Folinic acid 400 mg/m² IV, day 1 5-fluorouracil 400 mg/m² IV, day 1 5-fluorouracil 2400 mg/m² IV given over 46–48 h continuous infusion, days 1–2	14-d cycle
FOLFOX[54]	Oxaliplatin 85 mg/m² IV, day 1 Folinic acid 400 mg/m² IV, day 1 5-fluorouracil 400 mg/m² IV, day 1 5-fluorouracil 2400 mg/m² IV given over 46–48 h continuous infusion, days 1–2	14-d cycle
LV5FU2[54]	Folinic acid 400 mg/m² IV, day 1 5-fluorouracil 400 mg/m² IV, day 1 5-fluorouracil 2400 mg/m² IV given over 46–48 h continuous infusion, days 1–2	14-d cycle
Capecitabine[59]	Capecitabine 1000 mg/m² po bid, days 1–14	21-d cycle

Abbreviation: IV, intravenous.

advanced disease will die within a year of diagnosis. Therefore, continued research will be necessary to better understand the biology of pancreatic cancer and to intelligently integrate new agents into current treatment programs for the benefit our patients today and in the future.

REFERENCES

1. Siegel R, Ma J, Zou Z, et al. Cancer statistics, 2014. CA Cancer J Clin 2014;64(1): 9–29.
2. Rahib L, Smith BD, Aizenberg R, et al. Projecting cancer incidence and deaths to 2030: the unexpected burden of thyroid, liver, and pancreas cancers in the United States. Cancer Res 2014;74(11):2913–21.
3. Burris HA 3rd, Moore MJ, Andersen J, et al. Improvements in survival and clinical benefit with gemcitabine as first-line therapy for patients with advanced pancreas cancer: a randomized trial. J Clin Oncol 1997;15(6):2403–13.
4. Conroy T, Desseigne F, Ychou M, et al. FOLFIRINOX versus gemcitabine for metastatic pancreatic cancer. N Engl J Med 2011;364(19):1817–25.
5. Von Hoff DD, Ervin T, Arena FP, et al. Increased survival in pancreatic cancer with nab-paclitaxel plus gemcitabine. N Engl J Med 2013;369(18):1691–703.

6. Hornick JL, Lauwers GY, Odze RD. Immunohistochemistry can help distinguish metastatic pancreatic adenocarcinomas from bile duct adenomas and hamartomas of the liver. Am J Surg Pathol 2005;29(3):381–9.

7. Tempero MA, Uchida E, Takasaki H, et al. Relationship of carbohydrate antigen 19-9 and Lewis antigens in pancreatic cancer. Cancer Res 1987;47(20): 5501–3.

8. Humphris JL, Chang DK, Johns AL, et al. The prognostic and predictive value of serum CA19.9 in pancreatic cancer. Ann Oncol 2012;23(7):1713–22.

9. Boeck S, Haas M, Laubender RP, et al. Application of a time-varying covariate model to the analysis of CA 19-9 as serum biomarker in patients with advanced pancreatic cancer. Clin Cancer Res 2010;16(3):986–94.

10. Ueno H, Okada S, Okusaka T, et al. Prognostic factors in patients with metastatic pancreatic adenocarcinoma receiving systemic chemotherapy. Oncology 2000; 59(4):296–301.

11. Szkandera J, Stotz M, Absenger G, et al. Validation of C-reactive protein levels as a prognostic indicator for survival in a large cohort of pancreatic cancer patients. Br J Cancer 2014;110(1):183–8.

12. Yachida S, White CM, Naito Y, et al. Clinical significance of the genetic landscape of pancreatic cancer and implications for identification of potential long-term survivors. Clin Cancer Res 2012;18(22):6339–47.

13. Biankin AV, Waddell N, Kassahn KS, et al. Pancreatic cancer genomes reveal aberrations in axon guidance pathway genes. Nature 2012;491(7424):399–405.

14. Huang P, Chubb S, Hertel LW, et al. Action of 2',2'-difluorodeoxycytidine on DNA synthesis. Cancer Res 1991;51(22):6110–7.

15. Grunewald R, Abbruzzese JL, Tarassoff P, et al. Saturation of 2',2'-difluorodeoxycytidine 5'-triphosphate accumulation by mononuclear cells during a phase I trial of gemcitabine. Cancer Chemother Pharmacol 1991;27(4):258–62.

16. Gelibter A, Malaguti P, Di Cosimo S, et al. Fixed dose-rate gemcitabine infusion as first-line treatment for advanced-stage carcinoma of the pancreas and biliary tree. Cancer 2005;104(6):1237–45.

17. Poplin E, Feng Y, Berlin J, et al. Phase III, randomized study of gemcitabine and oxaliplatin versus gemcitabine (fixed-dose rate infusion) compared with gemcitabine (30-minute infusion) in patients with pancreatic carcinoma E6201: a trial of the Eastern Cooperative Oncology Group. J Clin Oncol 2009;27(23): 3778–85.

18. Poplin E, Wasan H, Rolfe L, et al. Randomized, multicenter, phase II study of CO-101 versus gemcitabine in patients with metastatic pancreatic ductal adenocarcinoma: including a prospective evaluation of the role of hENT1 in gemcitabine or CO-101 sensitivity. J Clin Oncol 2013;31(35):4453–61.

19. Berlin JD, Catalano P, Thomas JP, et al. Phase III study of gemcitabine in combination with fluorouracil versus gemcitabine alone in patients with advanced pancreatic carcinoma: Eastern Cooperative Oncology Group Trial E2297. J Clin Oncol 2002;20(15):3270–5.

20. Cunningham D, Chau I, Stocken DD, et al. Phase III randomized comparison of gemcitabine versus gemcitabine plus capecitabine in patients with advanced pancreatic cancer. J Clin Oncol 2009;27(33):5513–8.

21. Herrmann R, Bodoky G, Ruhstaller T, et al. Gemcitabine plus capecitabine compared with gemcitabine alone in advanced pancreatic cancer: a randomized, multicenter, phase III trial of the Swiss Group for Clinical Cancer Research and the Central European Cooperative Oncology Group. J Clin Oncol 2007; 25(16):2212–7.

22. Ueno H, Ioka T, Ikeda M, et al. Randomized phase III study of gemcitabine plus S-1, S-1 alone, or gemcitabine alone in patients with locally advanced and metastatic pancreatic cancer in Japan and Taiwan: GEST study. J Clin Oncol 2013; 31(13):1640–8.

23. Colucci G, Labianca R, Di Costanzo F, et al. Randomized phase III trial of gemcitabine plus cisplatin compared with single-agent gemcitabine as first-line treatment of patients with advanced pancreatic cancer: the GIP-1 study. J Clin Oncol 2010;28(10):1645–51.

24. Heinemann V, Quietzsch D, Gieseler F, et al. Randomized phase III trial of gemcitabine plus cisplatin compared with gemcitabine alone in advanced pancreatic cancer. J Clin Oncol 2006;24(24):3946–52.

25. Louvet C, Labianca R, Hammel P, et al. Gemcitabine in combination with oxaliplatin compared with gemcitabine alone in locally advanced or metastatic pancreatic cancer: results of a GERCOR and GISCAD phase III trial. J Clin Oncol 2005;23(15):3509–16.

26. Rocha Lima CM, Green MR, Rotche R, et al. Irinotecan plus gemcitabine results in no survival advantage compared with gemcitabine monotherapy in patients with locally advanced or metastatic pancreatic cancer despite increased tumor response rate. J Clin Oncol 2004;22(18):3776–83.

27. Abou-Alfa GK, Letourneau R, Harker G, et al. Randomized phase III study of exatecan and gemcitabine compared with gemcitabine alone in untreated advanced pancreatic cancer. J Clin Oncol 2006;24(27):4441–7.

28. Oettle H, Richards D, Ramanathan RK, et al. A phase III trial of pemetrexed plus gemcitabine versus gemcitabine in patients with unresectable or metastatic pancreatic cancer. Ann Oncol 2005;16(10):1639–45.

29. Jain RK. Normalization of tumor vasculature: an emerging concept in antiangiogenic therapy. Science 2005;307(5706):58–62.

30. Kindler HL, Niedzwiecki D, Hollis D, et al. Gemcitabine plus bevacizumab compared with gemcitabine plus placebo in patients with advanced pancreatic cancer: phase III trial of the Cancer and Leukemia Group B (CALGB 80303). J Clin Oncol 2010;28(22):3617–22.

31. Van Cutsem E, Vervenne WL, Bennouna J, et al. Phase III trial of bevacizumab in combination with gemcitabine and erlotinib in patients with metastatic pancreatic cancer. J Clin Oncol 2009;27(13):2231–7.

32. Rougier P, Riess H, Manges R, et al. Randomised, placebo-controlled, double-blind, parallel-group phase III study evaluating aflibercept in patients receiving first-line treatment with gemcitabine for metastatic pancreatic cancer. Eur J Cancer 2013;49(12):2633–42.

33. Kindler HL, Ioka T, Richel DJ, et al. Axitinib plus gemcitabine versus placebo plus gemcitabine in patients with advanced pancreatic adenocarcinoma: a double-blind randomised phase 3 study. Lancet Oncol 2011;12(3):256–62.

34. Goncalves A, Gilabert M, Francois E, et al. BAYPAN study: a double-blind phase III randomized trial comparing gemcitabine plus sorafenib and gemcitabine plus placebo in patients with advanced pancreatic cancer. Ann Oncol 2012;23(11):2799–805.

35. Kindler HL, Richards DA, Garbo LE, et al. A randomized, placebo-controlled phase 2 study of ganitumab (AMG 479) or conatumumab (AMG 655) in combination with gemcitabine in patients with metastatic pancreatic cancer. Ann Oncol 2012;23(11):2834–42.

36. Philip PA, Benedetti J, Corless CL, et al. Phase III study comparing gemcitabine plus cetuximab versus gemcitabine in patients with advanced pancreatic

adenocarcinoma: Southwest Oncology Group-directed intergroup trial S0205. J Clin Oncol 2010;28(22):3605–10.

37. Ueda S, Ogata S, Tsuda H, et al. The correlation between cytoplasmic overexpression of epidermal growth factor receptor and tumor aggressiveness: poor prognosis in patients with pancreatic ductal adenocarcinoma. Pancreas 2004; 29(1):e1–8.

38. Moore MJ, Goldstein D, Hamm J, et al. Erlotinib plus gemcitabine compared with gemcitabine alone in patients with advanced pancreatic cancer: a phase III trial of the National Cancer Institute of Canada Clinical Trials Group. J Clin Oncol 2007;25(15):1960–6.

39. Wacker B, Nagrani T, Weinberg J, et al. Correlation between development of rash and efficacy in patients treated with the epidermal growth factor receptor tyrosine kinase inhibitor erlotinib in two large phase III studies. Clin Cancer Res 2007; 13(13):3913–21.

40. Van Cutsem E, Li CP, Nowara E, et al. Dose escalation to rash for erlotinib plus gemcitabine for metastatic pancreatic cancer: the phase II RACHEL study. Br J Cancer 2014;111(11):2067–75.

41. Karapetis CS, Khambata-Ford S, Jonker DJ, et al. K-ras mutations and benefit from cetuximab in advanced colorectal cancer. N Engl J Med 2008;359(17): 1757–65.

42. Eberhard DA, Johnson BE, Amler LC, et al. Mutations in the epidermal growth factor receptor and in KRAS are predictive and prognostic indicators in patients with non-small-cell lung cancer treated with chemotherapy alone and in combination with erlotinib. J Clin Oncol 2005;23(25):5900–9.

43. Heinemann V, Vehling-Kaiser U, Waldschmidt D, et al. Gemcitabine plus erlotinib followed by capecitabine versus capecitabine plus erlotinib followed by gemcitabine in advanced pancreatic cancer: final results of a randomised phase 3 trial of the 'Arbeitsgemeinschaft Internistische Onkologie' (AIO-PK0104). Gut 2013; 62(5):751–9.

44. da Cunha Santos G, Dhani N, Tu D, et al. Molecular predictors of outcome in a phase 3 study of gemcitabine and erlotinib therapy in patients with advanced pancreatic cancer: National Cancer Institute of Canada Clinical Trials Group Study PA.3. Cancer 2010;116(24):5599–607.

45. Boeck S, Jung A, Laubender RP, et al. KRAS mutation status is not predictive for objective response to anti-EGFR treatment with erlotinib in patients with advanced pancreatic cancer. J Gastroenterol 2013;48(4):544–8.

46. Gourgou-Bourgade S, Bascoul-Mollevi C, Desseigne F, et al. Impact of FOLFIRINOX compared with gemcitabine on quality of life in patients with metastatic pancreatic cancer: results from the PRODIGE 4/ACCORD 11 randomized trial. J Clin Oncol 2013;31(1):23–9.

47. Mahaseth H, Brutcher E, Kauh J, et al. Modified FOLFIRINOX regimen with improved safety and maintained efficacy in pancreatic adenocarcinoma. Pancreas 2013;42(8):1311–5.

48. Gunturu KS, Yao X, Cong X, et al. FOLFIRINOX for locally advanced and metastatic pancreatic cancer: single institution retrospective review of efficacy and toxicity. Med Oncol 2013;30(1):361.

49. Neuzillet C, Tijeras-Raballand A, Cros J, et al. Stromal expression of SPARC in pancreatic adenocarcinoma. Cancer Metastasis Rev 2013;32(3–4):585–602.

50. Neesse A, Frese KK, Chan DS, et al. SPARC independent drug delivery and anti-tumour effects of nab-paclitaxel in genetically engineered mice. Gut 2014;63(6): 974–83.

51. Zhang Y, Hochster HS, Stein S, et al. Second-line gemcitabine plus nab-paclitaxel (G+A) for advanced pancreatic cancer (APC) after first-line FOLFIRI-NOX: Single institution retrospective review of efficacy and toxicity. ASCO Meeting Abstracts 2014;32(3_suppl):344.

52. Zaniboni A, Bertocchi P, Abeni C, et al. Gemcitabine plus nab-paclitaxel as second line and beyond for metastatic pancreatic cancer (MPC): A single institution retrospective analysis. ASCO Meeting Abstracts 2014;32(15_suppl): e15202.

53. Oettle H, Riess H, Stieler JM, et al. Second-line oxaliplatin, folinic acid, and fluorouracil versus folinic acid and fluorouracil alone for gemcitabine-refractory pancreatic cancer: outcomes from the CONKO-003 trial. J Clin Oncol 2014; 32(23):2423–9.

54. Gill S, Ko Y-J, Cripps MC, et al. PANCREOX: a randomized phase 3 study of 5FU/LV with or without oxaliplatin for second-line advanced pancreatic cancer (APC) in patients (pts) who have received gemcitabine (GEM)-based chemotherapy (CT). ASCO Meeting Abstracts 2014;32(15_suppl):4022.

55. Von Hoff D, Li CP, Wang-Gillam A, et al. O-0003NAPOLI-1: randomized phase 3 study of mm-398 (nal-iri), with or without 5-fluorouracil and leucovorin, versus 5-fluorouracil and leucovorin, in metastatic pancreatic cancer progressed on or following gemcitabine-based therapy. Ann Oncol 2014;25(suppl 2):ii105–6.

56. Hurwitz H, Uppal N, Wagner SA, et al. A randomized double-blind phase 2 study of ruxolitinib (RUX) or placebo (PBO) with capecitabine (CAPE) as second-line therapy in patients (pts) with metastatic pancreatic cancer (mPC). ASCO Meeting Abstracts 2014;32(15_suppl):4000.

57. Bramhall SR, Schulz J, Nemunaitis J, et al. A double-blind placebo-controlled, randomised study comparing gemcitabine and marimastat with gemcitabine and placebo as first line therapy in patients with advanced pancreatic cancer. Br J Cancer 2002;87(2):161–7.

58. Van Cutsem E, van de Velde H, Karasek P, et al. Phase III trial of gemcitabine plus tipifarnib compared with gemcitabine plus placebo in advanced pancreatic cancer. J Clin Oncol 2004;22(8):1430–8.

59. Kulke MH, Blaszkowsky LS, Ryan DP, et al. Capecitabine plus erlotinib in gemcitabine-refractory advanced pancreatic cancer. J Clin Oncol 2007;25(30): 4787–92.

Novel Therapeutics for Pancreatic Adenocarcinoma

Maeve A. Lowery, MD, Eileen M. O'Reilly, MD*

KEYWORDS

- Pancreatic adenocarcinoma • Novel therapeutics • Immunotherapy • BRCA
- Stromal targeting • KRAS

KEY POINTS

- Pancreatic ductal adenocarcinoma (PDAC) is characterized by relative genomic complexity, a desmoplastic microenvironment with exclusion of immune effector cells, and intrinsic therapy resistance.
- Therapeutic benefit to date in PDAC has largely ensued from cytotoxic therapy, and future progress will likely continue to include cytotoxic therapy as a mainstay.
- Multiple novel targeted approaches are in development, including evaluation of stromal modulation, immunotherapeutic approaches, and targeting effectors of key signaling pathways, along with evaluation of novel cytotoxic formulations.
- Ongoing challenges include biomarker identification and validation and optimal therapy selection on an individual patient basis.

IMMUNOTHERAPY

The development of kirsten rat sarcoma viral oncogene homolog (KRAS)-driven mouse models of PDAC that recapitulate the evolution from low-grade to high-grade pancreatic intraepithelial neoplasia (PanIN) to invasive carcinoma observed in human disease has increased the understanding of the complex immunologic changes involved in the development of PDAC (**Table 1**).[1] Invasive pancreatic cancer, rather than being poorly immunogenic as was previously considered, is associated with a dynamic immune response; early-stage PanINs promote an inflammatory response that in turn promotes further dysplasia, whereas the established tumor microenvironment is immunosuppressive, facilitating immune evasion.[2]

Gastrointestinal Oncology Service, Department of Medicine, Rubenstein Center for Pancreatic Cancer Research, Memorial Sloan Kettering Cancer Center, Weill Medical College of Cornell University, 300 East 66th Street, New York, NY 10065, USA
* Corresponding author.
E-mail address: oreillye@mskcc.org

Hematol Oncol Clin N Am 29 (2015) 777–787
http://dx.doi.org/10.1016/j.hoc.2015.04.006
0889-8588/15/$ – see front matter © 2015 Elsevier Inc. All rights reserved.
hemonc.theclinics.com

The accumulation of genetic alterations including KRAS and SMAD4 result in the secretion of additional factors, including interleukin 8 and transforming growth factor (TGF) β, which further promote an inflammatory immune response.[3] An established pancreatic tumor therefore typically has an immunosuppressive microenvironment, containing increased number of tumor-associated macrophages with immunosuppressive phenotype, increased numbers of Treg cells and myeloid-derived suppressor cells, and reduced numbers of CD4+ and CD8+ T cells.[4] The challenge remains, however, to translate these insights into the complex pathways with many inhibitory and stimulatory signals into the development of effective therapeutic strategies for PDAC.

GVAX, CRS207 VACCINES

Multiple vaccine-based immunotherapeutic approaches to PDAC have been developed during the last decade, including peptide vaccines,[5] recombinant microorganism-based vaccines,[6] and whole-cell vaccines,[7] with limited activity overall. Encouraging data were presented from a phase 2 trial evaluating the allogeneic whole-cell vaccine, granulocyte-macrophage colony-stimulating factor (GM-CSF) gene-transfected tumor cell vaccine (GVAX), given in combination with low-dose cyclophosphamide alone or followed by live-attenuated listeria monocytogenes–expressing mesothelin (CRS207), an attenuated *Listeria* strain modified to express mesothelin, an antigen expressed by most PDACs, but with limited expression in normal tissues. Ninety patients with metastatic PDAC with eastern cooperative oncology group performance status (ECOG) 0 to 1 performance status previously treated and some with stable disease at enrollment were randomized 2:1 to either cyclophosphamide/GVAX followed by CRS-207 or cyclophosphamide/GVAX. The primary end point was overall survival. Results demonstrated an improvement of 6 months in survival in the CRS-207 group versus 3.4 months in the cyclophosphamide/GVAX group; $P = .0057$, hazard ratio (HR) 0.4477, and there was a suggestion of increased benefit in more heavily pretreated patients, possibly representing both tumor biology and patient selection. Both vaccines were well tolerated.[8] An ongoing randomized phase 2 trial (ECLIPSE [Safety and Efficacy of Combination Listeria/GVAX Pancreas Vaccine in the Pancreatic Cancer Setting]) is enrolling patients with previously treated metastatic PDAC to evaluate CRS207 alone or in combination with cyclophosphamide/GVAX, with a third arm randomized to investigators' choice of several single-agent cytotoxic agents or erlotinib (NCT02004262).

HYPERACUTE VACCINATION

Other strategies under evaluation include an allogeneic pancreatic cancer vaccine algenpantucel-L; composed of 2 human PDAC cell lines (HAPa-1 and HAPa-2) that have been genetically modified to express αGal by using retroviral transfer of the murine αGT gene. Antibodies against αGal are produced by human intestinal bacterial flora continuously and are the mediators of hyperacute rejection, thereby potentially inducing an antitumor immune stimulatory response. A recently published single-arm non–phase 2 trial evaluated the addition of algenpantucel-L to standard therapy in patients with resected pancreas cancer and showed encouraging survival in treated patients compared with historical data.[9] Ongoing phase 3 studies are evaluating the efficacy of Algenpantucel-L in patients with locally advanced/borderline resectable and resected PDAC (NCT01836432, NCT01072981).

CHECKPOINT BLOCKADE

The monoclonal antibody ipilimumab, which blocks binding to cytotoxic T-lymphocyte antigen-4 (CTLA-4), has shown significant activity in clinical trials of patients with advanced melanoma, and thus evaluation has proceeded in other malignancies including PDAC. Binding of CD28 on the T-cell surface to B7-1 and B7-2 receptors on antigen-presenting cells provides a costimulatory signal, which in combination with major histocompatibility complex binding to the T-cell receptor, results in T-cell activation.[10] Inhibition of CTLA-4 therefore prevents the development of immune tolerance, allowing maintenance of T-cell activation in response to tumor-associated antigen presentation. Initial evaluation of ipilimumab in a phase 2 trial of patients with advanced PDAC showed limited activity by conventional response criteria, but 1 patient was observed to have a delayed response.[11] Ongoing trials are evaluating novel checkpoint inhibitors of PD1 alone and in combination with CTLA-4 blockade and inhibitors of PDL1 in patients with advanced pancreatic cancer (NCT01693562, NCT01928394).

IMMUNE MICROENVIRONMENT

Although these strategies are under early evaluation, it is likely that given the complexity of the PDAC microenvironment, combination strategies of immune checkpoint blockade with stromal depleting agents, vaccines, or agents targeting other components such as macrophages and tumor-associated fibroblasts will be required for significant responses to be observed. Several preclinical studies have shown promising results in preclinical models of PDAC. Feig and colleagues[12] found that depletion of cancer-associated fibroblasts (CAFs) expressing fibroblast activation protein (FAP) allowed control of pancreatic tumors by anti-CTLA 4 and anti-PD-L1. In addition, FAP + CAFs were found to secrete the chemokine CXCL12, and administration of the CXCL12 receptor inhibitor, plerixafor (AMD3100), acted synergistically with anti-PDL1 to induce significant tumor regression. Early phase 1 assessment of this strategy in advanced solid tumor malignancies and PDAC is scheduled to start in the near future.

T-CELL MANIPULATION

Another immunotherapeutic strategy with potential promise is utilization of modified T cells that are genetically engineered to express a chimeric antigen receptor, targeting in solid tumor malignancies, mesothelin, a tumor antigen significantly expressed in PDAC. An ongoing phase 1 trial is evaluating the safety and early efficacy signal of this approach in PDAC (NCT01897415).

Immunotherapeutic approaches are also beginning to be investigated in combination with cytotoxic therapy and as a maintenance strategy in PDAC. An example of the former is the evaluation of indoleamine 2,3-dioxygenase inhibitors in conjunction with a standard cytotoxic regimen (NCT02077881), the rationale in part based on preclinical data demonstrating synergy with chemotherapy.

BRCA-RELATED THERAPIES AND POLY-ADP RIBOSE POLYMERASE INHIBITORS

Although most cases of PDAC are sporadic, up to 1 in 10 cases occur in the setting of a hereditary cancer predisposition syndrome, the most common of which is a germline BRCA1 or 2 mutation.[13,14] The lifetime risk of PDAC in a *BRCA1/2* mutation carrier is estimated at between 2 and 3.5 times that of the general population.[15] Among patients with more than 3 family members affected with pancreatic cancer, the prevalence of germline breast cancer 2 early onset (*BRCA2*) mutations was found to be 17%, whereas in a study of European families with at least 2 first-degree relatives with pancreatic cancer, 12% were found to harbor a *BRCA2* mutation.[14,16] In Ashkenazi Jewish patients, mutations in *BRCA1/2* are more prevalent and are usually 1 of 3 founder mutations; breast cancer 1 early onset (*BRCA1*) 185delAG and 5382insC and *BRCA2* 6174delT. In a series of patients of Ashkenazi ancestry unselected for family history from Memorial Sloan Kettering Cancer Center (MSKCC) with resected pancreatic cancer, 5.5% were found to be *BRCA1/2* mutation positive.[17] In a subsequent series evaluating 211 Ashkenazi Jewish patients with a personal history of breast cancer and a family history of PDAC, 30 (14.2%) were found to harbor a mutation in *BRCA*, 14 (47%) in *BRCA1*, and 16 (53%) in *BRCA2*.[18] Germline mutations in the gene *PALB2*, which encodes a protein critical for the initiation of homologous recombination, have also been identified in patients with pancreatic cancer and a personal or family history of breast cancer.[19]

Overall, this population represents a small but significant number of patients with PDAC, in whom the identification of an inherited cancer predisposition syndrome may be potentially exploited for therapeutic benefit. DNA double strand breaks (DSBs) may be induced during cell replication by stalled replication forks and are optimally repaired by homologous recombination; in the absence of functional BRCA1/ BRCA2 or PALB2, however, these DSBs are repaired by the error-prone nonhomologous end joining pathway leading to genetic instability.[20] Poly ADP-ribose polymerase (PARP) inhibitors (PARPis) block repair of single strand breaks and induce DSBs. They have been developed for treatment of cancers deficient in homologous recombination, which are unable to accurately repair DSBs and so maintain genomic integrity, resulting in cell death via a synthetic lethal effect.[21] Similarly, BRCA-deficient cells demonstrate increased susceptibility to platinum drugs because of induction of interstrand cross-links, which require repair by the homologous repair pathway. Several retrospective series have described significant response to platinum agents and PARPis in patients with known BRCA1/2 mutations and pancreatic cancer.[22,23] A prospective phase 2 study of the PARPi olaparib in patients with BRCA1/2-associated malignancy enrolled 23 patients with pancreatic cancer, of whom 22% showed either complete or partial response to treatment with single agent olaparib. In addition, 35% of patients with pancreatic cancer demonstrated stable disease for at least 8 weeks. Overall survival after 1 year was 41% for patients with BRCA1/2 mutation-associated pancreatic cancer treated in the study.[24]

At MSKCC, in collaboration with the National Cancer Institute (NCI) and other sites in the United States, Israel, and Canada, the authors are conducting several trials evaluating the safety and activity of platinum drugs and PARP inhibition in this subpopulation of BRCA and PALB2 mutated PDAC by combining the PARPi veliparib with the cytotoxic backbone of cisplatin and gemcitabine. Results of the phase 1b portion of this study were presented at the American Society of Clinical Oncology in 2014; 17 patients were enrolled, 9 of whom had known BRCA1/2 mutations. The main grade 3 to 4 toxicities were fatigue and hematologic events. The recommended phase 2 dose of veliparib in combination with gemcitabine and cisplatin was identified to be 80 mg by mouth twice a day from day 1 to 12 every 3 weeks.[25] Significant activity was observed in all BRCA/12 mutation carriers treated. A randomized phase 2 trial evaluating cisplatin and gemcitabine with or without the addition of veliparib in BRCA1/2 or PALB2 mutation carriers is underway. An additional phase 2 protocol evaluated the use of single agent veliparib, at a dose of 400 mg daily, as second-line or third-line therapy in patients with previously treated BRCA- or PALB2-mutated pancreas cancer is complete and results are pending (NCT01585805).

MOLECULARLY TARGETED THERAPIES

PDAC is characterized by several key genetic alterations, which accumulate during the development of invasive adenocarcinoma from precursor lesions initially in KRAS, CDKN2A, and later in SMAD4 and p53. It has become clear that established PDAC continues to accumulate genetic alterations resulting in molecular subclones with considerable genetic heterogeneity.[26] Despite this interpatient and intrapatient variation in genetic alterations, the functional implications of these mutations seem to converge on several key signaling pathways, including cell cycle regulation, DNA repair, apoptosis, and Wnt/Notch signaling.[27,28] Agents targeting one or ideally combinations of these common pathways offer potential to overcome the difficulties posed by the molecular heterogeneity that has long been considered a major contributing factor to the therapy-resistant phenotype of PDAC.

TARGETING KRAS

Despite the ubiquitous finding and central importance of mutant KRAS as a molecular driver in the initiation and maintenance of invasive PDAC, direct therapeutic targeting of constituently active KRAS has proved ineffective to date. Newer generations of KRAS-targeting therapies, for example, small allosteric inhibitors of ras (G12C), which block in the GDP state and inhibit downstream signaling, have shown promising activity in preclinical studies and are under clinical evaluation in non–small cell lung cancer, as are combination strategies targeting downstream effectors of mutant RAS.

Reolysin is a naturally occurring, nonpathogenic reovirus, which replicates preferentially in cells with an activated RAS pathway. Preclinical studies have shown accumulation of viral products and initiation of apoptosis in KRAS-mutant pancreas cancer models[29]; however, a phase 2 randomized trial of carboplatin and paclitaxel with or without the addition of Reolysin in patients with previously untreated advanced PDAC showed no benefit to the addition of Reolysin to chemotherapy (median progression free survival [PFS] 4.63 vs 5.1 months; HR, 1.07; $P = .81$).[30]

Other approaches include the development of small interference RNA (siRNA) against G12D mutant KRAS, using a novel delivery system of a biodegradable polymeric matrix, siRNA LODER, to protect siRNA from degradation and facilitate local release within the tumor for prolonged periods.[31] Encouraging preclinical results led to initial evaluation in combination with gemcitabine or 5-fluorouracil, oxaliplatin, irinotecan, leucovorin (FOLFIRINOX) in a phase 1 trial of 15 patients with untreated locally advanced PDAC, with safety demonstrated.[32] A randomized phase 2 trial evaluating the addition of siRNA LODER to chemotherapy in this population is planned.

Activating mutations in KRAS result in constitutive signaling through the RAS-RAF-MEK-ERK pathway, providing opportunity for therapeutic targeting of downstream effectors of the mutant oncogene; this provides the rationale for development of inhibitors of MEK1/2 in treatment of pancreatic cancer, although a recent phase 2 trial demonstrated no benefit to the addition of the MEK1/2 inhibitor trametinib to gemcitabine in patients with previously untreated advanced PDAC.[33] It is likely given the potential for resistance to a single targeted therapy via activation of redundant pathways and feedback signaling loops that combination strategies will be required to see antitumor activity with these agents. Combination approaches under evaluation include a phase 1B trial of combined inhibition of phosphoinositide 3-kinase and MEK1/2 (BYL719 and MEK162, NCT01449058) in KRAS or BRAF mutant tumors. An NCI-sponsored Southwest Oncology Group (SWOG) randomized phase 2 trial evaluated FOLFOX compared with MEK1/2 and AKT inhibition (selumetinib/MK2206) as second-line therapy in patients with advanced PDAC (NCT01658943). One hundred and thirteen patients were enrolled, there was no benefit seen to the combination are. Median overall survival was shorter in the selumetinib/MK2206 arm (median OS 4.0 vs 7.5 months, HR 1.46), while more patients in the FOLFOX arm went on to receive additional therapy.[34]

JAK-STAT PATHWAY AND INFLAMMATION

Activation of the janus kinase/signal traducer and activator of transcription (JAK-STAT) pathway, in which constitutive activation of STAT3 through phosphorylation by the JAK family of tyrosine kinases leads to up regulation of a variety of cellular processes promoting cell proliferation and an inflammatory response, has been associated with poor clinical outcomes both in resected and advanced PDAC.[35]

A recently presented randomized, double-blind, placebo-controlled phase 2 trial (RECAP [Study of Ruxolitinib in Pancreatic Cancer Patients]) evaluated capecitabine with or without the addition of the JAK1/2 inhibitor, ruxolitinib, in 138 patients with progressive PDAC following prior gemcitabine therapy. The trial failed to meet its primary end point of overall survival improvement in all patients (HR, 0.79; $P = .12$); however, in a preplanned subgroup analysis of patients with evidence of systemic inflammation as measured by elevated levels of C-reactive protein (CRP), there was a significant improvement in overall survival (HR, 0.47; $P = .005$) and a 6-month overall survival of 42% versus 11% compared with those without elevated levels of CRP. A benefit was also observed in patients with a modified Glasgow prognostic score (mGPS), a composite score related to serum albumin and CRP, of 1 or 2 compared with those with mGPS of 0 (HRs 0.91, 0.71, 0.49 for mGPS 0, 1, 2, respectively).[36] Based on these data, 2 phase 3 randomized trials of capecitabine with ruxolitinib/placebo as second-line therapy in patients with advanced PDAC are underway (JANUS1 and JANUS2 [JAK INhibition with RUxolitinib combined with Capecitabine for Adenocarcinoma of the PancreaS]; NCT02117479, NCT02119663).

AUTOPHAGY

Autophagy, the process of degradation and recycling of cellular contents, has been shown to be required for growth of pancreatic cancer cells and may have a chemoprotective effect.[37] Inhibitors of autophagy, including hydroxychloroquine, offer potential to overcome chemoresistance, and several ongoing trials are evaluating their use in combination with cytotoxic therapy (NCT01506973, NCT01978184).

NOTCH AND STEM CELL TARGETING

The notch signaling pathway has been shown to be upregulated in PDAC cells early in development and seems to interact with the MEK/ERK pathway activation through increased expression of notch target gene Hes1. The importance of the notch pathway in the initiation and maintenance of PDAC is supported by results of large-scale sequencing studies.[38] It has also been identified that notch signaling plays a key role in the maintenance of PDAC stem cells and that therapeutic targeting of notch may deplete this population.[39] A phase 1b study of the notch 2/3 inhibitor, OMP-59R5 (tarextumab), in combination with gemcitabine and nab-paclitaxel has demonstrated safety and encouraging activity, and an ongoing double-blind, placebo-controlled randomized phase 2 trial will evaluate the activity of OMP-59R5 in combination with standard cytotoxic therapy in patients with untreated metastatic PDAC (NCT01647828).[40]

STROMAL TARGETING THERAPIES

PDAC is characterized by a dense, desmoplastic stroma comprising a cellular component including fibroblasts, endothelial cells, and immune cells contained in a protein-rich extracellular matrix.[41,42] A complex tumor-stroma interaction facilitates the development, growth, and metastatic spread of PDAC and contributes to the relative therapy resistance of PDAC in part through impairing efficient drug delivery. An increased understanding of stromal biology, aided by preclinical study of accurate genetically engineered mouse models (GEMMs) of PDAC, has elucidated several potential therapeutic targets within the tumor microenvironment.

Although initial encouraging preclinical studies indicated targeting of the developmental hedgehog pathway as a strategy to deplete stroma and increase drug delivery, a subsequent randomized phase 2 study of hedgehog inhibitor, vismodegib, in combination with gemcitabine in patients with advanced PDAC did not show improvement compared with treatment with gemcitabine alone.[43] However, stromal targeting remains a major therapeutic strategy for treatment of PDAC, and several promising agents are under clinical evaluation.

PEGPH20

Hyaluron is a glycosaminoglycan abundant in the extracellular matrix of PDAC, which may be degraded by the enzyme hyaluronidase. The recombinant hyaluronidase enzyme, pegylated recombinant human hyaluronidase (PEGPH20), was found in preclinical studies to degrade hyaluronan, reduce interstitial fluid pressure, and increase vascular permeability to enhance drug delivery. Combination therapy with PEGPH20 and gemcitabine was found to inhibit tumor growth and prolong survival in a GEMM of PDAC.[44,45] Two ongoing randomized trials are evaluating the addition of PEGPH20 to standard chemotherapy for patients with advanced PDAC. The SWOG S1313 trial is a phase 1b/2 trial evaluating the addition of PEGPH20 to modified FOLFIRINOX in 138 patients with advanced untreated PDAC (NCT01959139), with a primary end point of overall survival, whereas HALO-109-202 is a randomized phase 2 trial evaluating the addition of PEGPH20 to nab-paclitaxel and gemcitabine in a similar patient population (NCT01839487). Both studies have experienced a recent pause due the observation of increased thromboembolic events in the PEGPH20 experimental arm, and modifications have been effected to include primary anticoagulation prophylaxis and both studies have now reopened.

TH302

TH302 is a prodrug activated only in the hypoxic conditions typical of the PDAC microenvironment, where it releases bromoisophosphoramide mustard (Br-IPM), a DNA alkylating agent. Once activated in hypoxic tissues, the active Br-IPM can then diffuse into adjacent oxygenated tissue to exert further cytotoxic effect.[46,47] Encouraging results from a randomized phase 2 study evaluating the addition of TH302 to gemcitabine in patients with advanced untreated PDAC[48] led to the development of a phase 3 trial (MAESTRO [Clinical Trial Testing TH-302 in Combination With Gemcitabine in Previously Untreated Subjects With Metastatic or Locally Advanced Unresectable Pancreatic Adenocarcinoma]), which will enroll 660 patients with untreated PDAC, randomized to gemcitabine and placebo versus gemcitabine and TH302 (NCT01746979).

NECUPARANIB

Heparin sulfate proteoglycans bind to growth factors in the tumor microenvironment and modulate their activity, including those of several key signaling proteins involved in PDAC tumor stromal signaling such as fibroblast growth factor 2, platelet-derived growth factor, and TGFs. The heparin sulfate mimetic M402 (necuparanib) acts to modulate tumor-stromal interactions, modify angiogenesis, and attenuate signaling pathways involved in PDAC tumor progression. Encouraging preclinical studies in GEMM model of PDAC showed prolonged survival in combination with gemcitabine,[49] and phase 1 clinical study in combination with gemcitabine and nab-paclitaxel has completed accrual; a randomized phase 2 study of the addition of M402/placebo to nab-paclitaxel and gemcitabine in patients with untreated advanced PDAC is underway (NCT01621243).

NOVEL CYTOTOXIC FORMULATIONS

Recently presented data confirmed activity of the nanoliposomal bound form of irinotecan, MM398, in patients with advanced PDAC. The novel formulation allows increased accumulation of the active metabolite SN38 at the tumor site and more prolonged circulation of drug than conventional irinotecan. Encouraging phase 2 data led to completion of a randomized phase 3 trial in 417 patients with advanced PDAC who had previously received gemcitabine. Three treatment arms were evaluated, including treatment with 5 fluorouracil (5FU)/leucovorin (LV) alone, MM-398 alone, or combination 5FU/LV/MM-398. The median overall survival was 6.1 months in the MM-398 plus 5FU/leucovorin group compared with 4.2 months in the group receiving standard treatment with 5FU/leucovorin alone (HR, 0.67; $P = .012$). Progression-free survival also improved significantly, from 1.5 months with the standard therapy to 3.1 months in patients receiving MM-398 plus 5FU/leucovorin (HR, 0.56; $P<.001$). MM-398 alone did not provide any additional survival benefit over standard therapy. The US Food and Drug Administration is evaluating these data for consideration of approval, although it remains unclear if MM-398 is more active in this setting than irinotecan.[50]

Table 1			
Selected ongoing randomized trials of novel therapy for advanced PDAC			
Trial	**Trial Design**	**N**	**Target**
NCT01839487	Gemcitabine + nab-paclitaxel ± PEGPH20	132	Hyaluron
NCT01959139	FOLFIRINOX ± PEGPH20	138	Hyaluron
NCT01621243	Gemcitabine + nab-paclitaxel ± M402	148	Antistromal
NCT01647828	Gemcitabine + nab-paclitaxel ± OMP-59R5	140	Notch, Stem cells
NCT01746979	Gemcitabine ± TH-302	660	Hypoxia
NCT01728818	Gemcitabine ± afatinib	117	EGFR, Her2, 4
NCT01585805	Gemcitabine, cisplatin ± veliparib	70	PARP (BRCA+)
NCT02004262	CRS-207± cyclophosphamide/GVAX vs chemotherapy	240	Mesothelin (vaccine)
NCT02117479	Capecitabine ± ruxolitinib	310	JAK/STAT
NCT01016483	Gemcitabine ± MSC1936369B	174	MEK

Abbreviations: BRCA, breast cancer 1/2 early onset; CRS 207, live-attenuated listeria monocytogenes–expressing mesothelin; EGFR, epidermal growth factor receptor; FOLFIRINOX, 5-fluorouracil, irinotecan, oxaliplatin, leucovorin; GVAX, granulocyte-macrophage colony-stimulating factor (GM-CSF) gene-transfected tumor cell vaccine; JAK/STAT: janus kinase/signal traducer and activator of transcription; MEK, mitogen-activated protein kinase; PARP, poly ADP-ribose polymerase; PEGPH20, pegylated recombinant human hyaluronidase.

SUMMARY

Over the last several years a substantially enhanced understanding of the molecular pathogenesis and underpinnings of PDAC has accrued, along with incremental improvements in cytotoxic therapies for this disease, and increasing public health recognition of the challenges that PDAC poses collectively account for a renewed focus on novel therapeutic strategies in this disease (**Table 1**). Current research directions include the integration of molecularly targeted, stromal-modulation, varied immunotherapeutic approaches and revisiting ras targeting. The challenges are steep; however, the ultimate rewards are high, and there is a sense of optimism that meaningful impacts will ensue from current research endeavors.

REFERENCES

1. Clark CE, Hingorani SR, Mick R, et al. Dynamics of the immune reaction to pancreatic cancer from inception to invasion. Cancer Res 2007;67:9518–27.
2. Goggins M, Kern SE, Offerhaus JA, et al. Progress in cancer genetics: lessons from pancreatic cancer. Ann Oncol 1999;10(Suppl 4):4–8.
3. Evans A, Costello E. The role of inflammatory cells in fostering pancreatic cancer cell growth and invasion. Front Physiol 2012;3:270.
4. Zheng L, Xue J, Jaffee EM, et al. Role of immune cells and immune-based therapies in pancreatitis and pancreatic ductal adenocarcinoma. Gastroenterology 2013;144:1230–40.
5. Bernhardt SL, Gjertsen MK, Trachsel S, et al. Telomerase peptide vaccination of patients with non-resectable pancreatic cancer: a dose escalating phase I/II study. Br J Cancer 2006;95:1474–82.
6. Gulley JL, Arlen PM, Tsang KY, et al. Pilot study of vaccination with recombinant CEA-MUC-1-TRICOM poxviral-based vaccines in patients with metastatic carcinoma. Clin Cancer Res 2008;14:3060–9.
7. Lutz E, Yeo CJ, Lillemoe KD, et al. A lethally irradiated allogeneic granulocyte-macrophage colony stimulating factor-secreting tumor vaccine for pancreatic adenocarcinoma. A phase II trial of safety, efficacy, and immune activation. Ann Surg 2011;253:328–35.
8. Le DT, Wang-Gillam A, Picozzi V. A phase 2, randomized trial of GVAX pancreas and CRS-207 immunotherapy versus GVAX alone in patients with metastatic pancreatic adenocarcinoma: updated results. J Clin Oncol 2014;32 (Suppl 3; abstract: 177).
9. Hardacre JM, Mulcahy M, Small W, et al. Addition of algenpantucel-L immunotherapy to standard adjuvant therapy for pancreatic cancer: a phase 2 study. J Gastrointest Surg 2013;17:94–100 [discussion: 100–1].
10. Hoos A, Ibrahim R, Korman A, et al. Development of ipilimumab: contribution to a new paradigm for cancer immunotherapy. Semin Oncol 2010;37:533–46.
11. Royal RE, Levy C, Turner K, et al. Phase 2 trial of single agent ipilimumab (anti-CTLA-4) for locally advanced or metastatic pancreatic adenocarcinoma. J Immunother 2010;33:828–33.
12. Feig C, Jones JO, Kraman M, et al. Targeting CXCL12 from FAP-expressing carcinoma-associated fibroblasts synergizes with anti-PD-L1 immunotherapy in pancreatic cancer. Proc Natl Acad Sci U S A 2013;110:20212–7.
13. Klein AP, Brune KA, Petersen GM, et al. Prospective risk of pancreatic cancer in familial pancreatic cancer kindreds. Cancer Res 2004;64:2634–8.
14. Hahn SA, Greenhalf B, Ellis I, et al. BRCA2 germline mutations in familial pancreatic carcinoma. J Natl Cancer Inst 2003;95:214–21.

15. Iqbal J, Ragone A, Lubinski J, et al. The incidence of pancreatic cancer in BRCA1 and BRCA2 mutation carriers. Br J Cancer 2012;107:2005–9.
16. Murphy KM, Brune KA, Griffin C, et al. Evaluation of candidate genes MAP2K4, MADH4, ACVR1B, and BRCA2 in familial pancreatic cancer: deleterious BRCA2 mutations in 17%. Cancer Res 2002;62:3789–93.
17. Ferrone CR, Levine DA, Tang LH, et al. BRCA germline mutations in Jewish patients with pancreatic adenocarcinoma. J Clin Oncol 2009;27:433–8.
18. Stadler ZK, Salo-Mullen E, Patil SM, et al. Prevalence of BRCA1 and BRCA2 mutations in Ashkenazi Jewish families with breast and pancreatic cancer. Cancer 2012;118:493–9.
19. Jones S, Hruban RH, Kamiyama M, et al. Exomic sequencing identifies PALB2 as a pancreatic cancer susceptibility gene. Science 2009;324:217.
20. Jasin M, Rothstein R. Repair of strand breaks by homologous recombination. Cold Spring Harb Perspect Biol 2013;5:a012740.
21. Cavallo F, Graziani G, Antinozzi C, et al. Reduced proficiency in homologous recombination underlies the high sensitivity of embryonal carcinoma testicular germ cell tumors to cisplatin and poly (ADP-ribose) polymerase inhibition. PLoS One 2012;7:e51563.
22. Golan T, Kanji ZS, Epelbaum R, et al. Overall survival and clinical characteristics of pancreatic cancer in BRCA mutation carriers. Br J Cancer 2014;111(6):1132–8.
23. Lowery MA, Kelsen DP, Stadler ZK, et al. An emerging entity: pancreatic adenocarcinoma associated with a known BRCA mutation: clinical descriptors, treatment implications, and future directions. Oncologist 2011;16:1397–402.
24. Kaufman B, Shapira-Frommer R, Schmutzler RK. Olaparib monotherapy in patients with advanced cancer and a germ-line BRCA1/2 mutation: an open-label phase II study. J Clin Oncol 2013;31 (Suppl; abstract: 11024).
25. O'Reilly EM, Lowery MA, Segal MF. Phase IB trial of cisplatin (C), gemcitabine (G), and veliparib (V) in patients with known or potential BRCA or PALB2-mutated pancreas adenocarcinoma (PC). J Clin Oncol 2014;32:5s (Suppl; abstract: 4023).
26. Makohon-Moore A, Brosnan JA, Iacobuzio-Donahue CA. Pancreatic cancer genomics: insights and opportunities for clinical translation. Genome Med 2013;5:26.
27. Biankin AV, Waddell N, Kassahn KS, et al. Pancreatic cancer genomes reveal aberrations in axon guidance pathway genes. Nature 2012;491:399–405.
28. Jones S, Zhang X, Parsons DW, et al. Core signaling pathways in human pancreatic cancers revealed by global genomic analyses. Science 2008;321:1801–6.
29. Carew JS, Espitia CM, Zhao W, et al. Reolysin is a novel reovirus-based agent that induces endoplasmic reticular stress-mediated apoptosis in pancreatic cancer. Cell Death Dis 2013;4:e728.
30. Bekaii-Saab T, Noonan AM, Lesinski G. A multi-institutional randomized phase 2 trial of the oncolytic virus Reolysin in the first line treatment metastatic adenocarcinoma of the pancreas. Ann Oncol 2014;25(5):1–41.
31. Zorde Khvalevsky E, Gabai R, Rachmut IH, et al. Mutant KRAS is a druggable target for pancreatic cancer. Proc Natl Acad Sci U S A 2013;110:20723–8.
32. Talia Golan AH, Shemi A. Novel KRAS-directed therapy in combination with chemotherapy for locally advanced pancreatic adenocarcinoma. J Clin Oncol 2014;32 (Suppl 3; abstract: 270).
33. Infante JR, Somer BG, Park JO, et al. A randomised, double-blind, placebo-controlled trial of trametinib, an oral MEK inhibitor, in combination with gemcitabine for patients with untreated metastatic adenocarcinoma of the pancreas. Eur J Cancer 2014;50:2072–81.

34. Chung VM, McDonough SL, Philip PA, et al. SWOG S1115: Randomized phase II trial of selumetinib (AZD6244; ARRY 142886) hydrogen sulfate (NSC-748727) and MK-2206 (NSC-749607) vs. mFOLFOX in pretreated patients (Pts) with metastatic pancreatic cancer. Chung et al, J Clin Oncol 33, 2015 (suppl; abstr 4119).

35. Denley SM, Jamieson NB, McCall P, et al. Activation of the IL-6R/Jak/stat pathway is associated with a poor outcome in resected pancreatic ductal adenocarcinoma. J Gastrointest Surg 2013;17:887–98.

36. Hurwitz H, Uppal N, Wagner SA. A randomized double-blind phase 2 study of ruxolitinib (RUX) or placebo (PBO) with capecitabine (CAPE) as second-line therapy in patients (pts) with metastatic pancreatic cancer (mPC). J Clin Oncol 2014; 32:5s (Suppl; abstract: 4000).

37. Hashimoto D, Bläuer M, Hirota M, et al. Autophagy is needed for the growth of pancreatic adenocarcinoma and has a cytoprotective effect against anticancer drugs. Eur J Cancer 2014;50:1382–90.

38. Tremblay I, Pare E, Arsenault D, et al. The MEK/ERK pathway promotes NOTCH signalling in pancreatic cancer cells. PLoS One 2013;8:e85502.

39. Abel EV, Kim EJ, Wu J, et al. The Notch pathway is important in maintaining the cancer stem cell population in pancreatic cancer. PLoS One 2014;9:e91983.

40. O'Reilly EM, Smith LS, Bendell JC. Phase Ib of anticancer stem cell antibody OMP-59R5 (anti-Notch2/3) in combination with nab-paclitaxel and gemcitabine (Nab-P+Gem) in patients (pts) with untreated metastatic pancreatic cancer (mPC). J Clin Oncol 2014;32 (Suppl 3; abstract: 220).

41. Stromnes IM, DelGiorno KE, Greenberg PD, et al. Stromal reengineering to treat pancreas cancer. Carcinogenesis 2014;35:1451–60.

42. Rucki AA, Zheng L. Pancreatic cancer stroma: understanding biology leads to new therapeutic strategies. World J Gastroenterol 2014;20:2237–46.

43. Catenacci DV, Bahary N, Edelman MJ, et al. A phase IB/randomized phase II study of gemcitabine (G) plus placebo (P) or vismodegib (V), a hedgehog (Hh) pathway inhibitor, in patients (pts) with metastatic pancreatic cancer (PC): interim analysis of a University of Chicago phase II consortium study. J Clin Oncol 2012; 30 (Suppl; abstract: 4022).

44. Jacobetz MA, Chan DS, Neesse A, et al. Hyaluronan impairs vascular function and drug delivery in a mouse model of pancreatic cancer. Gut 2013;62:112–20.

45. Provenzano PP, Cuevas C, Chang AE, et al. Enzymatic targeting of the stroma ablates physical barriers to treatment of pancreatic ductal adenocarcinoma. Cancer Cell 2012;21:418–29.

46. Sun JD, Liu Q, Wang J, et al. Selective tumor hypoxia targeting by hypoxia-activated prodrug TH-302 inhibits tumor growth in preclinical models of cancer. Clin Cancer Res 2012;18:758–70.

47. Duan JX, Jiao H, Kaizerman J, et al. Potent and highly selective hypoxia-activated achiral phosphoramidate mustards as anticancer drugs. J Med Chem 2008;51: 2412–20.

48. Ryan DP, Reddy SG, Bahary N, et al. TH-302 plus gemcitabine (G+T) versus gemcitabine (G) in patients with previously untreated advanced pancreatic cancer (PAC). J Clin Oncol 2013;31 (Suppl 4; abstract: 325).

49. Schultes BC, Lolkema MP, Chu CL. M402, a heparan sulfate mimetic and novel candidate for the treatment of pancreatic cancer. J Clin Oncol 2012;30 (Suppl; abstract: 4056).

50. Von Hoff D, Li CP, Wang-Gillam A. NAPOLI-1: randomized phase 3 study of MM-398 (nal-iri), with or without 5-fluorouracil and leucovorin, versus 5-fluorouracil and leucovorin, in metastatic PAC. Ann Oncol 2014;25(Suppl_2):ii105–17.

Index

Note: Page numbers of article titles are in **boldface** type.

Hematol Oncol Clin N Am 29 (2015) 789–798
http://dx.doi.org/10.1016/S0889-8588(15)00096-9
0889-8588/15/$ – see front matter © 2015 Elsevier Inc. All rights reserved.

Moving?

Make sure your subscription moves with you!

To notify us of your new address, find your **Clinics Account Number** (located on your mailing label above your name), and contact customer service at:

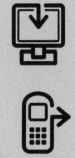

Email: journalscustomerservice-usa@elsevier.com

800-654-2452 (subscribers in the U.S. & Canada)
314-447-8871 (subscribers outside of the U.S. & Canada)

Fax number: 314-447-8029

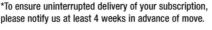

Elsevier Health Sciences Division
Subscription Customer Service
3251 Riverport Lane
Maryland Heights, MO 63043

*To ensure uninterrupted delivery of your subscription, please notify us at least 4 weeks in advance of move.

Printed and bound by CPI Group (UK) Ltd, Croydon, CR0 4YY

03/10/2024

01040492-0002